Sports Injuries Guidebook

Lear~
Ser~

Robert S. Gotlin, DO

Editor

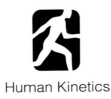

Human Kinetics

Library of Congress Cataloging-in-Publication Data

Sport injuries guidebook / Robert Gotlin, editor.
   p. cm.
  Includes bibliographical references.
  ISBN-13: 978-0-7360-6339-5 (soft cover)
  ISBN-10: 0-7360-6339-0 (soft cover)
  1. Sports injuries--Handbooks, manuals, etc. I. Gotlin, Robert S.
  RD97.S6888 2008
  617.1'027--dc22

                         2007021398

ISBN-10: 0-7360-6339-0 (Print)
ISBN-13: 978-0-7360-6339-5 (Print)
ISBN-10: 0-7360-6339-0 (Adobe PDF)
ISBN-13: 978-0-7360-6339-5 (Adobe PDF)

This publication is written and published to provide accurate and authoritative information relevant to the subject matter presented. It is published and sold with the understanding that the author and publisher are not engaged in rendering legal, medical, or other professional services by reason of their authorship or publication of this work. If medical or other expert assistance is required, the services of a competent professional person should be sought.

The Web addresses cited in this text were current as of June 2007, unless otherwise noted.

Acquisitions Editors: Martin Barnard and Jana Hunter; **Developmental Editors:** Julie Rhoda and Heather Healy; **Assistant Editor:** Carla Zych; **Copyeditor:** John Wentworth; **Proofreader:** Kathy Bennett; **Permission Manager:** Carly Breeding; **Graphic Designer:** Nancy Rasmus; **Graphic Artist:** Tara Welsch; **Cover Designer:** Keith Blomberg; **Photographers (cover):** © Photodisc (runner), Tom Roberts/© Human Kinetics (basketball players and tennis player); **Photographer (interior):** Neil Bernstein, unless otherwise noted; **Visual Production Assistant:** Joyce Brumfield; **Art Manager:** Kelly Hendren; **Associate Art Manager:** Alan L. Wilborn; **Illustrator:** Jason McAlexander, unless otherwise noted; **Printer:** Seaway Printing

Human Kinetics books are available at special discounts for bulk purchase. Special editions or book excerpts can also be created to specification. For details, contact the Special Sales Manager at Human Kinetics.

Printed in the United States of America   10   9   8   7   6   5   4   3   2

Human Kinetics
Web site: www.HumanKinetics.com

United States: Human Kinetics
P.O. Box 5076
Champaign, IL 61825-5076
800-747-4457
e-mail: humank@hkusa.com

Canada: Human Kinetics
475 Devonshire Road Unit 100
Windsor, ON N8Y 2L5
800-465-7301 (in Canada only)
e-mail: info@hkcanada.com

Europe: Human Kinetics
107 Bradford Road
Stanningley
Leeds LS28 6AT, United Kingdom
+44 (0) 113 255 5665
e-mail: hk@hkeurope.com

Australia: Human Kinetics
57A Price Avenue
Lower Mitcham, South Australia 5062
08 8372 0999
e-mail: info@hkaustralia.com

New Zealand: Human Kinetics
P.O. Box 80
Torrens Park, South Australia 5062
0800 9 222 062
e-mail: info@hknewzealand.com

E3688

Sports Injuries
Guidebook

CONTENTS

PREFACE

Participation in recreational sports and physical activities is at an all-time high. While the benefits of such participation are evidenced by our increased longevity and well-being, staying physically fit and athletically active does have its consequences. Fortunately, most of the negative consequences—injuries—are minor setbacks and not season-ending tragedies. With this in mind, the *Sports Injuries Guidebook* details the most common injuries from head to toe that are experienced by athletes from the weekend warrior to the pro.

Many approaches exist for the treatment of athletic injuries, and this book does not include every method or philosophy. Rather than overwhelm you with confusing options, our goal was to create a simple yet thorough user-friendly guidebook compiled by the best physicians and sports medicine professionals in the business.

The result is outstanding. We have put into print the "how to" for identifying, assessing, and treating injuries so you can get back in action as quickly and safely as possible, or even avoid being sidelined in the first place. In fact, you will be able to treat many injuries on your own. You'll be surprised how useful good old common sense can be in treating many of the injuries received in sports participation and how straightforward other treatments can be. But, most important, you'll learn to identify when it's time to seek professional medical care.

The injuries are arranged by body region, so easy identification is only a flip of the pages away. The color illustrations and concise sections on identification and treatment will help you conquer that which ails you, but the detailed and descriptive injury explanations will put it all into context and, in some cases, help prevent the injury next time. The contributors were carefully selected, each possessing areas of sport-specific expertise, each with a lengthy track record of injury management, and each with a keen knack for making it all read easily. The knowledge you will gain from their expertise will keep you on the field, on the court, on the slopes—in short, on track to enjoy your athletic pursuits and stay healthy in the process.

ACKNOWLEDGMENTS

I cannot thank the entire Human Kinetics family enough for their dedicated professional and personal assistance in preparing this book. Their constructive criticism, creative advice, and, most important, total dedication to making this project a success deserves the utmost praise and gratitude.

Every project has a "right hand man." Grant Cooper is much more than a right hand man. Not only did he contribute an eloquent, well-written chapter for this book, he also provided continual personal assistance throughout the project. Without his relentless effort in gathering information, acquiring data, and ensuring that deadlines were met, this book might not have been possible.

I thank all the contributors for sharing their expertise and giving of their time to make this book a comprehensive yet easy-to-read success.

And to my family, my pride and joy—thank you for allowing me time to create this product. You patiently remain in my corner, supportive and loving, every day and always.

INJURY FINDER

Injury	TYPE OF PAIN						LOCATION OF PAIN		SWELLING	COLOR OF SKIN			ACTIVITY SYMP-TOMS			PAGE
	Acute onset	Gradual onset	Dull	Throbbing	Constant	During weight-bearing	Topical	Below skin		Red	White	Blue	Weakness in muscle or joint	Limited range of motion	Unable to bear weight	
CHAPTER 4 CONCUSSIONS AND HEAD INJURIES																
Concussion	✓		✓	✓			✓	✓	*	✓						57
Ear Trauma	✓		✓	✓	✓		✓	✓	*	✓						65
Eye Injuries	✓			✓	✓		✓	✓								66
Nasal and Mandible Fractures	✓			✓	✓		✓	✓	✓	✓						64
Skull Fracture	✓			✓	✓		✓	✓	✓	✓			*	*		63
Subdural and Epidural Hematoma	✓		✓		*			✓					*	*		62
CHAPTER 5 NECK AND CERVICAL SPINE INJURIES																
Burners	✓			✓	✓			✓					✓	*		70
Cervical Disc Injury		✓			*		*	✓					*	*		72
Cervical Fracture	✓			✓	✓		*	✓	*				*	*		76
Cervical Osteoarthritis		✓	✓		*		*	✓					*	*		71
Cervical Stenosis		✓	✓		*		*	✓					*	*		74
Whiplash	✓				✓		*	✓						*		69
CHAPTER 6 SHOULDER INJURIES																
Acromio-clavicular Joint Injury	✓		*		*		*	✓	*					*		88
Biceps Tendon Rupture	✓				*	✓	*	✓					*	*		92
Bicipital Tendinitis		✓	✓		*		*	✓					*			94

* = characteristic may or may not be present

Injury	TYPE OF PAIN						LOCATION OF PAIN		SWELLING	COLOR OF SKIN			ACTIVITY SYMPTOMS			PAGE
	Acute onset	Gradual onset	Dull	Throbbing	Constant	During weight-bearing	Topical	Below skin		Red	White	Blue	Weakness in muscle or joint	Limited range of motion	Unable to bear weight	
Collar Bone Fracture	✓			✓	✓		*	✓	*	✓			*	✓		79
Deep Vein Thrombosis	*	*	✓	✓	✓			✓	✓	*		*		*	*	98
Labral Injury	*	*	✓		*			✓						*		86
Recurrent Shoulder Dislocation	✓		✓	✓	✓			✓						*		82
Rotator Cuff Tear		✓	✓		*			✓					✓	✓		89
Shoulder Dislocation	✓	*	✓	✓	✓			✓						✓		80
Shoulder Impingement		✓			*			✓					*	*		90
Shoulder Subluxation	*	*	*		*		*	✓						*		84
Suprascapular Nerve Injury		✓	*		✓			✓					*			96
CHAPTER 7 ARM AND ELBOW INJURIES																
Cubital Tunnel Syndrome		✓	*	*	*			✓					*			116
Elbow Dislocation	✓		✓	✓	✓			✓	*	✓		*	*	✓		118
Golfer's Elbow		✓	✓	✓	*			✓					*			104
Humeral Stress Fracture	✓		✓	✓	✓			✓								117
Little League Elbow	*	*	✓		*			✓					✓	*		112
Olecranon Bursitis	✓			✓	✓		✓	✓	✓	✓				*		120

(continued)

Injury	TYPE OF PAIN						LOCATION OF PAIN		SWELLING	COLOR OF SKIN			ACTIVITY SYMPTOMS			PAGE
	Acute onset	Gradual onset	Dull	Throbbing	Constant	During weight-bearing	Topical	Below skin		Red	White	Blue	Weakness in muscle or joint	Limited range of motion	Unable to bear weight	
CHAPTER 7 ARM AND ELBOW INJURIES (CONTINUED)																
Osteochondritis Dissecans		✓	✓					✓								114
Posterior Interosseous Nerve Syndrome		✓	✓		*		✓	✓								107
Pronator Syndrome	*	✓			*			✓					✓			108
Radial Tunnel Syndrome		✓			*		✓						*			106
Tennis Elbow		✓		*	*		*	✓	*				*			101
Ulnar Collateral Ligament Tear	✓			✓	✓			✓					✓			110
CHAPTER 8 WRIST AND HAND INJURIES																
Carpal Tunnel Syndrome		✓	*	*	*		✓						*			126
Finger or Thumb Dislocation	✓			✓	✓			✓	✓				*	✓		133
Finger or Thumb Fracture	✓			✓	✓			✓	✓				*	✓		134
Finger Sprain	✓		*	*	*			✓	*					*		132
Hand Fracture	✓		*	*	*			✓	✓				✓	✓		130
Mallet Finger	*	*	✓		*			✓						✓		135
Thumb Sprain	✓	✓						✓	*							131
Wrist Fractures	✓			✓	✓			✓	✓				✓	✓		123
Wrist Sprain	✓				✓			✓	*				✓			124
Wrist Tendinitis		✓			✓			✓	*				✓			128

Injury	TYPE OF PAIN						LOCATION OF PAIN		SWELLING	COLOR OF SKIN			ACTIVITY SYMPTOMS			PAGE
	Acute onset	Gradual onset	Dull	Throbbing	Constant	During weight-bearing	Topical	Below skin		Red	White	Blue	Weakness in muscle or joint	Limited range of motion	Unable to bear weight	
CHAPTER 9 CHEST AND ABDOMINAL INJURIES																
Abdominal Trauma	✓		✓	⋆	⋆		✓	✓								146
Bladder, Kidney, or Ureter Injury	⋆	⋆	✓	⋆	⋆	⋆		✓								148
Commotio Cordis	✓						✓	✓				⋆				140
Costochondritis	⋆	⋆	✓	✓	✓			✓								145
Hemothorax	✓						✓	✓								139
Rib Fracture	✓			⋆	⋆	⋆	✓	✓	⋆	⋆		⋆				142
Sternal Fracture	✓			✓	✓			✓	⋆							144
Testicular Injury	✓		✓	✓	✓	⋆	✓	✓	⋆							147
CHAPTER 10 LOWER-BACK INJURIES																
Annular Tear	⋆	⋆	⋆		⋆	⋆		✓							⋆	156
Burst Fracture	✓			✓	✓	✓		✓					⋆	⋆	⋆	159
Compression Fracture	⋆	⋆	⋆	⋆	⋆	✓		✓						⋆	⋆	158
Facet Joint Pain		✓	✓		⋆	⋆		✓						✓	⋆	163
Herniated Disc	✓			✓	✓	⋆		✓					⋆	⋆	⋆	154
Lumbar and Thoracic Area Contusion	✓	✓	⋆		⋆			✓	⋆	⋆		⋆				151
Lumbar Degenerative Disc Disease		✓	⋆		⋆	⋆		✓						⋆		164

(continued)

Injury	TYPE OF PAIN						LOCATION OF PAIN		SWELLING	COLOR OF SKIN			ACTIVITY SYMPTOMS			PAGE
	Acute onset	Gradual onset	Dull	Throbbing	Constant	During weight-bearing	Topical	Below skin	SWELLING	Red	White	Blue	Weakness in muscle or joint	Limited range of motion	Unable to bear weight	PAGE
CHAPTER 10 LOWER-BACK INJURIES (CONTINUED)																
Lumbar Sprain or Strain	✓		*	✓	*	*		✓								152
Sacroiliac Joint Dysfunction		✓	*		*	*		✓								162
Spondylolysis and Spondylolisthesis		✓	✓		*	*		✓						*		160
Transverse Process Fracture	✓		✓	*	*	*		✓	*	*		*		*		157
CHAPTER 11 HIP INJURIES																
Adductor Canal Syndrome	*	*	*	*	*	*		✓								176
Adductor Strain	✓		*	*	*	*		✓								173
Adductor Tendinosis		✓	*			*		✓						*		167
Coccyxgeal Fracture	✓		✓	✓	✓			✓	*	*						185
Greater Trochanteric Bursitis	*	*	*	*	*	*		✓	✓	*				*		170
Hip Labral Tear	*	*	*		*	✓		✓						*		174
Hip Pointer	✓			✓	✓			✓	*	*		*				180
Iliopsoas Tendinitis	*	*			✓	*		✓								172
Osteitis Pubis and Athletic Pubalgia	*	*	*	*	*	*		✓	*						*	182

Injury	TYPE OF PAIN						LOCATION OF PAIN		SWELLING	COLOR OF SKIN			ACTIVITY SYMPTOMS			PAGE
	Acute onset	Gradual onset	Dull	Throbbing	Constant	During weight-bearing	Topical	Below skin		Red	White	Blue	Weakness in muscle or joint	Limited range of motion	Unable to bear weight	
Osteoarthritis		✓	✓		*	*	✓	✓						*		168
Pelvic Avulsion Fractures	✓		*	*	*	✓		✓	*				*	*	*	178
Pelvic Nerve Injury	*	*		*				✓					*			190
Pelvic Stress Fracture	*	*	*		*	✓		✓						*	*	177
Sacroiliac Joint Injury	*	*	*		*	*		✓						*	*	188
Snapping Hip Syndrome		✓		*	*			✓								179
Sports Hernia		✓	✓	*	*			✓							*	186
CHAPTER 12 THIGH AND HAMSTRING INJURIES																
Compartment Syndrome	✓		✓		✓	✓	✓	✓	✓				*			204
Femoral Stress Fracture	✓		*	*	*	✓		✓							✓	198
Hamstring Avulsion	✓			✓	✓	✓		✓	*				✓	✓	✓	193
Hamstring Strain	✓		*			✓		✓	*				✓	*		194
Myositis Ossificans		✓	✓		*	*		✓								203
Quadriceps Contusions	✓		✓	✓	*	✓		✓	*	*		*	*	*		200
Quadriceps Strain	✓		✓	*		✓		✓	*				*	*		202
CHAPTER 13 KNEE INJURIES																
Anterior Cruciate Ligament Tear	✓				✓			✓	✓	✓				✓		214

(continued)

Injury	TYPE OF PAIN						LOCATION OF PAIN		SWELLING	COLOR OF SKIN			ACTIVITY SYMPTOMS			PAGE
	Acute onset	Gradual onset	Dull	Throbbing	Constant	During weight-bearing	Topical	Below skin		Red	White	Blue	Weakness in muscle or joint	Limited range of motion	Unable to bear weight	
CHAPTER 13 KNEE INJURIES *(CONTINUED)*																
Iliotibial Band Syndrome		✓			*	*		✓								208
Lateral Collateral Ligament Tear	✓				*	*		✓	✓							217
Medial Collateral Ligament Tear	✓				*	*		✓	*							212
Meniscal Tear	*	*	✓			✓		✓						*	*	210
Osgood-Schlatter's Syndrome	✓		✓	✓	✓	✓		✓	*						*	221
Osteochondritis Dissecans		✓	✓		*	*		✓							*	222
Patella Fracture	✓			✓	✓	✓		✓	✓				✓	✓	✓	219
Patellar Tendinitis	*	*	*		*	✓		✓	*							218
Patellofemoral Instability	*	*				✓		✓						*		220
Patellofemoral Pain		✓	*	*	*	✓		✓	*					*		207
Posterior Cruciate Ligament Tear	✓					*		✓	*					*		216
CHAPTER 14 LOWER-LEG AND ANKLE INJURIES																
Ankle Fracture	✓			✓	✓	✓		✓	✓				✓	✓	✓	232
Ankle Sprain	✓			*	*	✓		✓	✓					✓	*	231
Achilles Tendinitis	*	*	*		*	✓		✓	*					*	*	230

Injury	TYPE OF PAIN						LOCATION OF PAIN		SWELLING	COLOR OF SKIN			ACTIVITY SYMPTOMS			PAGE
	Acute onset	Gradual onset	Dull	Throbbing	Constant	During weight-bearing	Topical	Below skin		Red	White	Blue	Weakness in muscle or joint	Limited range of motion	Unable to bear weight	
Achilles Tendon Rupture	✓			✓	✓	✓		✓	✓				✓	✓	✓	229
Bone Spurs on the Ankle		✓	✓		*	✓		✓	*							234
Calf Strain or Tear	✓		*	*	*	✓		✓	✓				✓	*	*	228
Lower-Leg Compartment Syndrome	✓			✓		✓	✓	✓	✓				*			226
Lower-Leg Stress Fracture	*	*		✓	✓	✓		✓	*						✓	227
Posterior Tibial Tendinitis	*	*	*		*	✓		✓	*							233
Shin Splints	*	*	✓	✓	✓	✓		✓								225
CHAPTER 15 FOOT AND TOE INJURIES																
Bunions		✓	✓	✓		✓		✓								248
Corns		✓	✓			✓	✓									253
Fifth Metatarsal Fractures	✓		✓	✓	✓	✓		✓	✓					✓	*	245
Forefoot Neuromas		✓		✓	*	✓		✓								252
Freiberg's Disease		✓	✓	*		✓		✓								251
Fungal Infections		✓					✓									254
Hallux Rigidus		✓	*	✓	✓	✓		✓	*					✓		246
Lisfranc's Sprain		✓			✓			✓						✓	*	243

(continued)

Injury	TYPE OF PAIN						LOCATION OF PAIN		SWELLING	COLOR OF SKIN			ACTIVITY SYMPTOMS			PAGE
	Acute onset	Gradual onset	Dull	Throbbing	Constant	During weight-bearing	Topical	Below skin	SWELLING	Red	White	Blue	Weakness in muscle or joint	Limited range of motion	Unable to bear weight	PAGE
CHAPTER 15 FOOT AND TOE INJURIES (CONTINUED)																
March or Dancer's Stress Fracture	✓		✓	✓	✓	✓		✓	*					✓	*	244
Painful Accessory Navicular Bone		✓	✓			*		✓								241
Plantar Fasciitis		✓		✓	✓	✓		✓							*	238
Purple Toe		✓		✓		*	✓					✓				257
Navicular Bone Stress Fracture	*	*	✓	✓	✓	✓		✓							*	242
Sesamoid Injury	*	*	✓		*	✓		✓	*						*	249
Shoelace Pressure Syndrome	✓		*	*		✓	✓	✓							*	256
Stone Bruise		✓	✓	✓		✓		✓	*						*	240
Talon Noir												✓				258
Tarsal Tunnel Syndrome		✓	✓		*	✓		✓								255
Tennis Toe		✓		✓		*	✓									250
Turf Toe	✓		✓	✓	✓	✓		✓							*	247

CHAPTER 1

Body Conditioning and Maintenance

Evan M. Chait, PT, ARTC, CPCS

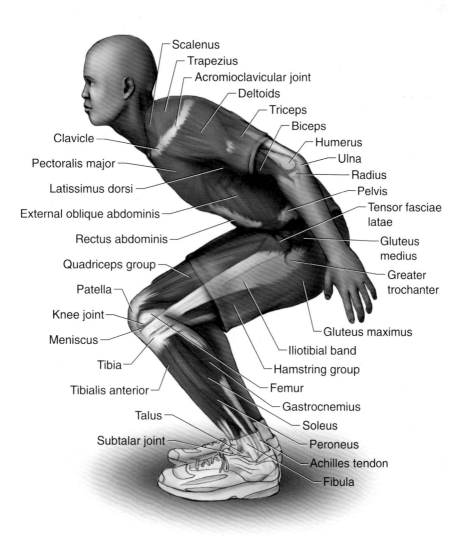

An inherent connection exists between proper conditioning and injury prevention. Conditioning prepares and trains the body for sport and everyday tasks. The more efficient and better conditioned the athlete, the less likely it is that an injury will occur. Thus an exercise program must balance the goal of conditioning the body with the goal of preventing injury. Athletes must have a purpose for entering and performing a specific exercise program, but they must also have an appreciation of the essential components of conditioning.

Unfortunately, many people take an impractical and poorly planned approach to exercise. They focus on training and pushing their bodies to the limit to reach a particular result, be it to lose weight or to improve sport-specific speed. But in training this way they overlook the long-term consequences of physical activity—that is, until an injury occurs.

To reach an ideal balance of conditioning that will allow them to achieve their goals while preventing injury, athletes must learn to condition the body functionally. Functional conditioning consists of exercises that incorporate balance, flexibility, stability, acceleration, and deceleration. In essence, functional conditioning trains movements rather than isolated muscles.

This chapter explains the concept of functional conditioning and introduces the elements involved in it. It also explores the roles these elements play in preventing injury and provides a guide for using the information presented to create an effective warm-up and exercise program. An understanding of the complexities of human activity is essential for engaging in appropriate conditioning and preventing injuries.

Understanding Functional Conditioning

According to Gary Gray (2000), a respected physical therapist and trainer, function is the "interaction between muscles, nerves, and joints, working together simultaneously to decelerate, accelerate, and stabilize both external and internal forces." Simply put, function is the outcome of any activity. Everyday functional movements include running, biking, throwing, walking, carrying a child, tying shoelaces, getting out of bed, and even switching from a sitting to a standing position. Thus, the benefits of functional conditioning are not limited to athletics. Its movements occur in some form in work, home, and sport environments. To perform these tasks, a chain reaction involving muscles, nerves, and joints occurs. If this chain reaction is interrupted because of inadequate flexibility or lack of strength in part of the chain, a breakdown results, leading to a decrease in performance and to possible injury.

Exercises to help condition the body for functional movements must meet all four of these criteria:

1. They must include movements in all three planes (sagittal, frontal, and transverse).

2. They must properly condition the body's nerves and muscles to develop muscle memory and help make movements "automatic."

3. They must condition for responding to external forces, allowing the body to make best use of outside influences such as gravity, ground reaction forces, and momentum.

4. They must condition biomotor abilities (flexibility, strength, power, endurance, agility, or coordination).

A quick look at these four criteria comfirms that functional conditioning works beyond the realm of physical fitness and benefits the body during the activities that most people, athletes and nonathletes alike, do every day.

Moving in Multiple Planes

To help prevent injury and to function effectively, conditioning must occur in the sagittal, frontal, and transverse planes (figure 1.1). An exercise that exemplifies movement in all three planes is the 3-D lunge, also known as the lunge matrix, which includes a forward and lateral lunge as well as a lunge with a rotational movement. The standard forward lunge works the sagittal plane. This requires taking a big step forward with one leg and squatting straight downward until the other knee almost touches the floor before returning to the starting position. In the lateral lunge the athlete stands straight up and steps out to the side with one leg, bending the stepping leg's knee while keeping the other leg relaxed. The transverse plane is emphasized in the 3-D lunge, in which the athlete adds a rotational movement by twisting the back while performing a forward lunge. Many motions in everyday life require postural control through multiple planes of motion and at different speeds. For example, a mother carrying a newborn baby requires postural control to keep the child securely in her arms.

Moving forward and backward, such as running, works the sagittal plane. Side-to-side movement, such as sidestepping or shuffling, uses the frontal plane. Rotational movements, such as the twisting motion of throwing or hitting a baseball, occur in the transverse plane.

Unfortunately, most exercise conditioning programs and equipment focus primarily on the sagittal plane (forward and backward). For example,

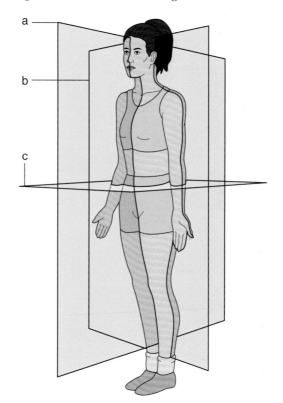

Figure 1.1 Conditioning movements occurring in the (a) sagittal, (b) frontal, and (c) transverse planes improve performance and help prevent injuries.

Adapted, by permission, from E. Harman, 2000, The biomechanics of resistance exercise. In *Essentials of strength training and conditioning*, 2nd ed., edited by T.R. Baechle and R.W. Earle (Champaign, IL: Human Kinetics), 34.

the hamstring curl is performed on a fixed piece of equipment. The athlete lies down and inserts the heel under the pull pad, lifts up the foot, angles the knee, and then lowers the leg down to its initial position to repeat the process. The exercise targets the hamstring muscles. Although performed on a machine, the exercise is not useless or ineffective. Such a piece of equipment can supplement a workout by strengthening the hamstrings. However, training with a hamstring curl machine alone is not functional conditioning because lifting the legs up and down allows only the targeted muscle and joint to operate within the sagittal plane. This means the hamstring curl has little carryover in improving overall sport-specific performance. For instance, the hamstring curl might benefit a bodybuilder trying to increase the muscle size of the hamstring, but because the exercise isolates the hamstring, it does not develop the athlete's quickness, speed, body control, awareness, and overall athletic performance. Likewise, research indicates that most injuries occur in the transverse plane during eccentric, decelerating muscle contractions (National Academy of Sports Medicine 2003). Examples include tearing the ACL (anterior cruciate ligament) upon landing after shooting a basketball lay-up and throwing the back out while bending over to pick up an object.

Whether you are playing basketball or doing yardwork, multiplanar condition-ing movements play an integral role in avoiding injury. All foundational functional movement patterns, such as throwing, running, leaping, squatting, crawling, jump-ing, hopping, pushing, pulling, lifting, twisting, and carrying, are multiplanar and involve multiple joints. Conditioning the body in this fashion and conditioning the foundational movement patterns is essential for preventing injury, rehabilitating an injury, and improving athletic development.

Conditioning the Neuromuscular System

Functional conditioning requires the training of the nervous system. For example, when someone bends down to pick an object off the ground, he or she is unaware of *how* the body executes this movement. The flexing and rotating of the spine, hips, knees, and ankles are not premeditated actions. Rather, the nervous system plays an integral role in this process. The body's nerves send messages to the muscles, telling them when, how, and at what speed to move. To clarify how this occurs, we should examine the neurological mechanisms of the nervous system that are used during movement and their relation to functional conditioning and preventing injury.

The brain learns movement by developing motor programs. According to physi-cal therapist Gray Cook, motor programs are ways that the brain stores information about movement. So, every time someone learns how to shoot a basketball or ride a bike, the brain creates a motor program that allows the athlete to repeat the activity without relearning the mechanics each time (Cook 2003). This is the nervous system's way of running efficiently. Improving the way the body develops motor programs and helping the neuromuscular system operate to its highest potential require con-ditioning the neural network through repeated functional movements.

Conditioning the nervous system through repetitive functional movements improves the feedback of proprioceptors to the muscles in the body. Propriocep-tors are sensory receptors located within joints, muscles, and tendons. They deal with the physical state of the body, constantly informing the central nervous system about muscle tone and the coordination of certain movements. Likewise, the way the body senses both touch and movement is referred to as proprioception, which means "sense of self." Through proprioception, the body communicates with itself at a subconscious level. For example, people do not have to think about maintaining a particular posture or how to position body parts during a particular movement. Their proprioceptors govern the spatial and temporal relations of their body and limbs in space, freeing the conscious mind to focus on other matters.

Two of the most important proprioceptors are muscle spindles and the Golgi tendon organs (GTOs; figure 1.2). Muscle spindles keep the muscle in a state of readiness by monitoring the strength, length, and tension of the muscle in which they are embedded so the muscle can relax or contract to permit proper movement. Also, these sensors initiate a muscle's contraction in order to reduce stretch in the muscle. Spindles make muscle activation possible. Meanwhile, the GTOs inhibit muscle activation to protect the muscle from a perceived injury by responding to tension within the tendon by sending signals to the spine to convey the change in tension. When the tension goes beyond a certain threshold, a reaction is triggered

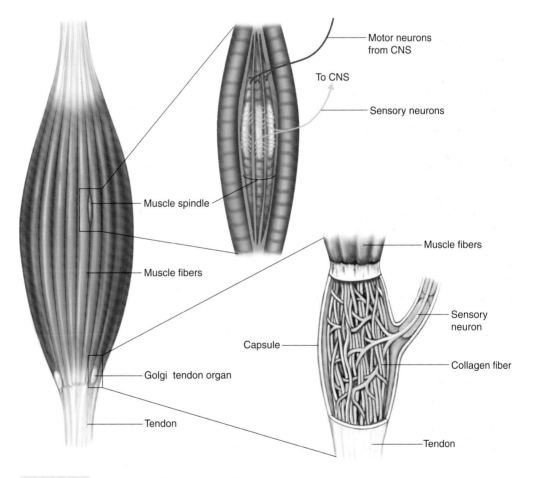

Figure 1.2 Muscle spindles and Golgi tendon organs monitor muscle tension and initiate contraction and relaxation, respectively.

Fig. 13.3, p. 388 from HUMAN PHYSIOLOGY, 2nd ed. by Dee Unglaub Silverthorn. Copyright © 2001 by Prentice-Hall, Inc. Reprinted by permission of Pearson Education, Inc.

that inhibits muscles from contracting and causes them to relax. Overall, these sensors are responsible for function itself.

With conditioned proprioceptors, an athlete is in better position to react, as joints and muscles respond automatically to protect the body from injury and other physical problems (Cook 2003). For instance, someone with highly conditioned proprioception can slip on ice and land on the ground without turning an ankle. According to Mark Verstegen, founder and president of Athletes' Performance, using a physioball (also known as a Swiss, balance, or stability ball) in exercise routines helps to condition proprioceptors (Verstegen and Williams 2004; figure 1.3). For example, a sit-up performed on a physioball relies on different parts of the neuromuscular system than a regular sit-up does. The unstable surface forces the athlete to maintain balance, which calls the muscles into action, enabling the athlete to help control and stabilize the body. Physioball exercises develop strength and stability in the shoulders, hips, and core and improve the activation and elongation of muscles. As a result, enhancement occurs in both the physical and neurological realms. Essentially, to improve the nervous system's response to movement, it is necessary to implement a conditioning

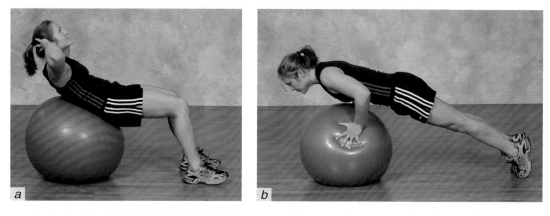

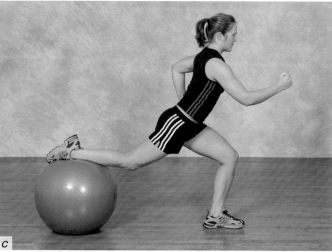

Figure 1.3 Physioball exercises such as the *(a)* crunch, *(b)* push-up, and *(c)* split squat condition the neuromuscular system.

program that stimulates and challenges the muscular, skeletal, and nervous systems. Increasing the stimulus of the proprioceptors with physioball and single-leg exercises will improve balance, coordination, flexibility, stability, and strength.

Conditioning for External Forces

Proprioception is the process of the body's muscular, skeletal, and nervous systems working together to perform everyday tasks on both conscious and subconscious levels. This process of working together is further demonstrated through the way muscles react to external forces such as gravity, ground reaction forces, and momentum. One of the best ways to condition the neuromuscular system to use these outside forces to mechanical advantage is by conditioning the muscles' stretch-shortening cycle.

The human body relies on outside forces to begin, engage, and enhance movement. Specific reflexes occur during movement that allow for suitable responses in function. Muscles react and interact with the environment to allow the body to rotate, run, jump, bend, and perform other types of movements. Basically, the stretch-shortening cycle is a process muscles go through in reaction to contact with outside forces. First, the muscles pronate. Pronation is a movement in which the muscle lengthens, the body decelerates, and the force exerted by the muscle decreases. Generally, pronation is associated with the foot and ankle, but pronation actually occurs throughout the entire body with ground reaction forces. Then, as a result of pronation, supination occurs. Supination is the opposite of pronation; in supination the muscle shortens, the body accelerates, and more force is produced. A good example of the pronating–supinating process is the stretching of a rubber band. Pronation is the rubber band stretching, and supination is the rubber band returning to its original shape.

Pronation and supination make up the stretch-shortening cycle. The stretch-shortening cycle is when two types of muscle actions (eccentric and concentric) occur simultaneously in combinations of muscle function. Eccentric muscle action refers to the lengthening of a muscle. If impact on a muscle is greater than its internal tension force, the muscle lengthens in an eccentric contraction. This allows the muscle to slow down, or decelerate, skeletal movements. Eccentric lengthening (before rapid concentric shortening) produces the greatest force and power capabilities in skeletal muscle because of chemical, mechanical, and neurological factors that influence the force and stiffness of the contracting muscle (Radcliffe and Farentinos 1999). Then, the muscle shortens during concentric (acceleration) action. For instance, when the foot hits the ground during walking, the muscles in the body, including but not limited to the hip rotators, quadriceps, deep muscles in the calf, and abdominal muscles, go through the stretch-shortening cycle. This sequence occurs during most natural movements, including running, walking, and jumping.

Consider the action of the quadriceps muscle of the thigh while moving up and down a staircase. As the knee straightens (extends) to ascend the staircase, the quadriceps concentrically contracts (shortens). As the knee bends (flexes) to descend the staircase, the quadriceps muscle eccentrically contracts (lengthens) and controls the speed of flexion. Without this action, the knee would rapidly bend and likely collapse under the load of the weight of the body.

An important element of the stretch-shortening cycle is the stretch reflex. As humans load, or apply force, to the joints, muscles, and nerves, they subconsciously elicit a stretch-shortening reflex in the center of each involved muscle. Its purpose is to monitor the length of the muscle and prevent it from overstretching. If the muscle is overstretched, a strain in the muscle fiber might occur. The stretch-shortening reflex occurs in all planes of motion and at every joint during function. This allows humans to decelerate, stabilize, and accelerate all movement. The stretch-shortening reflex is evident during the knee-jerk test performed at a doctor's office, when the leg swings in response to the knee being hit with a reflex hammer. This kind of subconscious response occurs with all functional movement.

Conditioning the stretch-shortening cycle so that it is more efficient improves both muscular and neurophysiological mechanisms. Training this feature stimulates changes in the neuromuscular system by enhancing the ability of the nervous system to recruit muscle groups and to respond to both slight and rapid changes in muscle length more quickly and powerfully (Radcliffe and Farentinos 1999). Training muscles in this fashion increases the power of movements, using the muscles' and tendons' elastic elements in addition to the stretch reflex. Also, it makes it possible for a muscle to reach maximal force in the shortest possible time and involve the stretch-shortening cycle (Potach and Chu 2000).

Several exercises can be done to improve the stretch-shortening cycle, including jumping drills and stability training, such as single-leg squats, standing bench press with cables, three-directional lunge, and standing shoulder press (see figure 1.4, *a* and *b*). Like all exercises, stretch-shortening conditioning depends on coordination of movement and variations of speed.

The stretch-shortening cycle is also improved through plyometrics (see figure 1.4 *c*), which increase the power of movements through the use of the elastic elements

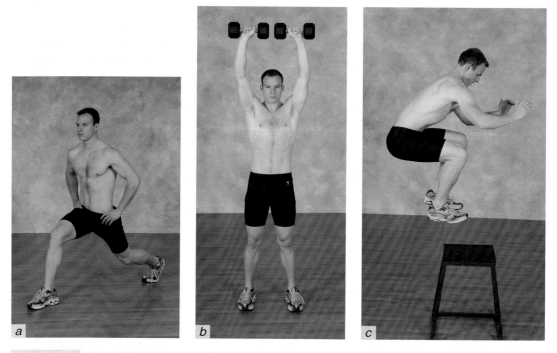

Figure 1.4 Condition the stretch-shortening cycle with exercises like *(a)* lunges, *(b)* the standing shoulder press, and *(c)* plyometrics.

of muscles and tendons and the stretch reflex. Various sorts of jumps—high-hurdle jumps, jumping side to side, clapping in the air while performing push-ups—are all examples of plyometrics. When performing these exercises, athletes should land in a prestretched position (arms and legs bent and on the ball of the feet). Plyometric training is efficient in that it recruits most, if not all, motor units and their corresponding fibers and increases the firing rate of motor neurons (Bompa 1999). This method of conditioning allows faster and more powerful changes in direction (Radcliffe and Farentinos 1999). When used properly, plyometrics not only result in quicker movements but also help prevent injury because they train the nervous system for demands placed on the body during sport and exercise.

Conditioning Biomotor Abilities

Biomotor abilities consist of flexibility, strength, power, endurance, agility, and coordination. Tudor Bompa, one of the world's leading specialists in training and fitness, refers to the ability to perform an exercise as both a basic, natural ability and an outcome of these biomotor abilities. Biomotor abilities are interdependent; there is a relationship between strength, speed, and endurance. During the initial years of training, all of these abilities must develop in order to build a solid foundation for more specialized training. Furthermore, when developing an exercise program, conditioning the neuromuscular system and soft tissue adaptation cannot be neglected without running the risk of injury or poor motor development. Including biomotor abilities helps determine how functional an exercise is and if the movements are applicable to everyday tasks. Being aware of functional characteristics when creating a conditioning program helps to train the body in a healthy manner.

Before developing any performance program, athletes should assess their biomotor systems to determine their strengths and deficiencies. An excellent assessment program is included in physical therapist Gary Gray's *Functional Video Digest Series* (2002). Prominent corrective and high-performance exercise expert Paul Chek recommends determining which biomotor abilities are required in an athlete's sport, work, and leisure environments before beginning an exercise program (2002b). Using a machine for stabilization can prohibit the development of biomotor abilities (Chek 2000). Rather than improve balance, agility, and coordination, machines isolate certain muscles, allow only simplistic movements, and hinder the development of movement patterns. Developing strength through functional movement patterns, such as those shown in figure 1.5 on page 10, generates proper movement with greater power for longer periods of time. This increase in endurance provides more opportunity for motor learning during conditioning and skill training. Overall, biomotor abilities are the key components to creating long-term and effective conditioning programs.

Implementing Functional Conditioning

Now that you understand how functional conditioning can aid injury prevention, we can look at how the four elements just discussed can be applied within a workout program. There is much more to preventing injury than proper stretching and breathing techniques. Optimal injury prevention requires improving parts of the body invisible

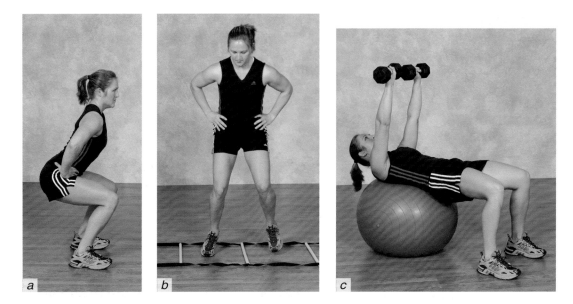

Figure 1.5 The biomotor abilities of endurance, speed, and strength can be trained with *(a)* body-weight squats, *(b)* ladder drills, and *(c)* the physioball bench press, respectively.

to the human eye. With so many exercises to choose from, the greatest challenge in creating a conditioning program is choosing which ones to do and what order to do them in. Before selecting exercises and their placement in your program, ensure that you understand everything involved in creating a conditioning program.

For starters, you need to create a movement preparation program to prepare the nervous system, muscular system, and joint complexes for the demands of exercise. After this, your actual workout occurs within a movement conditioning program that consists of fundamental movement patterns, as noted by nationally recognized exercise specialist Lenny Paracino in a 2005 telephone interview by Evan Chait:

- Push: bench press on a physioball with dumbbells
- Pull: seated or squatting lat pull-down
- Press: shoulder press with dumbbells
- Squat: with straight bar or dumbbells
- Lunge: preferably in three directions
- Step up and down: preferably in three directions
- Core stability training: crunches on ball or standing; chopping in three directions
- Complex variations: Olympic lifts (e.g., cleans)
- Isolated variations: machine training; traditional strength training; biceps curls or knee extension machine

The following program should give you an idea of how to prepare the body for the demands of exercise through a sequence of movements and activation drills. A basic template is provided with a suggested progression to help monitor essential elements as conditioning improves. The examples here provide a basic guideline for an injury-preventive functional training program. Because each sport and athlete requires an individual approach and progression to a conditioning program, the examples might need to be modified to meet particular needs.

Movement Preparation

Both physiologically and mentally, the beginning of a practice or a game sets the tone for the rest of the performance. By "turning on" the different components of athletic movement, we can expect considerably higher levels of performance and optimally absorbed training effects. Using the movement preparation protocol as an athlete's warm-up optimizes the body's ability to adapt to a given training stimulus. Besides enhancing performance and preventing injuries, the benefits of following a movement preparation sequence include the following:

1. Helps maximize the gains in performance enhancement and injury prevention by preparing the musculoskeletal and neurological components for the demands of the sport training
2. Ensures the multilateral development of flexibility, strength, balance, speed, and agility
3. Accelerates recovery and prevents overtraining

Movement preparation typically replaces the traditional warm-up of 5 to 15 minutes of aerobic activity, such as jogging, followed by a series of static stretches. Movement preparation is a kind of "high-tech" warm-up and occurs in the beginning of each conditioning session. It takes about 15 to 30 minutes. The preparation component consists of four kinds of training: flexibility, coordination, plyometric, and activation.

• **Flexibility training.** The goal here is to prepare the muscle and connective tissue for active movement. Traditional static stretching alone often fails to activate the body for athletic movement. Correctly chosen *dynamic* flexibility exercises "wake up" the proprioceptors that regulate the movement through the central nervous system. Some exercises also restore the muscles to their proper force production potential. A professionally planned and executed flexibility continuum helps reveal the true potential of the athletes and keeps them healthier for the whole season.

• **Coordination training.** This phase is used primarily to improve neuromuscular efficiency, dynamic stability, and coordination of movement. It prepares the neuromuscular system to do work. Particularly, the movements on a single leg prepare the whole kinetic chain for athletic movement. Coordination drills are also an essential part of injury prevention. The coordination phase helps the movement system respond to the demands of a game environment.

• **Plyometric training.** The stretch-shortening cycle that occurs in the muscles, tendons, and fascia during all movement must be turned on and optimized through plyometric exercises. Proper landing mechanics guide the musculoskeletal system to correctly load the whole kinetic chain. Effective loading and unloading of the chain results in powerful and controlled movement, whereas the inability to execute this cycle properly results in lack of speed, agility, and quickness. Proper technique, attention to detail, and the correct number of repetitions are important in making the plyometrics phase as beneficial as it can be.

• **Activation training.** This phase is used to develop an increase in neuromotor recruitment in movement patterns particular to sport or activity. As a last phase of the movement preparation, the activation segment is the closest to sport-specific performance. This phase transfers the benefits of the first three phases into the game. Activation is more subconscious than the other phases and enables the nervous system to "download" all the training benefits so they can be used within a sport situation. Activation also "switches on" the inner athlete, the mind and soul, and helps him or her approach tasks with the proper attitude and focus.

Movement Preparation Programming

The most important factor when creating a movement preparation program is exercise selection and purpose. Exercise selection and knowing when and how to use a push, pull, squat, or a complex movement can prevent an injury. All movements must have a purpose. Other factors influencing the training outcome include choosing the right acute variables, such as repetitions, sets, rest periods, intensity, and periodization (see Tudor Bompa's *Periodization Training for Sport* (1999) for more information on these topics). Each movement preparation component requires well-thought-out planning in order to achieve an effective overall program.

• **Flexibility training programming.** What makes a good flexibility program is the selection of the muscle groups you are stretching and the type of stretching technique you use. Essentially, there are three types of flexibility techniques: static, active, and dynamic. Static flexibility (see figure 1.6a) consists of holding a position for a period of time between 20 and 30 seconds. An example of this is holding the position during the track stretch for stretching the calves. This stretching technique is most effective after a conditioning program and is not recommended prior to exercising. Static flexibility inhibits the excitation of the muscle and "turns the muscle off." Performing static stretches before activity increases the risk of injury during the activity.

Active flexibility involves moving a particular body region into a new range of motion and holding the position for two to five seconds. An example is lying on your back with a strap around your ankle and lifting your leg up toward the ceiling (see figure 1.6b). Only use the strap at the end range to facilitate and increase in the new range of motion, and be sure to hold the position for two to five seconds. Active flexibility is effective before or after a conditioning program.

Finally, dynamic flexibility involves moving into a new range of motion without a hold in the position. It increases the body's core temperature and prepares the neuromuscular and proprioceptive systems better than either static or active flexibility. Examples include walking lunges, inchworms (see figure 1.6c), leg swings, and jumping jacks. Dynamic flexibility is most effective before a conditioning program.

To learn more about flexibility techniques, check out *The Whartons' Stretch Book*, Gary Gray's *Functional Video Digest Series*, Ann and Chris Frederick's *Stretch to Win*, or Jay Blahnik's *Full-Body Flexibility*.

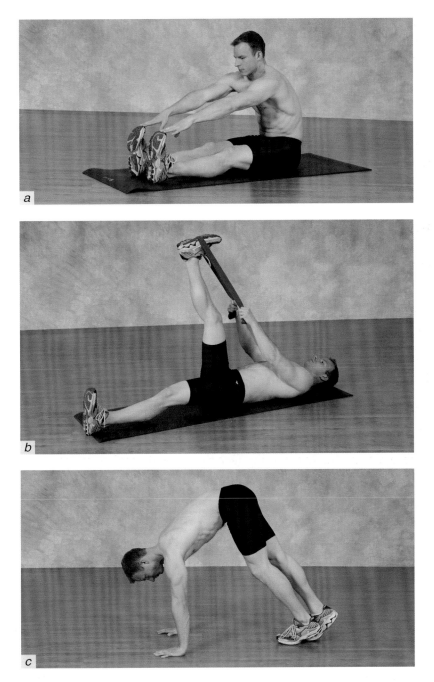

Figure 1.6 *(a)* Static flexibility, *(b)* active flexibility, and *(c)* dynamic flexibility.

• **Coordination training programming.** Coordination training is the most neglected component in conditioning programs. Examples of coordination training include single-leg balance, single-leg squat touch down, single-leg balance on an airex pad with a ball toss, and single-leg hip rotation. This type of training challenges an athlete's ability to remain upright when challenged by external forces or put in situations where he or she is off balance. Often simply raising one lower limb while attempting to balance on the other can be extremely difficult. Consider the relative ease of standing upright on solid ground when there is no wind blowing and there are no ambient challenges versus the extreme difficulty of standing on a mobile surface, such as on a balance board or rock board. For more information on coordination training, see Robert Gotlin's "The Lower Extremity" chapter in *Sports Medicine: Principles of Primary Care* or Michael Boyle's *Functional Training for Sports*.

• **Plyometric training programming.** Plyometric training techniques include squat jumps, lunge jumps, box jumps, single hops, and multiplanar jumps and hops. Selection and periodization is extremely important in creating a plyometric training program. A linear progression must be practiced in order to prevent injury and enhance performance. Start with foundational movement patterns, such as landing technique and squat jumps with holds for three to five seconds. For additional information on exercise selection and periodization of plyometric training, refer to Donald A. Chu's *Jumping Into Plyometrics.*

• **Activation training programming.** This phase is the most sport-specific phase of conditioning. It involves understanding speed mechanics, running mechanics, acceleration–deceleration mechanics, and change-of-direction mechanics. Examples include speed training and repeats, speed ladder training, and change-of-direction exercises. More information on activation training can be found in *The Pose Method of Running* by Dr. Nicholas Romanov, *Athletic Development* by Vern Gambetta, and *Training for Speed, Agility, and Quickness* by Lee E. Brown and Vance A. Ferrigno.

CHAPTER 2

Prevention and Treatment Toolbox

Elise Weiss, MD; Todd D. Hirsch, MS, ATC; Grant Cooper, MD

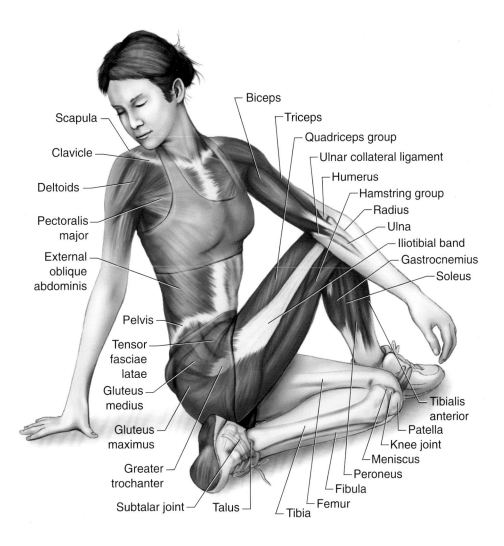

njuries lower an athlete's fitness level, impair competitive performance, and predispose him or her to long-term musculoskeletal problems. The two best predictors of injury are a history of past damage (such as a previous ankle sprain increasing the likelihood of a future ankle sprain) and the number of consecutive days spent training (the higher the number of consecutive days, the greater the incidence of injury). Many sports injuries, whether acute (occurring suddenly or caused by sudden trauma) or chronic (of a long duration or recurring) can be prevented through proper training before participation in the sport and with appropriate action taken after the initial harmful event. This chapter presents ways to prevent injuries, treat acute injuries, and manage chronic injuries.

Prevention Strategies

Injury prevention begins before an athlete steps onto the playing field. It involves adhering to a comprehensive conditioning program that includes a complete warm-up and cool-down routine, stretching, aerobic training, and sport-specific strength training. This is the way to create well-balanced and flexible muscles. For many sports, proper and well-fitted equipment is also required. Finally, eating properly plays a key role in preventing injury; eating right makes athletes less susceptible to being injured, and an anti-inflammatory diet may minimize the impact and duration of an injury.

Creating a Balanced Program

Proper conditioning for a sport allows for greater enjoyment, safer participation, and better performance. It reduces injury risk and allows athletes to reach their maximum potential. Contrary to popular belief, being properly conditioned doesn't necessarily require extensive training. Rather, what is required is a customized training program targeted to the style and level of activity at which the athlete wishes to perform.

An athlete's conditioning program should address several areas, including a proper warm-up and cool-down for each session and a balance of strength and endurance training. While many specific philosophies exist, conditioning should take into account two important training principles: progressive overload and periodization. *Progressive overload* ensures that the initial program is tolerable in terms of intensity and volume and that these components are adjusted appropriately throughout the program to lead to a targeted goal. The intensities of several workout variables can be adjusted to apply this concept and reduce the risk of overuse injury. The acronym FITT highlights the four variables at play in developing a conditioning program: frequency, intensity, time, and type (Krivickas 1999). Two important parts of adhering to a progressive overload program are to match any increase in training with an increase in rest and to precede any increase in overall load with an increase in strengthening (Schwellnus 2003).

An important companion to progressive overload is the concept of *periodization*, which is the planned variation of a training program over time. Research supports this variation as key to optimizing and safely performing physical training (Frontera 2003). To periodize a program, the total training time in a season (called a macrocycle) is divided into smaller time periods (called mesocycles), each with a specific goal. An example of a mesocycle goal would be to build a solid strength base or to develop sport-specific skills. The ultimate goal of periodized training is being prepared for competition. When setting mesocycle goals, integrate rest into the program to allow time for recovery and reduce injury risk. Please refer to Frontera's *Rehabilitation of Sports Injuries: Scientific Basis* for more detailed readings on this subject.

Warm-Up and Cool-Down

Warming up prior to any workout improves performance by increasing blood flow, warming the muscles, and preventing rapid alterations in body physiology that might occur if an athlete simply started participating at full speed (Kraemer 2003). For any sport or activity, a warm-up program should follow the movement preparation program described in chapter 1. At the least, a warm-up should include 5 to 10 minutes of slow jogging to increase body temperature, followed by 10 to 15 minutes of sport-specific drills.

Many experts also advocate 10 to 15 minutes of stretching to reduce muscle stiffness before activity. Those who recommend stretching at this point in a warm-up assert that muscle stiffness is directly related to muscle injury and that stretching should be included in all warm-up routines. If stretching is used as part of a warm-up, it should focus on dynamic stretches that decrease muscle stiffness (Mujika and Padilla 2001). An example of a dynamic stretch is 8 to 12 repetitions of controlled leg swings, arm swings, or torso twists (Kibler and Chandler 1994). Do not confuse dynamic stretching with ballistic stretching, which involves forcing a part of the body beyond its natural range of motion. There are no such movements in dynamic stretching.

After a workout or game, a cool-down helps dissipate metabolic waste products (such as lactic acid) from muscle, reduce the potential for muscle soreness, and reduce the chances of dizziness or fainting caused by pooling of venous blood in the extremities (Krivickas 1999). Cooling down should include 5 to 10 minutes of jogging or walking followed by 5 to 10 minutes of static stretching exercises. Static stretches help muscles relax and improve their range of movement. Generally, a static stretch is held for 30 to 60 seconds with continuous tension on the target muscle. Because static stretches slowly ease the muscle into position, they produce far fewer instances of muscle soreness, injury, or damage to connective tissues than dynamic or ballistic stretches do. Keep in mind that static stretches are best as a cool down; they do not prepare muscles for activities as well as dynamic stretching.

Flexibility Training

All athletes require a degree of flexibility, which is derived through stretching. Stretching should include all major muscle groups regardless of their degree of involvement in the athlete's particular sport. Stretching has become so important in the minds of some trainers and coaches that many advocate specific routines. Some insist that athletes must stretch *before* any workout or contest and *after* an initial warm-up. Many studies from the 1980s and early 1990s support this idea. More recently, other studies suggest that preexercise stretching does not prevent injury and might in fact hinder performance. Proponents of this theory believe that postexercise stretching provides more benefit and that, before a workout, light warm-up activities, such as easy jogging, are enough to reduce muscle stiffness.

Why are the older studies at odds with the newer studies? Part of the reason might be that many of the injuries suffered by athletes today are caused by circumstances that stretching cannot prevent. For instance, increasing mileage, resistance, or intensity too quickly; improper use of equipment; and poor biomechanics lead to injuries that cannot be prevented through stretching. More investigative work needs to be done to determine the exact benefits obtained from stretching and when stretching should be done to maximize its benefits.

Despite ongoing debate about the effectiveness of stretching in preventing sports-related injuries, stretching after exercise is known to be an effective way to increase flexibility. By definition, flexibility reduces tension and resistance in muscle tissue (Fleck and Kraemer 1997). Because a muscle that causes movement (agonist) can contract only as forcefully as its antagonist (the muscle that works in opposition to the agonist) can relax, it makes sense that flexibility of an antagonistic muscle increases the force, power, and speed of its agonist. For example, an agonist muscle whose function is to flex is restricted by the antagonist muscle whose function is to extend the same muscle—therefore improving the flexibility of the extensor improves the peformance of the flexor. In addition, stretching plays an important role in maintaining healthy joints because it increases tissue temperature, blood supply, and joint lubrication (Mujika and Padilla 2001).

Some experts advocate stretching as a part of a training regimen apart from any other workout. For maximum gains in flexibility in the shortest possible time, the proprioceptive neuromuscular facilitation (PNF) technique may be most appropriate. In the PNF technique, the athlete assumes the stretch position while a partner holds the limb in place. The athlete then contracts the stretched muscle against partner-supplied resistance for 6 to 10 seconds. The partner then moves the limb further into the stretched position and the contraction is repeated for 6 to 10 seconds. This resetting of the stretch is performed three to four times. The effectiveness of PNF is based on the observation that agonist muscle relaxation increases after its own contraction. When done in conjunction with antagonist muscle contraction, however, stretching this way carries a greater risk of overstretching than other methods do (Frontera 2003). The microscopic muscle tears that result from overstretching ultimately lead to scar formation and reduction of muscle elasticity. If PNF is to be performed, it must be done with a trusted partner who is aware of the potential dangers of the technique.

Endurance Training

In general, aerobic endurance training should occur three to five times per week at an intensity of 60 to 85 percent of maximum heart rate (maximum heart rate can be approximated by subtracting the athlete's age from 220). Sessions of endurance training should usually last from 20 to 60 minutes. There are several different methods of endurance training. Endurance work is generally broken into either long, steady-duration sessions or interval training sessions. Long-distance training is used for preparation in all sports. It is characterized by long sessions at below race or competition intensity. Duration is usually between 30 minutes and two hours and intensity is below 80 percent of maximum heart rate. Although this type of training offers endurance-building benefits, it is often not sport-specific. Also, because it is done at a lower than maximal intensity, relying too heavily on it could have slowing effects on pace during competition (Fox, Bowers, and Foss 1988; Gaesser and Wilson 1988). As a result, general consensus supports alternating long, steady-duration training with interval training while including appropriate rest days. Interval training involves short bursts of activity for 3 to 5 minutes followed by a recovery period and then a return to high-intensity activity. Interval training can be tailored to improve endurance or speed. To improve endurance, short rest periods follow high-intensity sessions. For speed development, longer rest periods follow short, very intense work intervals. Because this type of training is so demanding, sessions are limited to 30 to 45 minutes. An additional benefit of this type of training is that it can be highly sport specific. A soccer player can intersperse sprints, while dribbling a ball, with long runs along the area of a soccer field and finish with a shot on goal. A tennis player can sidestep along the baseline of a tennis court before running sprints along the court and end with a simulated forehand shot.

Strength Conditioning

When just beginning, athletes should have someone supervise the strengthening program to ensure that they are performing a comprehensive routine and using proper technique. It is easy to become injured during strength training. The importance of proper technique cannot be overemphasized.

Most athletes should balance endurance training with resistance training. Many injuries are caused by weak muscles that cannot handle the demands of a sport; for example, a runner with a persistent hip injury tends over time to adopt a running style that helps him accommodate the pain. In this style of running, in which one side is favored over another because of pain, the hip extensors are not used effectively, and the runner's stance is more flexed than upright. Such a runner would benefit from a weight-training program aimed directly at the hip extensors. Strengthening the hip flexors would help the runner more evenly distribute the work of running over the leg muscles and would make running more efficient and less painful. This kind of specific training improves motor function and control. The same can be said of a tennis player with a weak back. Strengthening the muscles that support the back can correct the weak link and allow optimal connection between the muscles that generate the forces needed for the sport and the racket.

Each strengthening session should begin with a warm-up session (see p. 17). As with general conditioning, follow the concept of progressive overload by adding more load and more repetitions as the athlete's level of strength improves. A general rule is to increase the training load by no more than 10 percent per week and to train two to three times per week, allowing a day or two for recovery between sessions. Several variables can be periodized in a strengthening program, including exercise order, frequency, load, intensity, speed, and amount of rest between sets. Additionally, programs can include open exercises (such as seated knee extensions using an ankle weight), in which the end of the exercised limb is free to move in space, or closed exercises (such as the leg press), in which the end of the limb is fixed to the ground or another surface. Kinetic chain exercises can be used while alternating between free weights and machines.

Muscle contraction falls into three categories: isotonic, isometric, and isokinetic. Isotonic contractions shorten muscle, producing movement. Most consider these contractions the easiest to perform. A biceps curl is one example. Holding the curl static at 90 degrees is an example of an isometric contraction. In isometric contraction, there is no movement through a range of motion. An isokinetic contraction occurs when the contraction is performed at a particular speed and the resistance varies according to how fast the limb is moved. Isotonic contractions have the benefit of strengthening a muscle throughout its range of movement, but they tend to do so unevenly, and these types of contraction are most likely to result in muscle soreness. Isometric contractions do not shorten muscle and thus develop static strength. They don't require equipment and are relatively quick and easy to perform, but the muscle gains strength only at the exercise angle performed. Plus blood flow to the muscle stops during an isometric contraction, blood pressure rises, and there is less venous return to the heart. This means that isometric exercises are the most physiologically taxing and should be performed with caution by people with preexisting medical conditions. In isokinetic contractions, a muscle contracts and shortens at constant speed, thus, special equipment is needed to sense the speed of the muscle. This equipment is expensive but may allow the fastest method of increasing muscle strength. Keep in mind, however, that isokinetic strengthening may not equate to functional training because a constant speed is maintained; this is not the case in many functional movements.

The relation between muscles around a joint is known as muscle balance. Recall that muscle use can be separated into agonist and antagonist actions. For instance, the biceps (agonist) flexes the elbow while the triceps (antagonist) extends the elbow. Muscles can also be separated into the categories of stabilizers or mobilizers. Functionally, mobilizers tend to perform quick actions, whereas stabilizers are involved in posture maintenance. An imbalance can occur if the mobilizers, with their tendency to tighten and shorten, overtake stabilizers (Kraemer 2003).

A strengthening program must include stabilizer strengthening. For example, in a biceps curl, the stabilizer is the deltoid, which must be trained with a separate exercise aimed at the deltoid. In a shoulder press, the legs are the stabilizers. In a squat, the trunk muscles stabilize. When an athlete lifts free weights, the body must stabilize the movement; when an athlete uses a machine, the machine stabilizes for the body. This is one of the reasons many trainers advocate the use of free weights over machines.

Cross-Training

Cross-training—training in a sport other than your own—is a popular method of reducing injury risk because it takes pressure off constantly worked joints and can promote muscular balance. But choosing a cross-training activity can be difficult for athletes who are training for a specific event. For a runner, nothing can substitute for running. However, activities can be chosen to supplement running in way that maintains training volume while reducing the load on overstressed joints.

Cross-training is particularly appropriate during maintenance workouts in the off-season or during rest workouts. Endurance and strength dissipate at more rapid rates than those at which they are gained. Therefore, training programs should limit periods of complete inactivity to no more than two to three weeks. Athletes who choose a cross-training activity can achieve an effective rest for specifically stressed joints while maintaining overall endurance.

Periodic Assessment

To ensure that a training program is dynamic and changes with their increasing abilities (rather than remaining static with a consequent loss of effectiveness), athletes should have a fitness assessment done every two to three months. Such an assessment determines athletes' training needs and helps them make choices in developing their program based on the concept of progressive overload discussed earlier in the chapter. Things to note during these assessments may include training unit (speed, endurance, strength), load (mileage, sets/repetitions), and intensity (maximal heart rate achieved, weight lifted). Assessment and progress can be monitored with standardized time trials, endurance testing, and evaluation of maximum strength. Adjustments can be made to the program based on progress and desired outcome. For example, if a runner is not on his or her desired race pace, a greater amount of time might be devoted to interval training with emphasis on speed.

Using Proper Technique and Equipment

Biomechanics, the study of internal and external forces that affect the body, plays a crucial role in efficient and safe participation in any activity. Faulty biomechanics result from either static anatomical abnormalities or from functional abnormalities (Renstrom 1993). Although static abnormalities can be addressed by compensatory devices such as orthotics, the functional changes that result from both the abnormality and its correction must be addressed in training. Functional abnormalities are usually easier to change because they are often a result of injury, improper technique, or poorly adjusted equipment.

Two issues should be addressed in regard to equipment. The first is a proper fit. Ill-fitting equipment negatively affects biomechanics. The second is protection. Wearing or using proper protective equipment during training and competition significantly reduces the risk of injury.

The sport of cycling illustrates the role of properly fitted equipment in promoting good biomechanics. The bike minimizes the negative effects of both the repetitive motion of cycling and the static position that the body maintains. When seated on a bike with hands on the handlebars, the hands, shoulders, and front axle should all be in line, and the reach should be set so that the rider has slight elbow flexion with hands relaxed on the brake hoods (Kibler and Chandler 1994). This allows the rider to hold the wrist in a neutral position. If alignment is not correct and the wrist bears weight in an extended position, the rider might damage the ulnar nerve (the nerve that runs from the upper arm to the pinky side of the hand). This damage can be prevented if the build of the bike is fitted to the athlete. Specification of the bike to the rider also ensures that seat placement is correct. Seat height is critical to proper pedaling biomechanics. If a seat is too high, muscles must work beyond their optimal length-tension range. If a seat is too low, knee flexion is increased as is stress on the knee joints.

Proper footwear has a similar effect on biomechanics. Using our cycling example, shoes need to be both comfortable and rigid to transfer power from the pedal to the leg. If the transfer is inefficient, strain on the lower limb and lumbar spine is increased. In general, footwear should support the foot, absorb impact, and provide traction. The optimal shoe for an athlete is one that matches his or her biomechanical features and answers the demands of the sport. When appropriate, a simple foot orthotic can correct anatomical abnormalities.

The use of protective equipment is usually recommended as a result of research by health professionals that identifies a high risk of injury in a particular sport or recreational activity. Protective equipment includes personal equipment such as mouth guards and headgear as well as external equipment such as padding around the goal posts on an American football field. Such equipment must be used for its intended purpose, fit well, be comfortable, allow unrestricted movement, and be worn or used whether the athlete is at practice or in competition. It should be replaced when worn out or damaged and must comply with the rules of the sport for which it is intended. Protective equipment should not be shared among players of different sizes and should be appropriate to the player's gender, covering areas most likely to come into contact with other players or equipment.

Helmets have proven effective in preventing or reducing the severity of brain injuries in sport. Sport-specific helmets are designed to address the different risk factors particular to each sport. Risks vary from sport to sport because of distance to the ground, playing surface, playing equipment, and speed of movement. Regardless, the helmet should be firm, comfortable, and fitted to the athlete. A loose-fitting helmet might obstruct view or cause hyperextension of the cervical spine. Whereas hard helmets reduce the risk of head injury, soft headgear can help prevent serious abrasions to the scalp and ears. Helmets are either mandated or recommended for auto and motor sports, bicycling, boxing, equestrian, football, hockey, lacrosse, in-line skating, rugby, skateboarding, skiing, snowboarding, softball, and wrestling (Renstrom 1993).

Other protective gear includes eyewear and mouth guards. Protective eyewear standards currently exist for racket sports, women's lacrosse, paintball, and youth baseball. The Protective Eyewear Certification Council (PECC) assists consumers, sports organizations, and eye care professionals in choosing proper eyewear (Renstrom 1994). The PECC seal assures that equipment has been tested and certified to protect the eye from damage. Mouth protectors help prevent injury to the mouth, teeth, lips, cheeks, and tongue. They can cushion blows that might otherwise cause concussion or jaw fracture. Mouth guards should be worn by all athletes during contact and collision sports.

A concern related to protective equipment is the safety of the playing surface on which a sport is played. A hard surface generates more force to the musculoskeletal system than a soft surface. Additionally, traction plays a key role in the risk of injury. For example, in the case of American football, it has been found that dry fields increase the risk of anterior cruciate ligament injury because of the large amount of traction and the resulting forces transmitted to the knee during rapid movement and change of direction (Orchard et al. 2001). Watering down fields to soften them prior to play could reduce the risk of such injuries. Similarly, placing padding around goal posts to absorb impact and minimize trauma could reduce the severity of some types of injury.

Eating Nutritiously

Once injured, athletes typically turn to traditional treatment as their first intervention. That nutritional aspects of training and recovery are frequently overlooked before and after injury is a mystery to many sports nutritionists. After all, it is clear that training alters an athlete's nutritional requirements. A proper training diet is critical to optimal performance. To maintain their health, most athletes should follow a diet made up of 15 to 20 percent protein, 30 percent fat, and 50 to 55 percent carbohydrate. This is not a universal recommendation but rather a starting point from which to tailor a diet to the demands of athletic activity. A sports nutritionist could make specific determinations based on an individual athlete's needs.

An injury increases an athlete's already elevated nutritional needs. Consuming adequate calories while adhering to an anti-inflammatory diet might not only help prevent injury but also hasten recovery from an existing injury. Although inflammation serves as a protective process immediately after an injury, once it has done its job the body is better off without it.

If inflammation is not properly modulated, it continues unchecked. Inflammation is self-sustaining through the creation of free radicals, which are generated by the aerobic energy pathway itself. The more training an athlete does, the more free radicals the body produces. These free radicals damage muscle cells and trigger further inflammation and lipid peroxidation, thought to be the source of muscle soreness after rigorous training. Free radicals are also well-known culprits in blood vessel damage and many diseases.

Alcohol and caffeine consumption and tobacco use must also be addressed when targeting inflammation. These substances increase oxidation and free radical formation, which initiates the inflammatory process, which can exacerbate an otherwise minor injury. Athletes who consume alcohol and caffeine should do so in moderation, and they should avoid both smoking and chewing tobacco.

Carbohydrate

Muscle mass cannot be supported without sufficient carbohydrate. In the initial stages of exercise, 40 to 50 percent of the body's energy requirements are achieved through the metabolism of carbohydrate (Wilkinson 1997). Carbohydrate yields more energy per unit of oxygen consumed than fat, which supplies the remaining energy requirement. Because oxygen is often a limiting factor in duration events, it makes sense that the athlete first use the energy source that requires the least oxygen consumption.

During digestion, the body breaks down carbohydrate into glucose and stores it in the form of glycogen. During exercise, glycogen reverts to glucose and is used for energy. The ability to sustain exercise directly depends on the amount of glycogen stores. If an event's duration is under 90 minutes, standard muscle glycogen stores supply the energy needed. For events longer than 90 minutes, carbohydrate-loading over the three days before competition might be beneficial. Eating a diet composed of no more than 70 percent carbohydrate during this time fills all available glycogen stores while minimizing water retention associated with carbohydrate loading.

Not all carbohydrates are created equal; simple carbohydrates differ from complex carbohydrates. Simple carbohydrates such as honey and candy get most of their calories from sugar. These foods should make up less than 10 percent of an athlete's diet (Okuyama, Ichikawa, Fujii, and Ito 2005). Chemical reactions between sugar and protein produce proinflammatory advanced glycation end products (AGEs). In addition, the surge in blood sugar that results from eating these foods prompts a release of insulin from the pancreas, which increases inflammatory gene production. Also, contrary to popular belief, eating sugar before an event does not improve performance. Water is needed to absorb sugar into cells, and large glucose loads might increase dehydration. In addition, sugar leads to a large insulin surge, causing a drop in blood sugar, which in itself can compromise performance. The bulk of carbohydrate intake should be of complex carbohydrate, including fruits, vegetables, and whole grains. The insulin response from complex carbohydrates is not as significant as from simple carbohydrates, thus, blood sugar levels remain more steady.

Protein

The body works to recover after any event or training session by using protein synthesis to repair muscles. If inadequate amounts of protein are consumed to aid in this repair, muscle injury can occur. Generally, 1.0 to 1.5 grams per kilogram (1 kg = 2.2 lbs) of body weight per day of protein intake is recommended for regular training, with the higher end of the range intended for endurance athletes (Okuyama, Ichikawa, Fujii, and Ito 2005). Most athletes meet this protein requirement through a normal diet and do not require supplementation. The use of protein (powder) supplementation is rarely, if ever, required.

Essential Fat

To assure proper body function, athletes must consume fatty acids. Omega-6 and omega-3 fatty acids are particularly essential. Both are involved in the inflammatory process but in different ways. Arachidonic acid, an omega-6 fatty acid, is involved in the initiation of inflammation. For this reason, red meat and peanuts, which contain high levels of arachidonic acid, should be consumed in minimal amounts. Eicosapentaenoic acid, an omega-3 fatty acid, is critical in controlling inflammation.

Besides being an excellent source of protein, cold-water fish are rich in two omega-3 fatty acids: eicosapentaenoic (EPA) and docosahexaenoic (DHA). These potent anti-inflammatories are found in mackerel, salmon, trout, sardines, and tuna. Plant sources such as flaxseed, wheat germ, and walnuts can be converted into EPA and DHA, but the body's mechanism for this conversion is highly inefficient. Considerably larger amounts of plant-based omega-3 fatty acids must be consumed to meet the equivalent obtained from a fish source. Another way to get the essential fatty acids is to take fish oil supplements, which allow the body to bypass the conversion of alpha linolenic acid to EPA and DHA. Taking 3 grams of fish oil each day may be beneficial even if cold-water fish are consumed. On the down side, fish oil supplements might increase the risk of bleeding. Athletes should consult with a physician before embarking on this course, especially if they take blood thinners.

As the Western diet has become increasingly dependent on convenience, the ratio of omega fatty acids has shifted to favor the omega-6 variety. This is partly because of processed vegetable oils and food preservatives. To increase the shelf life of many products and reduce the amount of saturated fat in the diet, the food industry created trans fatty acids, which are partially hydrogenated oils. Unfortunately, a by-product of this innovation is an increase in the amount of omega-6 fatty acids in the diet and free radicals in the blood. In fact, many nutrition professionals believe that the Western diet, with its highly processed high-fat content, primes the body toward an inflammatory state. Additionally, trans fatty acids directly interfere in enzyme conversions to produce healthful EPA and DHA. Given the abundance of processed foods in the modern diet, direct supplementation of omega-3 fatty acids might be an effective strategy. As current media reports reflect, the use of trans fats in foods products is rapidly declining as consumers become more aware of the associated health concerns.

A well-known exception to the omega-6 fatty acid rule is gamma linolenic acid (GLA), which boosts prostaglandins that reduce inflammation. GLA is found naturally to varying extents in various plant seed oils (evening primrose seed oil, borage seed oil, black currant seed oil, and hemp seed oil). Olive oil, rich in omega-9 fatty oleic acid, is another non-omega-3 with anti-inflammatory properties. These two fatty acids, ingested directly or through supplementation, might help reduce inflammation in the body.

Antioxidants

Antioxidants are the body's natural mechanism to inhibit free radical damage. They neutralize the radicals, thereby inhibiting the lipid peroxidation process. The body has endogenous antioxidants that increase naturally after exercise. In addition, the body can use nutrient antioxidants.

Polyphenols, found in green tea, prune juice, and grape juice, are also important antioxidants. Drinking polyphenols is of particular benefit to athletes because the substances are rapidly absorbed after ingestion, allowing for maximum concentration in the blood during exercise. Green tea is the best source but should be consumed without milk because milk tends to bind flavonoids, allowing them to pass through the gastrointestinal tract without antioxidant benefit (Okuyama, Ichikawa, Fujii, and Ito 2005). Spinach, broccoli, blueberries, apples, cherries, and oranges are also rich in flavonoids. Many of these fruits and vegetables are also good sources of vitamins C and E, which have some benefit as antioxidants.

Vitamins and Minerals

Vitamin C is beneficial in the healing process for reasons other than its antioxidant properties. Vitamin C is a major component of connective tissue. It also boosts the growth of fibroblasts and chondrocytes (instrumental in production of connective tissue and cartilage). A dose of 1,000 milligrams of vitamin C a day is considered safe and effective.

Deficiencies of certain vitamins and minerals have been linked with injury. Calcium is critical in maintaining bone density and normal muscle contraction, and many experts recommend supplements for people with an insufficient dietary source. Others dispute whether calcium supplements provide the benefit of natural calcium, but as of this writing recommendations remain in place to supplement the diet to achieve a minimum of 1,200 milligrams of calcium a day. Because vitamin D facilitates absorption of calcium, many over-the-counter calcium supplements contain vitamin D.

Iron plays a role in the oxidative potential of muscles and is instrumental in hemoglobin function. Hemoglobin is the part of the blood that carries oxygen to the tissues. If iron levels are low, hemoglobin levels are adversely affected and oxygen delivery to tissues is decreased. Therefore, the body's more easily exhausted muscles are less able to support and stabilize joints. Some nutritionists believe that low iron levels might also slow the rate at which tissues are repaired, allowing what might have been a minor injury to mature into a significant one. Take iron supplements with caution because elevated blood counts of iron might be linked with an increased risk of heart attack and decreased absorption of zinc. Consult a doctor before starting an iron supplementation program.

Hydration

Another important component of eating nutritiously is adequate hydration. Dehydration has significant detrimental effects on sports performance. It decreases endurance during an activity and delays recovery after an activity. A general guideline to follow is to prehydrate two hours before exercise with 500 to 600 milliliters (17-20 oz) of fluid and to ingest an additional 500 milliliters (17 oz) of fluid 15 minutes before exercise. During exercise fluids should be taken as tolerated. In general, 150 to 350 milliliters (5-12 oz) of fluids should be ingested every 15 to 20 minutes (particularly during high-endurance exercise).

After exercise, 1 to 1.5 liters (or quarts) of fluids per kilogram (2.2 pounds) of body weight lost should be ingested to rehydrate. Rehydration can best be monitored through the production of clear or pale urine. Some important corollaries to these recommendations are that while plain water is appropriate for exercise lasting less than an hour, drinks containing 4 to 8 percent carbohydrate and 0.5 to 0.7 gram per liter of sodium are recommended for intense exercise that lasts longer than one hour (Bruckner and Karmim 1993). Athletes should avoid caffeine, energy drinks, and alcohol after exercise because they increase fluid loss.

Athletes must be aware of the condition known as hyponatremia (low salt), or more commonly as overhydration. Hyponatremia occurs when dehydration is addressed by replenishing with only pure water. The result is a relative dilution of the body's salt (sodium) concentration. This condition is dangerous and can be fatal as it can lead, rarely, to brain swelling and death. Rehydration should be carefully carried out as outlined above and a mixture of pure water and sports drinks is recommended.

Treatment Guidelines

Direct trauma is the cause of many injuries. Collision sports such as American football and high-velocity sports such as alpine skiing have the greatest risk for traumatic injuries. Sports such as basketball have a high incidence of sprains and strains. Sprains typically result from a sudden twisting or stretching movement. Strains may result from a sudden overexertion, stretching, or twisting movement. Other common sports injuries include bruises, lacerations (cuts through the skin), and abrasions (scrapes). Direct trauma to the affected body part causes many of these injuries. For example, a kick to the thigh may result in a bruise. A slide along a hard playing surface while wearing short pants may result in an abrasion. A swipe across the face with a hockey stick is likely to result in a laceration. The most important factors in controlling the extent of an injury are the steps taken immediately after the injury occurs.

At the moment of injury, chemicals are released from damaged cells, triggering the process of inflammation. Vessels at the injury site become dilated, and blood flow to the area increases to carry nutrients to the site of tissue damage. Within hours of injury, inflammatory cells travel to the injury site and begin to remove damaged cells and tissues. Within days, scar tissue is formed. Within three weeks, scar tissue begins to shrink and damaged tissues begin to regenerate. Despite the body's quick response, it will likely be several months before a traumatic injury is completely healed (Orchard, Seward, McGivern, and Hood 2001).

The role of inflammation as a healing and restorative process is widely recognized. Historically, inflammation was characterized by the five classical signs of dolor (pain), calor (heat), rubor (redness), tumor (swelling), and function laesa (loss of function). The physiology involved in inflammation accounts for the changes seen. The heat and redness are caused by increased movement of blood through dilated vessels. The swelling is the result of increased passage of fluid from dilated and permeable blood vessels into the surrounding tissues as well as the infiltration of inflammatory cells into the area. Pain is a result of pressure or chemical mediators stimulating pain-transmitting nerve fibers. The loss of function relates to the loss of mobility secondary to edema and pain or the replacement of functional tissue with scar tissue (Witvrouw, Mahieu, Danneels, and McNair 2004).

Initial Treatment

The primary goal of initial treatment is to reduce swelling and promote healing. PRICE is the acronym for the principles by which injury is initially managed (except in the case of a medical emergency that requires immediate care by a medical professional):

- **Protection.** When athletes suspect an injury, they should immediately stop doing whatever activity has caused the injury. Continued activity could cause further injury, delay healing, increase pain, and stimulate bleeding.

- **Rest.** In addition to discontinuing activity as needed, rest includes reducing weight bearing. If a leg is injured, the athlete should use a cane or crutch to minimize stress on the limb.

- **Ice.** An ice pack should be applied to the affected area as soon as possible after injury. Apply ice, alternating 5 to 10 minutes on and 5 to 10 minutes off for several cycles per treatment. The entire process should be repeated at least three times daily for the first two to three days after injury. Wrap the ice in a protective barrier such as a thin towel to prevent direct contact with the skin (hypothermic burns can occur when ice is placed directly onto the skin surface for long periods). Use ice with caution for those with circulatory deficiency or sensation deficits. Once skin tone turns pink for light-skinned athletes or darker for dark-skinned athletes, remove the ice to avoid overcooling or triggering ice burn. These changes in skin tone indicate that the proper level of cooling has been achieved. If skin turns blue or white, remove ice immediately to prevent serious harm (Okuyama, Ichikawa, Fujii, and Ito 2005).

- **Compression.** Apply compression to the injured area to help reduce swelling. Elastic wraps, special boots, air casts, and splints can be used. Compression must be performed carefully to assure that circulation is not compromised. If the athlete feels throbbing in the limb, the wrapping is probably too tight. Begin compression immediately or soon after the injury and apply ice through the wrapping. Taping and bracing to compress a joint are also useful for injury prevention and rehabilitation.

- **Elevation.** Finally, when possible, the limb should be elevated above the level of the heart to allow gravity to reduce swelling by returning fluids toward the heart. Elevation is obviously impractical in the case of a back injury but is appropriate for an arm or leg injury. At night, position a pillow for elevation to assist in the drainage of extra fluid from the affected area.

Along with following the PRICE principles, proper initial treatment of an injury includes avoiding several HARMful factors.

- **Heat** treatment, although helpful later in recovery, can delay healing if applied too soon after injury. If used too early, heat can increase internal bleeding and swelling.
- **Alcohol** can have the same effect. Alcohol use can also mask the pain of an injury and lead to inappropriate postponement of treatment.
- **Running** or any form of exercise should be avoided for 72 hours after injury unless a medical professional says otherwise.
- **Massage** may increase bleeding and swelling. Therefore, any deep massage should be avoided or performed cautiously for 72 hours after injury.

Although following the PRICE principles and avoiding the HARMful factors can be helpful in any sports injury, athletes should seek the advice of a medical professional if pain persists beyond a few days. What initially seems like a minor injury might prove to be a more serious one. Early identification and treatment can minimize long-term effects and lost participation time.

Follow-Up Treatment

After 48 to 72 hours, PRICE is replaced by MICE (movement replaces protection and rest). With the beginning of the repair process, scar tissue is incorporated into the damaged area. This tissue is made of collagen fibers, which have the capacity to contract. If these fibers are not exercised, an inevitable loss of flexibility occurs. This ultimately leads to pain, stiffness, and weakness. To prevent this from occurring, the athlete should start pain-free range-of-motion exercises within three days of the injury (assuming no complicating factors). Movements that gently stretch the scar tissue along the lines of force of the affected tissue allow for a stronger repair.

A good guide to determining when it is appropriate to restart movement is to perform the motion once. This movement should cause some discomfort but not pain. If the athlete has only discomfort and not pain with repeated performance of the movement, it is probably safe to continue. If pain is constant and persists after the movement, then the athlete likely has resumed the movement too soon, too vigorously, or both. In this case, resume PRICE for another 24 hours before attempting another movement trial.

In addition to ice, other modalities may be helpful (see table 2.1). In medicine, *modalities* generally refer to physical entities that can be applied to the body for a therapeutic purpose. For example, heat is a modality that can be applied to warm and loosen the underlying soft tissues. When using heat as a modality, it is generally best to use moist heat. Heat should only be used *24-36 hours after* an acute injury. Massage

Table 2.1   Treatment Modalities

Modality	Duration	Frequency	Intensity	Practical recommendations
Ice	5-10 min on/5-10 min off	Up to 3 × per day	N/A	Use in early stages of injury (first 24-36 hours) or after activity. Best to apply through a thin layer to avert freezing the skin.
Heat*	10-15 min	Up to 3 × per day	A tolerable temperature without being uncomfortable	Moist heat is preferred. Best to apply through a thin layer to avoid burning the skin.
Massage**	10-15 min	1-2 × per day	Should not cause discomfort	Always stroke toward the heart.
Whirlpool	20 min	1-2 × per day	Cold 55° F-60° F Hot 98° F-104° F	Use cold for acute injuries and hot for chronic injuries. Use active movement during treatment.

*Never use heat to treat an acute injury; wait 24-36 hours before applying heat.

**Never use massage to treat an acute injury; wait 72 hours before using massage.

and whirlpool are two other modalities that may be helpful. Massage should never be used for an acute injury. Begin massage only after 72 hours.

While modalities are generally safe, certain precautions must be taken. If you leave ice on for too long, a hypothermic burn can result. Similarly, leaving heat on for too long can result in a burn. Athletes must never fall asleep while heat or ice are being applied. If there is decreased feeling over a part of the body (from diabetic neuropathy or another medical condition that diminishes sensation), use modalities with caution. Follow the recommendations for use given in table 2.1. Additionally, the quick remedies presented in table 2.2 provide a guide to using modalities to manage the treatment of common injuries.

NSAIDs

Basic anti-inflammatory medications are commonly used in the treatment of acute sports injury. Nonsteroidal anti-inflammatory drugs (NSAIDs) such as ibuprofen may reduce the signs and symptoms of inflammation and provide pain relief. Given inflammation's role in healing, some controversy exists as to whether the risk involved in minimizing the inflammatory response by using such products outweighs the

Table 2.2   Quick Remedies

Injury	Treatment	Additional recommendations

Bruise	Initial:
	  Ice
	Follow-up:
	  Heat after 48 hours
		Discoloration initially appears dark blue or red and progresses to violet, green, and finally yellow, then fades away. Discoloration may travel due to gravity.
		Try to keep the bruise elevated above the heart. If no improvement in 2 weeks, call a physician.

Abrasion	Clean properly with appropriate cleanser, then apply antibiotic ointment and band-aid.	If the wound becomes tender and red, see a physician.
Laceration	Clean properly with appropriate cleanser, then apply antibiotic ointment and Band-Aid.	Any laceration that is 1/2 inch or more in length or greater than 1/10 of an inch in depth, continues to bleed, has jagged edges, or is in the face should be evaluated immediately by a physician to determine if stitches are required. If a wound of any size becomes tender and red, see a physician.

Sprain	Initial:
	  Ice
	Follow-up:
	  Heat after 48 hours
		Initial Care: Control swelling, immobilize if necessary, and limit weight bearing activity if injury is on lower extremity.
		Transitional Care: Begin using heat and mild range of motion. Increase activity as tolerated.
		Functional Return: Continue to increase activity as tolerated and consider using functional bracing.
		If recovery does not progress, see physician.

Strain	Initial:
	  Ice
	Follow-up:
	  Heat after 48 hours
		Initial Care: Control swelling, limit use of the injured area, and do not over-stretch.
		Transitional Care: Begin using heat and mild range of motion, increase activity as tolerated, and increase stretching as tolerated.
		Functional Return: Continue to increase activity as tolerated.
		If recovery does not progress, see a physician.

benefit. The general consensus is that NSAIDs are appropriate for most athletes in the early stages of inflammation, but they should be discontinued as soon as possible to minimize long-term negative effects. They should not be used in athletes with medical conditions such as heart or kidney ailments unless prescribed by a doctor. Acetaminophen (e.g., Tylenol) is *not* an anti-inflammatory but does relieve pain and is generally a safe medication to take as directed on the bottle. People with liver problems should take acetaminophen only after consulting a physician.

Return to Action

Often, the primary concern of an athlete is the duration of restricted participation. Traditionally, athletes have been allowed to return to activity when they demonstrate full range of motion and when the injured extremity exhibits 80 to 90 percent of full strength (Frontera 2003). In some instances consideration should be given to whether the athlete can perform sport-specific activities such as jumping or lunging without experiencing any problems. Athletes need to remember that adequate recovery is essential to ensure future pain-free performance.

Whereas acute management is considered routine, the long-term ramifications of injury are often ignored. A lack of attention to issues such as altered biomechanics, weakened anatomy, and appropriate rehabilitation can place a once-injured athlete at future risk.

Disregard for long-term management is one reason less dramatic overuse injuries make up the majority of sport-related injuries. Muscle imbalance, poorly fitted equipment, and repetitive motion alter normal biomechanics. The resulting microtrauma to the bone, tendon, ligament, and muscle initiates an inflammatory response. If the inflammatory response is not addressed, continued degradation leads to chronic pain and disability.

Splinting, Bracing, and Taping

For prevention and treatment of some injuries, techniques such as splinting, taping, and bracing are quite helpful. As is true for all other preventive or treatment protocols, certain principles need to be applied or the consequence of the use of these techniques could hinder the healing and recovery process.

Splinting

Splinting is a common technique for initial treatment of any suspected fracture or severe ligament injury. Use splinting to assist in safe transport for proper evaluation from a medical professional. Failure to properly secure the injured area with a splint could result in more severe damage to the area or might lead to shock (Meredith and Butcher 1997).

Commercial splinting materials are widely available but are not likely to be on hand unless a medical professional is present. Some smaller splinting materials can easily be added to most first-aid kits, but they are not typically included. Hand-moldable splints are compact enough to keep on hand and are useful for several areas of the body.

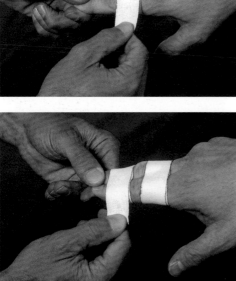

©Human Kinetics

©Human Kinetics

If you do not have a commercial splint, alternatives are available. An anatomical splint (using a healthy and uninjured area of the body to support an injured area) can be extremely helpful. Using a healthy finger to support an injured finger is common and is referred to as "buddy taping" (see figure 2.1).

Many rigid materials can be used as a splint. Items from the training or competition environment, including athletic equipment, might be used to support the injured area (Meredith and Butcher 1997). Splints should be secured to the injured area as well as to the joint above and below the injured area. For instance, when attempting to secure the lower leg for a potential fracture of the tibia or fibula, also secure the splint from the knee to the ankle so that both of those joints are immobile. Doing this helps minimize movement of the injured area. Splints can be secured with simple elastic wraps, if available, to cover the entire area. If elastic wraps are not available, a sock or t-shirt will do. Apply the wrap tightly enough to secure the splint without impeding circulation to the area (Meredith and Butcher 1999). An examiner should be able to feel a pulse in an area below the injured site.

Figure 2.1 Buddy taping supports the injured finger by securing it to the adjacent finger.

Bracing

Bracing can be broken down into two categories: prophylactic and functional. Prophylactic bracing is used as a preventive measure when no injury exists. Some researchers believe that such bracing reduces the risk of injury or at least reduces the severity of injury when injury occurs (Sharpe, Knapik, and Jones 1997; Verhagen, van Mechelen, and de Vente 2000; Arnold and Docherty 2004). The two most common areas of the body where prophylactic bracing is used are the ankle and the knee.

Many people believe that prophylactic bracing reduces the incidence of ankle sprains, whereas others are cautious and feel more research is needed to determine more specific effect on the joint (Wilkerson 2002; Fleck and Kraemer 1997; Frontera 2003).

Several types of over-the-counter ankle braces are available (see figure 2.2). The manner of construction determines the type and level of support they offer. A semi-rigid construction is a must in preventing ankle sprains. These braces have extra stirrup-like support to reduce excessive ankle inversion (i.e., turning the ankle), which is the most common cause of injury (Arnold and Docherty 2004). Use of these braces should be comfortable to the athlete and should not limit functional mobility

(Verhagen, van Mechelen, and de Vente 2000). Bracing is only one way to help prevent ankle injuries. Bracing does not substitute for a proper strengthening program that works on strength, balance, and proprioception (Arnold and Docherty 2004).

Braces for the knee differ in type as well. A knee sleeve is typically made of neoprene (a synthetic rubber) or a similar substance. Although such braces are successful in increasing warmth, offering proprioceptive feedback, and providing

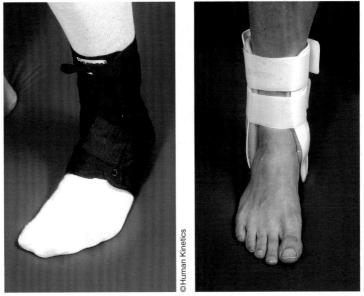

Figure 2.2 Common commercially available ankle braces.

compression, they should not be used in an attempt to increase the stability of a joint. A knee sleeve with a hole cut out over the knee cap (see figure 2.3), can assist in reducing symptoms of patellofemoral disorders (Martin and Committee 2001).

Other more rigid knee braces are used to add support to ligaments in the knee (see figure 2.4). Although braces have proven to decrease force applied to these ligaments, studies have not conclusively shown that they reduce the incidence of knee injuries. Because many questions remain unanswered regarding the effects braces have on the healthy knee, prophylactic bracing of the knee is not recommended, especially for younger athletes (Martin and Committee 2001).

Functional bracing is used for an existing or a recent injury. Functional braces provide additional protection to an injured area as it continues to heal and strengthen. Keep in mind that these are, in fact, the same braces that are used prophylactically. When used properly, they have been shown to reduce the incidence of reinjury. There are many braces available, with different features (see figure 2.5). Choose a brace that best protects the type of injury sustained. If unsure as to which brace to use, consult a physician or athletic trainer. Athletes might need to try a few different types before finding the right balance of comfort and adequate protection. Follow directions carefully when applying the brace because improper fit can

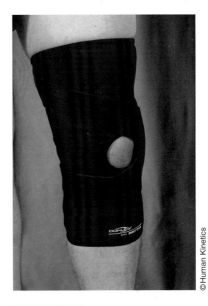

Figure 2.3 Knee sleeve with patellar opening and added support.

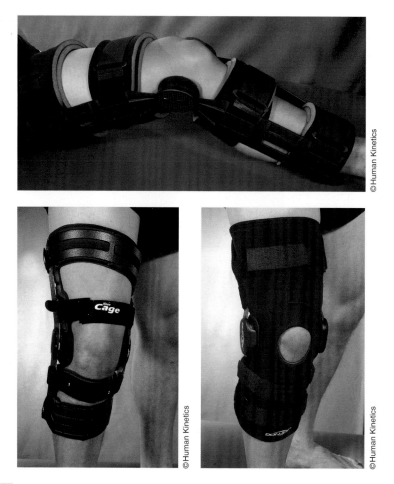

Figure 2.4 Common rigid knee braces.

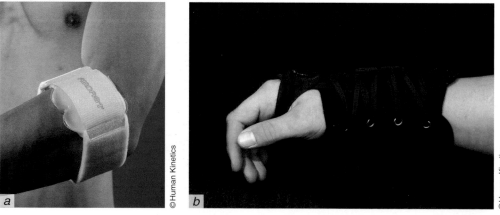

Figure 2.5 Commercially produced braces for *(a)* tennis elbow and *(b)* carpal tunnel syndrome can alleviate pain and protect the injured area as it heals.

lead to injury or reinjury. Using a brace for functional reasons is not a substitute for proper rehabilitation. Proper strength, balance, and proprioception must be returned to the area to assist in preventing reinjury (Arnold and Docherty 2004).

Taping

Bracing is quite popular, but taping techniques, ranging from the very simple to rather complex, are also useful for athletes. Specific taping techniques can be learned from a qualified health care professional or from one of the many books available on athletic taping. But before applying any particular taping skills, it is important to understand the basic principles of taping.

You might choose to use a particular taping technique for one of three reasons. The first reason is injury prevention (prophylactic taping), which comes into play when no current injury is present but when a high risk of injury exists or when an athlete has a history of injury to a particular area. Using tape for preventive measures might lower the chance of injury or, more likely, reduce the severity of injury (see figure 2.6). The use of prophylactic taping (or bracing) is constantly being reviewed for its efficacy. It seems to be most beneficial for use with athletes who have a history of injury.

A second use of taping is for an acute injury. In such a situation, the primary reason for taping *is not* to allow continued participation but rather to help stabilize and compress the injured area as a treatment technique. This practice falls under the fourth step of PRICE (compression), as discussed earlier.

A third use of taping is to assist in return to activity. Often, taping can help an athlete in the final stages of recovery or rehabilitation in his or her return to partial or full activity (see figure 2.7). The primary goal in this instance is to reduce likelihood of reinjury. Use taping along with proper rehabilitation to strengthen the injured area. As mentioned, taping should never be used as a substitute for medical attention.

Proper use of taping can be quite helpful, but it is important to recognize times when taping is not warranted, such as during the acute stages of an injury (unless done for compression). In the initial stages of an injury, taping to allow continued participation might exacerbate damage to the tissue and prolong healing. Check for swelling. If excess swelling exists in the injured area, or if swelling increases with even light activity, the athlete should rest the injury longer. Do not tape an area if there is any question about the nature or severity of the injury. In such cases, refer the athlete to a qualified medical professional for evaluation. Always err on the side of caution. If the athlete has functional limitations despite

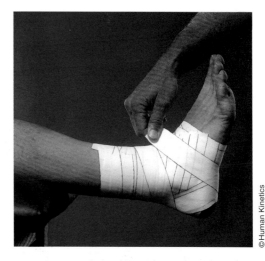

©Human Kinetics

Figure 2.6 Prophylactic taping of the ankle is commonly used to help prevent inversion sprains.

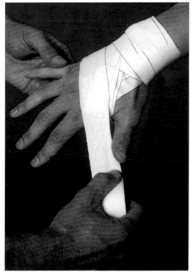

©Human Kinetics

Figure 2.7 Taping a previously injured area can reduce the stress placed on the affected bone, muscle, or ligament as an athlete returns to activity.

taping, he or she should postpone returning to activity. If he or she appears to have an awkward gait or is unable to perform simple functional movements (e.g., running, cutting, or jumping), do not use taping to allow return to play.

Strategies for Chronic Conditions

One reason athletes stop participating in their sport is fear of pain. It is intuitive to avoid that which is painful. Unfortunately, avoiding pain often does not improve a condition but rather exacerbates it. Obviously, exercising with acute lower-back pain or knee pain is not wise. But it is what athletes choose to do after the pain subsides that affects long-term recovery and wellness. Always consult a physician when starting or resuming a training program.

An active lifestyle strengthens bones, slows loss of muscle mass, and reduces joint and muscle pain. Becoming sedentary after being diagnosed with a chronic condition of the bones or joints will weaken surrounding support structures and ultimately lead to instability and increased pain. If one type of exercise causes pain, find an alternative activity. For instance, if running is no longer feasible, try aquatic training or bike riding, which should be less taxing to the knees, ankles, and hips. When starting a new training method, begin with short frequent sessions and increase duration as the body acclimates and tolerates the new activity. Remember that moderate intermittent activity is still effective in maintaining and improving health. Athletes need not be active for 60 minutes at a time. Instead try breaking up the exercise program into sporadic intervals throughout the day; this should provide many of the same benefits as a longer duration single program.

Regular exercise provides physical and psychological benefits that combat the process of aging. Chronic painful conditions might force a change in a training program, but pain should not cause anyone to avoid activity altogether. In some instances, adding weight training to what was primarily a cardiovascular regimen might restore the necessary muscle balance to allow pain-free activity. In other cases, an alternative program to replace the primary activity is a good idea. Cross-training is widely used to avoid overuse injuries, training plateaus, and muscle imbalance. Whatever strategy an athlete employs to combat a chronic musculoskeletal condition or injury, it must be one that allows him or her to remain active. A sedentary lifestyle only reinforces patterns that an injury provokes and creates a lasting negative influence on the mind and body.

Special Considerations for Young Athletes

Like adults, teenage athletes are at risk for repetitive use and traumatic injury. Unlike adults, teenagers have the additional concern of physical growth and development. Although many fears exist regarding intense athletic participation in teenagers, few of these are validated by scientific study. That said, it is important to address issues that logic dictates are particular to the not-yet-mature athlete. For the discussion here, children who are younger than 12 are considered preadolescent, and young people from 12 to 19 are considered adolescents.

Many adults intuitively believe that strength training places undue stress on the growth plates of young athletes and might lead to premature closure or injury with resulting growth disturbance. But with proper supervision and appropriate program design, there has been no adverse effect in growth, flexibility, motor performance, or development documented in maturing athletes who participate in weight-training exercise. In fact, weight training can begin in preadolescence so long as it is adapted for this age group and supervised by a knowledgeable adult. Athletes in this age group use lighter weights and do increased repetitions and sets. For instance, preadolescents would use a weight load that they can successfully (with proper mechanics) lift 12-15 times (repetitions) without undue stress or alteration in form. Before young athletes begin resistance training, they should visit a pediatrician for a full medical exam and be forewarned of the risks associated with anabolic steroids.

Teenagers who lift weights must be monitored closely and should adhere to established principles. For starters, Olympic-style and competitive weightlifting are dangerous for any age group and should be avoided. The American Orthopaedic Society for Sports Medicine recommends two or three weight-training sessions per week. The program should include 20 to 30 minutes of training with warm-up and cool-down periods. Weight resistance that allows three sets of 6 to 15 repetitions is a good starting point. Once a teen athlete has mastered three sets of 15 repetitions with appropriate technique and good control, weight can be increased slowly to allow for progression.

With other types of training, appropriate allowances should be made for the developing adolescent body. The lack of excessive risk associated with growth plate injury does not negate the presence and prevalence of overuse injuries. A study of 130 adolescent pitchers published in the June 2006 issue of *The American Journal of Sports Medicine* found that injured throwers pitched significantly more months per year, games per year, innings per game, pitches per year, and warm-up pitches before a game. With this information, Dr. James Andrews and coauthors recommended that adolescent baseball pitchers avoid pitching more than 80 pitches per game, avoid pitching competitively more than eight months per year, and avoid pitching more than 2,500 pitches in competition per year. Little League Baseball now requires monitoring of pitch counts (table 2.3) and periods of rest (table 2.4).

A concern to any athlete is malnutrition and its possible effects on training. An adolescent athlete has the additional risk of delayed maturation. The energy cost of activity in an adolescent is considerably higher than that in an adult. Dependence on adult recommendations may lead to a gross underestimation of the needs of the athlete. It should be noted that if any short-term discrepancy in training and nutrition is corrected, maturation will usually not be compromised. If there is doubt about an athlete's nutritional needs, he or she should consult a professional.

An implication of the elevated energy required by teenage athletes is the production of more metabolic heat and a faster increase in core body temperature caused by dehydration. Sweating effectively cools the body but also leads to fluid and electrolyte loss. Dehydration can be exacerbated by sports that promote voluntary fluid loss to make weight (e.g., wrestling). Both athletes and coaches should be educated on the effects of dehydration.

Children should arrive fully hydrated for a practice session or competition, and drink breaks should occur every 15 to 20 minutes during prolonged activities. Flavoring the drink and adding sodium chloride or carbohydrate to the beverage might prompt athletes to drink more fluids and will help prevent hyponatremia. Fluid consumption can be monitored by weighing the athlete before and after training. Athletes who do not drink enough to restore body weight to normal between practices or competitions should be required to rehydrate before being allowed to participate.

Table 2.3   Little League Pitch Count Limits

Age	Pitches allowed per day*
17-18	105
13-16	95
11-12	85
10 and under	75

*Limits established for the 2007 Little League Baseball season; subject to change.

Courtesy of Little League International, Williamsport, PA.

Table 2.4   Little League Pitching Rest Requirements

PITCHERS AGE 7-16	
Pitches per day	Required days of rest before pitching again
61 or more	3
41-60	2
21-40	1
20 and under	0
PITCHERS AGE 17-18	
Pitches per day	Required days of rest before pitching again
76 or more	3
51-75	2
26-50	1
25 and under	0

Source: Little League Baseball, Incorporated.

CHAPTER 3

Injury Types and Assessments

Paul M. Steingard, DO

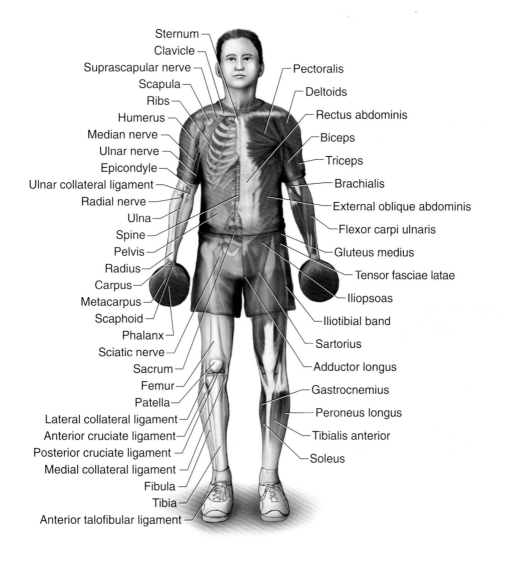

Sternum
Clavicle
Suprascapular nerve
Scapula
Ribs
Humerus
Median nerve
Ulnar nerve
Epicondyle
Ulnar collateral ligament
Radial nerve
Ulna
Spine
Pelvis
Radius
Carpus
Metacarpus
Scaphoid
Phalanx
Sciatic nerve
Sacrum
Femur
Patella
Lateral collateral ligament
Anterior cruciate ligament
Posterior cruciate ligament
Medial collateral ligament
Fibula
Tibia
Anterior talofibular ligament

Pectoralis
Deltoids
Rectus abdominis
Biceps
Triceps
Brachialis
External oblique abdominis
Flexor carpi ulnaris
Gluteus medius
Tensor fasciae latae
Iliopsoas
Iliotibial band
Sartorius
Adductor longus
Gastrocnemius
Peroneus longus
Tibialis anterior
Soleus

This chapter will help you classify some of the different types of injuries, some severe and others benign, that are discussed throughout the rest of the book. Various injury types are reviewed and defined, categorized by the type of tissue affected by the injury: bone, ligament, tendon, skin, or other. Although it is not possible to cover every injury in a single work, the most common sports injuries are discussed. This chapter also covers the diagnosis of sports injuries through such methods as self-testing as well as more invasive techniques.

In general, over a season, athletes spend far less time healthy than injured. That said, we must be aware that injuries can and do occur. Some injuries athletes have no control over, but with good equipment, good coaching, proper environment, and sensible exercise habits, athletes can count on being injury free most of the time.

Injuries by Structure or System

Bony injuries include various types of fractures, which are discussed in turn. An overview of injuries to ligaments and joints, muscles and tendons, skin injuries, and finally systemic disorders follows. Of all sports injuries, those to muscles, tendons, and ligaments are probably the most common. Naturally, the more physical a sport is and the more contact and high-energy collisions it involves, the greater the risk for injuries. American football and rugby are more likely to cause fractures, for instance, than tennis or basketball, in which ankle sprains tend to be more common.

Bone Injuries

One of the most common injuries that occurs to bones, particularly the longer bones of the arms and legs is a fracture, or a break in the bone. (A fractured bone and a broken bone are the same thing; one is not worse than the other.) Other common places for fractures are the bones of the wrist, ankle, and kneecap.

The many types of fractures include the following:

• **Simple** or **nondisplaced fractures** (see figure 3.1) are those in which a break is noted on an X-ray, but the bone is still in perfect position. These fractures are much less likely to require surgical intervention than displaced fractures are.

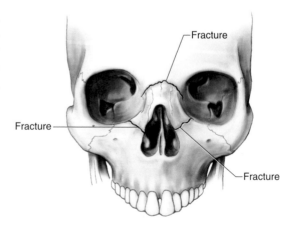

Figure 3.1 Simple fracture.

- **Displaced fractures** usually occur in the long bones of the body and typically result in severe trauma (see figure 3.2). These fractures involve either a separation or an angulation of the fracture segments. Displaced fractures frequently require surgery and often require metal plates to be inserted to add strength and preserve the length of the bone.

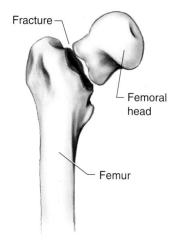

Figure 3.2 Displaced fracture.

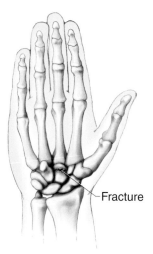

- **Comminuted** (involving fragmentation or splintering of the bone) **or impacted fractures** are those in which one part of the broken bone is pushing into the other, shortening the length of the bone (figure 3.3). This type of fracture is serious because loss of bone height can adversely affect the function of the bone. Such breaks are seen in fractures of the wrist. Wrist fractures become impacted when athletes instinctively try to break a fall with their hands. These dangerous injuries always relate to the falling action and are frequently seen in skiing, ice hockey, and in-line skating.

Figure 3.3 Impacted fracture.

- **Compound fractures** are complicated. Such fractures include multiple fractures with displacement of bones, comminuted sections, and even bone piercing skin (see figure 3.4). These fractures are usually related to severe trauma (e.g., motorcycle crashes) but can occur in any high-impact sport. Rodeo cowboys and football and rugby players are particularly susceptible to compound fractures.

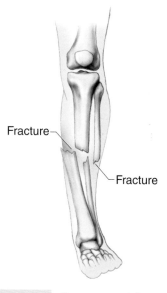

Figure 3.4 Compound fracture.

• **Fracture dislocations** are injuries that involve a break in a bone as well as damage to ligaments and muscles, causing the broken bone to dislocate at the joint (figure 3.5). These types of injuries are usually caused by the type of trauma seen in auto racing or parachuting.

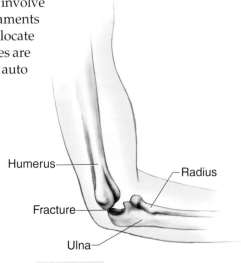

Figure 3.5 Fracture dislocation.

• **Epiphyseal fractures** are very serious injuries. The epiphyses, or growth centers, are seen in growing children. These growth centers are located near the ends of the long bones. The growth centers are soft and until they fuse do not have the strength of more mature bones. When fractures penetrate the growth centers (see figure 3.6), they can adversely affect future growth of the long bones. Such breaks must be handled with extreme care.

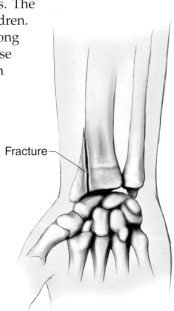

Classifications of epiphyseal fractures are called Salter type I through Salter type IV, depending on the location and severity of the fracture. The Salter classification relates to how involved the growth centers are in the injury. A mild separation is a type I, and severe breaks through the growth center are categorized as types II, III, or IV, with IV being the most severe. When the fracture is extensive through the growth center, the healing process can dangerously affect the future growth of the bone. Fortunately, epiphyseal fractures in children are rare, but occasionally a child will get hit by a baseball or a bat, for example, and receive a serious injury.

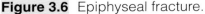

Figure 3.6 Epiphyseal fracture.

- **Stress fractures** are the most intriguing of all fractures (see figure 3.7). These injuries can be caused by overuse, poor training habits, and poor environmental or practice facilities. They result from an abnormal stress being placed upon a normal bone. Often, the diagnosis is not made until after healing has taken place and new bone has been laid down. Often no treatment other than rest is necessary. If a weight-bearing bone is affected, weight should not be placed on the bone while it is healing; for a leg bone injury, the athlete must use crutches for a time (three to four weeks for an adolescent, four to six weeks for an older athlete). The amount of rest required depends on the type and degree of stress fracture. Of course no one can predict when rest alone will be sufficient, so a diagnosis and additional treatment if needed is preferable. In some cases of stress fracture, X-rays might not show a break, so a nuclear bone scan, magnetic reasonance imaging (MRI), or computed tomography (CT) scan is needed for diagnosis.

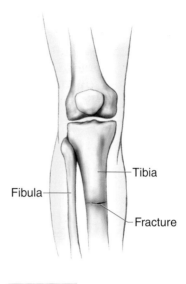

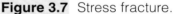

Figure 3.7 Stress fracture.

- **Avulsion fractures** are related primarily to torn ligaments or tendons. As a ligament or tendon tears, it may pull, or avulse, a small piece of bone with the ligaments or tendons as shown in figure 3.8. The soft tissue trauma rather than the fracture is the focus of treatment for these injuries. Avulsion is frequently seen in injuries to fingers. Baseball catchers are notorious for avulsions in the fingers.

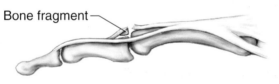

Figure 3.8 Avulsion fracture.

Fractures are suspected when swelling, pain, or a history of trauma is present and can be confirmed by X-ray, bone scan, CT scan, or MRI. Typically athletes experience pain with fractures for two reasons: the periosteum (the lining of the bone where the nerve endings lie) may be disrupted, or a bone contusion or bruise (not really a fracture) may be present. A bone bruise can be extremely painful and just as disabling as a fracture, and it often takes as long as a fracture to heal. Bruised shins and hip pointers (located near the hip joint) are common in American football. Bone bruises are diagnosed by taking a careful history and possibly an X-ray. In some instances a bone scan or MRI, which may reveal increased activity within the bone, can be helpful. A fracture must always be ruled out before calling an injury a bone bruise.

Other severe injuries resulting from trauma are compression injuries. Compression injuries are bone bruises with related bleeding in tight areas such as the shins or even the front of the thighs. The buildup of blood and the presence of the bone bruise can interfere with the normal blood supply, causing a breakdown of the surrounding tissue and interference with circulation.

Ligament and Joint Injuries

The area where two bones come together is called a joint. Joints are held together by tough but not very flexible tissues called ligaments. Many joints involve motion, such as the elbow, which is a hinge joint, or the shoulders and hips, which are ball and socket joints. Ligaments can surround a joint, acting as a capsule. Or they can be responsible for stability of a joint, as occurs in the cruciate ligaments of the knee. In either case, the main function of ligaments is to provide stability to a joint. At the joint, bones have surfaces covered by a very hard substance called articular cartilage. When a joint becomes arthritic, it is a breakdown of this articular cartilage that produces pain and disability. Lining the joint is the synovium, a thin tissue layer that secretes fluid which serves to lubricate the joint.

The most common joint and ligament injuries result from misuse or direct trauma. Fractures to the bones at the joint are rare because severe trauma is more likely to result in the ligaments being injured. However, preadolescents have very strong ligaments relative to bone strength and thus, a traumatic injury to the joint of a young athlete may result in an avulsion. Older athletes suffering a similar injury are more likely to sustain a ligament tear than a bony avulsion because of their relatively greater bone strength and relatively weaker ligament strength. Be aware, however, that both ligament and bony avulsion injuries can occur in both age groups.

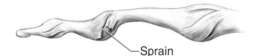

Figure 3.9 Ligament sprain related to a dislocation.

When a joint, such as a finger joint, dislocates, a straining or stretching occurs at the ligaments surrounding the joint as shown in figure 3.9. Remember that ligament tissue is not very elastic. Fracturing of the edge of the bones might also occur. This means that unless corrective action is taken, including rehabilitation, an easy pathway will exist for further dislocations at the same joint.

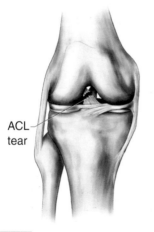

Figure 3.10 Ligament injury without joint involvement.

Ligaments can also be injured without joint involvement (see figure 3.10). The best-known injury of this type is the anterior cruciate ligament (ACL) knee injury common in so many sports (for more information see page

214 ACL tears). The ACL is the main stabilizer of the knee. When a running athlete suddenly stops and tries to cut, as athletes in many sports do, the force of that cut can cause the ACL to give out and tear. A very hard hit to the outside of the knee can cause the knee to cave inward, which can also strain the ACL. The majority of injuries to the ACL result from pivoting and cutting maneuvers and not from direct blows to the knee.

Ligament sprains and tears can occur anywhere in the body. Because of the inelasticity of ligaments, measures must be taken to prevent both initial and recurring injuries. Protective equipment and good body mechanics can make a significant difference.

Other joint injuries include subluxation, loose bodies, osteochondritis dissecans, chondromalacia, and osteoarthritis. Chondromalacia is discussed later in this chapter.

The patella (knee cap) is a stabilizer of the knee joint and glides through a groove created mutually by the femur and tibia. The patella is connected by the quadriceps tendon above the knee and by the patellar tendon below the knee. For various reasons the patella may sublux (that is, go to the edge of its groove) or dislocate. Probably the most common causes of these types of injury are a congenitally shallow groove for the patella to glide through and a lack of flexibility of the athlete.

Osteoarthritis is a problem, especially for runners. With this condition the athlete can develop spurs and loose bodies that are painful and that limit full range of motion. Can running cause osteoarthritis? Possibly yes, if the running involves nervous running, stopping, starting, or cutting. But in flexible runners running on a good surface, osteoarthritis is unlikely to be caused simply by running. However, any direct impact on a joint can contribute to osteoarthritis. Strengthening the surrounding muscles of a joint is one of the best ways to delay the onset and reduce the severity of the symptoms of osteoarthritis.

Tendon and Muscle Injuries

Tendons are the parts of muscles that attach to bones. The muscle–tendon unit (also called the musculotendinous unit) helps to stabilize the joint. A good example is the shoulder's rotator cuff, which actually forms a second capsule around the joint capsule. More significantly, the muscle–tendon unit is responsible for body movement and strength. The length and size of a body's muscle–tendon units depend largely on degree of training, heredity factors, and general health of the individual. Specific training can affect the size and function of the muscle–tendon unit.

Whereas stress injuries to ligaments are called *sprains,* injuries to tendons and the rest of the muscles are called *strains.* Strains to the muscles can be as minor as a mild spasm or can involve significant bleeding and swelling. Strains (also called pulled muscles) generally occur at the belly, or middle part, of a muscle and are graded on a scale of I to III based on the severity of injury to the muscle–tendon unit (see figure 3.11). In a grade I strain, a stretching and microtearing of the muscle fibers occurs, with minimal disability or loss of strength. Grade II strains result in partial tearing of the muscle–tendon unit, causing definitive functional deficits and a loss of strength. Grade III strains involve complete tearing of the muscle–tendon unit and result in severe functional deficits and significant weakness. Muscle bed injuries can involve strains, contusions, and tearing of the muscle.

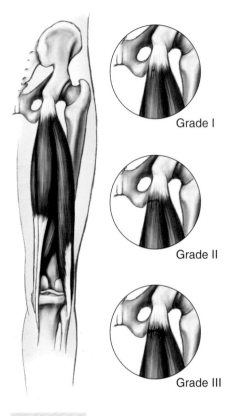

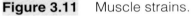

Figure 3.11 Muscle strains.

When a strain occurs at the origin or insertion of the muscles (at the site of the tendons, thus involving some inflammation of the tendons), the condition is called *tendinitis.* Tendinitis can be caused by a severe injury or can be a chronic condition. The chronic injuries—which are caused by overuse or poor body mechanics—are the most difficult to treat. A well-known sports injury, lateral epicondylitis (better known as tennis elbow; see p. 101), is a prime example of chronic tendinitis. As a result of overuse, playing too much tennis, or hitting with bad technique, many tennis players develop chronic tendinitis. Chronic problems of the tendons are very difficult to treat. Often the best treatments yield poor results.

Grade I: Minimal tearing of muscle fibers (<20%), mild tenderness, no joint instability

Grade II: Moderate tearing of muscle-tendon unit (20-70%), minimal to mild tenderness, mild joint instability

Grade III: significant tearing of muscle-tendon unit (>70%), moderate tenderness, moderate joint instability

Ruptured tendons can also occur and are classified in the same way muscle tears are classified (see p. 53).

Skin Injuries and Problems

Some serious sports-related problems can affect the skin. For example, skin infections (see figure 3.12); fungal, viral, and bacterial; are common in athletics and often present in athletic training rooms. Athlete's foot is a common fungal infection that can result from walking barefoot on dirty locker room floors or not changing socks frequently enough. It is best treated by maintaining good hygiene, keeping the feet dry, and applying appropriate powders or ointments for flares. If the nails appear eroded and are breaking down, a fungal infection of the nails may be present. This condition is more difficult to treat and may require systemic medications and removal of the affected nail(s).

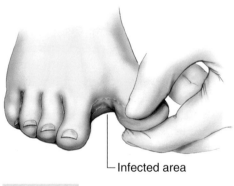

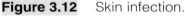
Infected area

Figure 3.12 Skin infection.

If symptoms of a fungal nail infection arise, professional medical care is warranted.

Methicillin resistant staph aureus (MRSA) is a serious skin infection that periodically appears in and around athletic training rooms. MRSA is very difficult to treat so proper sanitizing regimes are absolutely necessary to prevent it and other skin infections. Equipment must be wiped down with proper antiseptic solutions, sharing of dirty towels must be prohibited, and personal hygiene must be stressed.

Blisters—a common injury typically caused by overuse, poor fitting equipment, or improper mechanics—can undermine any athlete (see figure 3.13). Blisters might not look like much of a problem, but they can get infected or can get larger and become a big nuisance.

The same is true of chafing injuries and abrasions. Skin irritations must be kept clean and receive proper treatment. Chafing is fairly common in long-distance runners who wear shoes that do not fit. Chafing is also common among bicyclists who wear ill-fitting biker shorts or have poorly adjusted bicycle seats. Scrapes are particularly common among skateboarders and are also seen frequently in athletes who play soccer, American football, or baseball.

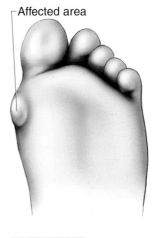

Affected area

Figure 3.13   Blister.

Many outdoor sports, including tennis, swimming, basketball, outdoor volleyball, and running, expose athletes to excess sunshine. Melanoma (a kind of skin cancer) has become more and more prevalent, especially in the Sunbelt states. Outdoor athletes must wear sunblock, shaded hats, and proper clothing for protection. Sunblock should protect against both UVA rays (which age the skin) and UVB rays (which burn the skin) and must be reapplied frequently (every two hours). When outdoors, athletes should seek shady areas when possible and drink plenty of fluids to prevent heat-related illnesses.

Other Systemic Injuries

Two injuries that can have catastrophic effects to systems throughout the body are heat injuries and sudden cardiac death. Various types of heat injuries occur and are differentiated by severity. Heat cramps (actually a form of dehydration) are probably the most painful and yet the least serious of heat-related injuries. A lack of fluids and essential minerals cause muscles, especially leg muscles, to cramp up. More serious heat exhaustion is caused by a higher degree of dehydration. Athletes with heat exhaustion become pale and lethargic and require quick treatment. The most serious kind of heat injury is heat stroke, in which the thermostat in the brain ceases to work. This is a true medical emergency and must be treated in a hospital.

To avoid heat injuries, athletes' bodies must be able to quickly and efficiently dissipate the heat generated by participating in sports. Athletes can dissipate body heat in four ways:

1. Moving to a cooler environment.

2. Moving air by moving the arms and legs. The movement of the arms and legs has a fanlike effect and prevents heat from mounting up.

3. Ingesting a cool drink (this provides only a little help).

4. Evaporation—and this is the most important. (However, evaporation can cause a loss of sodium, potassium, and fluids, which in turn can lead to dehydration and heat exhaustion.)

If these means aren't effective enough, the athlete might need to go to the emergency room, where IV fluids, cooling blankets, and other care can be provided.

Sudden cardiac death is thought to occur in 1 in 300,000 athletes. Although rare, cardiac death is obviously always tragic. About half the time, sudden death is due to a condition called hypertrophic cardiomyopathy (HCM), which is an enlarging of the heart. HCM is a congenital problem of atypical muscle that can be identified by electrocardiogram and echocardiogram. At this time it is not economically feasible to test everyone who wants to participate in sports, but the future holds promise that free clinics will spring up to screen all would-be athletes for this condition.

Injuries by Body Location

Obviously, location of an injury often depends on the sport or activity being performed. You would expect most baseball and tennis injuries to occur in the upper extremities. Conversely, basketball and track and field injuries would be more likely to involve the lower extremities.

Head and Neck Injuries

Head injuries (see chapter 4) are serious because they can cause death. The skull that houses the brain forms a hard protective capsule, but in the case of severe trauma the brain can be damaged by being shaken, or, in the event of a particularly severe blow, the skull might fracture.

Although fractures of the skull do occur, the most common injuries to the brain are concussions (see p. 57), which are seen most often in contact sports. Being hit in the head by a hockey puck or baseball has also been known to cause severe head injury or death. With a concussion, temporary disorientation or loss of consciousness can occur. A fairly common symptom of head injuries, especially concussions, is a brief "lucid period" immediately following the injury, during which the athlete is fine for a few minutes; shortly afterward the athlete becomes disoriented.

More serious than a concussion is a subdural hematoma (p. 62), in which a build-up of blood compresses the brain. This condition requires immediate professional care. And, recently, a "second-impact syndrome" (p. 59) has been identified as resulting in serious head injury. In this case, the individual suffers a head injury that might appear insignificant. Then later, after a week or two, another head injury occurs with disastrous results.

Lacerations can occur on the face, especially in ice hockey, and these often require suturing. Some facial fractures are also worthy of mention, including nasal fractures (p. 64) and orbital fractures (fractures of the bones surrounding the eyes), both of which frequently require surgical intervention. Orbital fractures can be difficult to diagnose, but they need to be recognized because an untreated orbital fracture might result in a "sinking" of the involved eye with a decrease or loss of vision. Jaw fractures are not common but obviously quite painful and disabling. Other less frequent but serious injuries include nose and teeth injuries. These are less common since protective devices have been upgraded in American football and other sports.

Cervical spine injuries (see chapter 5) can be classified as potentially catastrophic. These injuries are most often caused by lowering the head, which results in a straightening of the cervical spine. In such a position, if the head contacts an immovable object, such as another player or the ground, the cervical spine experiences a telescoping effect. Think of a trailer truck hitting a wall—the cab stops, the trailer continues on. Injury to the spinal cord can occur as a result of this impact, causing paralysis or even death. Cervical spine injuries are often tragic. American football and rugby players must be coached not to lower their heads during play. Other injuries to the spinal column can result in fractures, but the cervical spine injury is the most significant.

Upper Extremity Injuries

Problems in the upper extremities can occur in the shoulders, elbows, arms, hands, and wrists. Probably the most common **shoulder injuries** (see chapter 6) involve the rotator cuff (p. 89). The rotator cuff is made up of four muscles that form a second capsule around the shoulder. Injuries to the rotator cuff range from tendinitis to muscle strains or tendon sprains.

Probably the most interesting and difficult to treat rotator cuff injury is the impingement syndrome (p. 90) in which muscle tendons are pinched under a bridge in the anterior shoulder area formed by ligament and bone. The coraco-acromion ligament is the only one of its type in the body. It goes between two points on the same bone. Impingement syndrome is related to overhead motion and is most common in baseball pitchers, tennis and volleyball players, and freestyle swimmers. These athletes make violent overhead maneuvers in their respective sports. Impingement syndrome can be difficult to treat. Surgery, a last resort, often does not help. Many promising careers have ended prematurely as a result of shoulder impingement syndrome.

A shoulder injury often difficult to diagnose is the labrum tear. The cartilage around the cup of the shoulder joint is called the labrum. Labrum tears (p. 86) often produce symptoms that are identical to rotator cuff injuries and therefore sometimes cannot be identified without arthroscopic surgery.

Another interesting and not uncommon overuse injury that occurs in proximity to the shoulder joints is the rupture of the tendon of the long head of the biceps (p. 92), which gives the biceps a Popeye effect. When an athlete flexes the forearm, the biceps muscle balls up into what appears to resemble a big biceps muscle. Because the muscle has two tendinous attachments, functionally there is little interruption of activity. The Popeye syndrome causes very little discomfort and, because of the stronger other tendon, causes little or no disability.

Traumatic **elbow injuries** (see chapter 7) such as fractures and dislocation can occur and frequently result in significant deformity. This is because the elbow joint is such a precise joint that any trauma can and will result in loss of range of motion, even after healing. Although functionally we can survive loss of extension or flexion or even loss of pronation (internal rotation), loss of supination (external rotation) can significantly affect a person's everyday activities. Injuries to the elbow joint are treacherous and must be treated properly and vigorously.

There are two important chronic elbow injuries. The first, known as *Little League elbow* (p. 112) occurs in youngsters whose growth centers of the bones around the elbows have not closed yet. Because of excessive throwing, primarily pitching, the ulnar (inside) or radial (outside) epiphysis closes prematurely. This condition may not cause pain, but as growth continues, the growth of the humerus is adversely affected, as is the athlete's throw.

The other chronic problem is epicondylitis (p. 101), an overuse condition in which either the ulnar or, more commonly, the radial epicondyle is involved. The epicondyles are bony prominences on either side of the elbow. It is to these bony prominences that the tendons which extend and flex the forearms attach. We could very easily refer to these conditions as tendinitis because both the attachment of the tendons and the bony prominences, the epicondyles, are involved. What causes epicondylitis is that the bellies of the muscles of the forearm become spastic and shortened, which puts extra stress on the muscle tendons as they attach to the epicondyles of the humerus. This problem commonly occurs in racket sports when players hold the racket too tight and use a smaller grip than they should. When this is done repeatedly, the muscle tightens up, thus causing the problem. Epicondylitis can be very difficult to treat because not only must the irritation at the bony attachment be treated but also the tendinitis and the chronic muscle strains that tend to result from this problem.

Two common **wrist injuries** (see chapter 8) need to be mentioned. The first is a fracture of the radius and ulna (p. 123), which can occur when someone tries to break a fall with his or her hand. There is frequently deformity with these injuries, and they require surgery if the deformity cannot be corrected conservatively.

A second wrist injury, a fracture to the scaphoid bone (p. 123), is also significant. The scaphoid bone lies between the thumb and index finger and, when injured, might not show a fracture immediately. But if the pain persists, the possibility of fracture must be considered because an untreated scaphoid fracture can result in a "pseudojoint" or a nonunion (in which the two ends of the fractured bone fail to fuse). A nonunion can occur for several reasons but when it does occur, it can lead to chronic pain and loss of function. The pseudojoint acts like a joint, but there are no ligaments, and the edges are rough. This condition is not only painful but totally disrupts the mechanics of the affected body part. A nonunion is quite painful and ultimately requires complicated treatment, including surgery.

Fractures and dislocations of the fingers are relatively common **hand injuries** (see chapter 8). These injuries are sometimes belittled but in fact are every bit as significant as some larger injuries. In sports, with dislocations, there is a tendency to "bite the bullet," reduce the dislocation (that is, correct or relocate the disloca-tion), and continue playing. But doing this can lead to a marked deformity called the "boutonniere" deformity, in which the joint next to the knuckle bends while the last joint of the finger remains straight. The boutonniere deformity gets its name because it looks as if the proximal finger joint (proximal interphalangeal joint, or PIP) slips through the extensor tendon as if it were a button hole. Essentially, this deformity results in the PIP joint hyperflexing, and the distal interphlanageal (DIP) joint and metacarpophalangeal (MCP) joint hyperextending. These complications illustrate why dislocations, despite any self-corrections made by the athlete, need to be followed up on and treated.

Trunk and Lower-Back Injuries

Chest injuries (chapter 9) often occur during an impact to the chest, causing the ribs to break or the lungs to collapse. Less severe chest injuries may result in contusions or inflammation of the more superficial structures of the chest wall. For example, costochondritis (p. 145), an inflammation of the area where the rib meets the breastbone, is a benign condition but causes significant discomfort especially when the upper extremities are stretched above the head. Perhaps the most unusual chest injury is commotio cordis (p. 140), which occurs when an object suddenly hits a person in the chest, causing the heart to deviate from its regular rhythm, which can subsequently cause cardiac arrest and even death. This type of injury has been a factor in putting devices known as Automated External Defibrillators (AEDs) in public places and at sporting events. AEDs supply an electric shock to the heart and can save the life of a victim of cardiac arrest by shocking the heart back to a normal rhythm.

Abdominal injuries (see chapter 9) are relatively uncommon in sports, but when they occur they can be serious. Causes include high-speed collisions, such as a child riding a bicycle and being thrown into the handlebars. When significant abdominal pain occurs and persists, immediate medical care should be sought.

Lower-back injuries (see chapter 10), especially herniated discs, are common among athletes. To minimize the occurrence of such injuries, athletes—including weekend athletes—must work to develop and then maintain their flexibility. Many times refining the technique used in sports such as swimming, racquetball, or hurdling lowers the risk of a lower-back injury.

Lower-Extremity Injuries

Problems in the lower extremities might occur in the hips, thighs, hamstrings, knees, ankles, or feet. In addition to bruised hip pointers, discussed earlier in this chapter, several other **hip injuries** (chapter 11) are frequently seen in athletes. Often young runners (in their 20s) complain of pain in their hips. Both greater trochanteric bursitis (p. 170) and iliopsoas tendinitis (p. 172) can produce such pain. A rare but significant hip problem is the coccygeal fracture (p. 185), which can often be resolved without the services of an orthopedic surgeon.

Of the **thigh injuries** (chapter 12), muscular injuries to the quadriceps (muscles on front of the thigh) are quite common. Because these muscles are responsible for extension (straightening the leg) in locomotion, they are among the largest and strongest muscles. They can be strained and torn and combined with contusions such injuries can be serious. When an athlete is hit hard enough in front of the thigh, bleeding within the thigh can occur. This injury is commonly experienced as a charley horse—a pain, cramping, or stiffness in the muscle as a result of a strain or bruise. However, if a second blow occurs in the same area, bleeding could become severe enough to warrant surgery.

The hamstring muscles (muscles on the back of the thigh) are the flexors of the lower extremities. The hamstring muscles help to propel the body forward during locomotion. Hamstring contusions do occur, but the most common injuries to these muscles are strains. Highly trained athletes often succumb to hamstring injuries, and they take a long time to heal.

When it comes to the lower extremities, the most common injuries are **knee injuries** (chapter 13); this is because the knee carries the weight of the whole body and is involved in locomotion, including running and pivoting.

A common knee injury is the rupture of the anterior cruciate ligament (ACL, see p. 214). Because of modern methods of surgery and rehab, an ACL injury is not the career-ender it used to be. The ACL functions to prevent the lower leg (tibia) from gliding too far forward on the upper leg (femur). Interestingly, females are much more prone to ACL injuries than males. There are many theories regarding the four- to six-fold higher incidence of ACL injuries, including female knee anatomy, hormonal influences, and other physiological differences but none has proven to be the definitive explanation. Currently one of the more widely accepted theories is that females tend to be more quadriceps dominant (as opposed to having balanced hamstrings and quadriceps), which raises the risk of an ACL strain. When quadriceps-dominant females contract their quads, they tend to put undue pressure on the front of the knee, pulling the tibia forward and causing increased stress on the ACL. In contrast, males are more hamstring dependent, so when they contract their quads, they tend to pull the tibia posteriorly, relieving pressure from the ACL.

Equally as disabling as ACL tears are patella dislocations (p. 220), in which the patella (kneecap), which normally glides along a groove formed by the femur (and to a lesser extent the tibia), suddenly "falls off the groove." On either end are tendons and ligaments that stabilize the patella. In the case of a muscle imbalance the patella might not track accurately, causing the under surface to become chronically irritated. In the case of trauma, the patella might dislocate. Another injury affecting the patella is patellar tendinitis (p. 218), which can produce pain during jumping, running, or stair climbing.

Knee problems can also be caused by the menisci, the half-moon-shaped bits of cartilage that serve as pads or "shock absorbers" and also deepen the surface for the femur to sit on the tibia. The menisci tear rather easily, and the knee can actually lock if a piece of the meniscus gets caught in the joint (p. 210). For the vast majority of athletes, a torn meniscus requires surgical attention. Fortunately, with arthroscopic surgery, meniscus injuries are not as serious as they once were.

Another well-known knee injury is Osgood-Schlatter's syndrome, which causes pain on the front of the leg bone directly below the knee. Pain is noted over the "bump" that is easily felt below the knee. This bump is called the tibial tubercle and is where the patella tendon (the area where the physician taps to elicit the knee reflex) attaches onto the tibia. Osgood-Schlatter is common in children who are active in sports at a young age. In these young athletes, the tendons and ligaments are actually stronger than the epiphyses, so they pull a small piece of bone away from the epiphysis. Later, when the growth center closes, the piece of bone that has been pulled away becomes prominent.

Injuries to the lower leg (see the **lower-leg and ankle injuries** in chapter 14) include such acute problems as ruptured Achilles tendons as well as chronic conditions such as tendinitis, shin splints, (p. 225), and stress fractures (p. 227). Shin splints is an injury that produces pain and tightness in the front (and sometimes the medial side) of the legs, usually caused by an inflammation of the sheath that surrounds and attaches to the bone. Shin splints is a chronic problem in running sports. Causes include poor practice habits, playing or running on improper surfaces, and what might be called "chromosomal poverty," such as the reduced flexibility resulting from an inherited high arch that causes the impact of the foot hitting the ground to be transmitted to the legs. High-arch athletes are also more prone to Achilles tendinitis and plantar fasciitis.

One of the most common injuries in sports is the sprained ankle (p. 231), which occurs most frequently on the outside of the ankle. This injury is likely when athletes come down on another player's foot or step into a divot or a hole. Sprains run from mild stretching of the ligaments (grade I) to complete rupture of the ligaments (grade IV), which requires surgery. Grade I ankle sprains are mild, stable, and without significant deformity, and may trigger mild swelling. Walking on this type of sprain as tolerated is not only okay but recommended to expedite recovery. With a more serious sprain, the ankle typically swells over the first few days, and there might be some discoloration of the foot, which usually disappears within a day or so. If the discoloration doesn't disappear or if significant swelling, instability, or pain develops, avoid putting weight on the ankle and consult a physician.

Trainers and physicians sometimes try to prevent sprained ankles by taping (see chapter 2 for information on taping). Unfortunately, not everyone knows how to tape an ankle properly, but there are stockinglike devices with straps available that might give adequate support and proprioceptive feedback (to improve joint stability).

Injuries to the weight-bearing surface of the body, the foot, (see **foot and toe injuries** in chapter 15) are extremely common in athletics. One of the most common conditions, plantar fasciitis, sometimes means months of disability. Whether related to body weight and habit or to biological flaws or footwear, it can be extremely painful and may severely limit athletic participation. Plantar fasciitis and other injuries to the foot such as stress fractures, neuromas, and ligament strains can be managed with subtle changes in weight bearing, specific strengthening exercises, and sometimes surgery. Unfortunately, the affected athlete must often restrict weight bearing on the injured foot to allow for healing. This can be tedious and frustrating but it does help to ensure a positive outcome.

Assessing Injuries

When assessing injuries, use your eyes and ears. Common sense will take you a long way. Obviously, a certain amount of knowledge is necessary, but many conditions or symptoms will be apparent. For instance, you can recognize a dislocated shoulder by the athlete's obvious discomfort and deformity of the shoulder. A displaced or compound fracture of the tibia and fibula can be easily differentiated from a benign contusion. Rapid swelling of an injured part is more ominous than no swelling. Inability to bear weight on an extremity is also an ominous sign. A pale person has heat exhaustion, whereas a ruddy complexion might indicate heat stroke. An athlete who has injured a knee and mentions hearing a pop probably has a torn anterior cruciate ligament. Someone with a concussion might be fine right after the blow and five minutes later not know what day it is.

Certain "red flag" signs should prompt emergency medical evaluation. These signs include disorientation following a head injury, inability to walk or move extremities following a collision or fall, inability to bear weight following a collision, and an obviously dislocated body part (e.g., shoulder, toe). Medical care should also be sought for athletes who do not improve after one to two weeks and when an injury cannot be diagnosed with certainty.

Among the most helpful instruments for assessment and diagnosis, particularly for fractures and other injuries to the skeletal system, are X-rays. X-rays cannot help with soft tissue structures, such as ligaments or cartilage, but they work great for bones, with the exception of subtle fractures, such as fresh stress fractures, which might not show up well on an X-ray. X-rays do involve a minimal amount of radiation exposure, so they should be used only when necessary. They are relatively inexpensive compared to other imaging methods and are widely available.

The CT or "CAT" scan is an X-ray study that, through the use of computers, is able to take "slices" of the involved areas, thus giving a more precise diagnosis. Although they require more radiation than an X-ray, CT scans are very useful in helping to diagnose questionable fractures. They can give doctors an accurate read on concussions and can help to rule out subdural hematomas. CTs are also very good in looking for chest and abdominal injuries. Compared to X-rays, CT scans entail considerable more radiation exposure and should be used only when necessary.

MRI has become quite useful and popular because of its ability to identify injuries in soft tissues such as ligaments and muscles. Instead of radiation, MRI uses magnets, radio waves, and computers to produce a literal picture of the body part being looked at. No longer do athletes with possible disc problems have to go through the misery of a myelogram. MRI can gather the same information with virtually no discomfort. In sports, MRI is particularly useful in diagnosing ACL tears. But compared to X-rays and CT scans, MRI is fairly expensive.

Nuclear bone scans are useful for looking at all the bones in the body. In this test, a dye is injected into the body that is picked up by metabolic activity in bones. Bone scans are particularly good for looking at inflammation and activity within bones. They can identify stress fractures even before the fractures show up on X-rays.

CHAPTER 4

Concussions and Head Injuries

Josh Krassen, DO

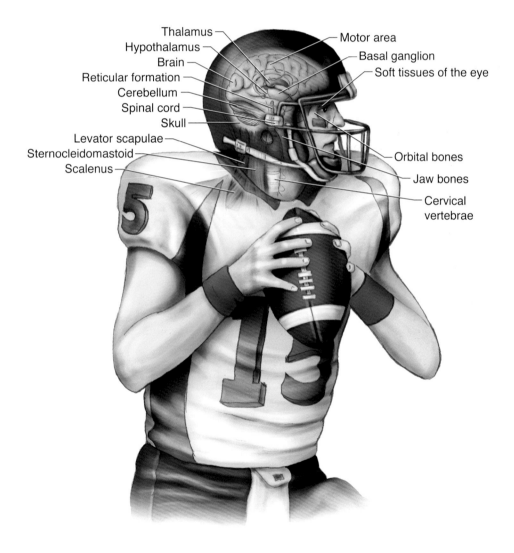

Thalamus
Hypothalamus
Brain
Reticular formation
Cerebellum
Spinal cord
Skull
Levator scapulae
Sternocleidomastoid
Scalenus

Motor area
Basal ganglion
Soft tissues of the eye

Orbital bones
Jaw bones
Cervical vertebrae

Proper diagnosis and management of head injuries are essential skills for any sports medicine practitioner. Head injuries (as well as neck and cervical spine injuries, discussed in chapter 5) have a high incidence of critical injury and death and must always be treated seriously. Athletes and those who work with them must be educated on head injuries, knowledgeable about the proper safety equipment and rules and regulations that can prevent such injuries, and aware of how to assess an athlete's risk for returning to play. Determining when an athlete who has sustained a head injury can return to play should be based on a careful medical evaluation of the athlete. Often the decision is based on limited observation of an athlete and a brief sideline evaluation. Often, pressure from a player or coach complicates or even influences a decision. Obviously, in the case of a head injury, the return-to-play decision must always be in the best interest of the athlete.

This chapter looks at several head injuries in terms of their causes, identification, and treatment. Included are injuries to the ear, jaw, nose, and eye as well as concussions and other related head injuries.

Head Injuries

CONCUSSION

Common Causes

An impact to the head with an acceleration–deceleration force may result in a concussion (note that a cervical spine injury should also be suspected with such an injury; see chapter 5).

Identification

A concussion is a traumatically induced alteration in mental status, such as confusion or amnesia, that may or may not involve a loss of consciousness (Kelly, Nichols, Filley, et al. 1991). Concussion affects approximately 300,000 athletes annually (Guskiewicz, Weaver, Padua, et al. 2000). This injury most commonly occurs in football during tackling or blocking but also occurs in other sports, such as in soccer when a player heads the ball.

Consciousness

First, evaluate an athlete's level or loss of consciousness. Neurological exams should be performed by a medical professional every five minutes until the athlete responds normally. If the results of such tests are deemed abnormal, repeat the exam every five minutes for the first hour, then hourly for the first day, and then daily after that until the athlete returns to normal. Loss of consciousness is defined as unresponsiveness to external stimuli for any amount of time and is seen in fewer than 10 percent of head injuries. An athlete's level of consciousness is often determined by the Glasgow Coma Scale (GCS), a numerical scale that corresponds to various levels of consciousness; this scale is used frequently by medical personnel. The Glasgow Coma Scale includes assessments of eye opening, motor response, and visual response (table 4.1). An injured athlete receives a score for each assessment, and the sum of the individual scores determines the head injury classification.

Concussions are often graded on two widely used scales: the Cantu Grading Scale and the American Academy of Neurology (AAN) Scale. Each grades a concussion on a scale from 1 to 3. The Cantu scale is based on loss of consciousness, posttraumatic amnesia, and postconcussive signs and symptoms. In a grade 1 concussion, the athlete experiences no loss of consciousness, posttraumatic amnesia occurs for no longer than 30 minutes after the injury, and postconcussion symptoms last from 15 to 30 minutes. A grade 2 concussion indicates a loss of consciousness shorter than five minutes; the athlete experiences posttraumatic amnesia and postconcussion symptoms 30 minutes to 24 hours after the injury. In a grade 3 concussion, the athlete loses consciousness for more than five minutes, posttraumatic amnesia occurs 24 hours after the injury, and postconcussion symptoms continue for up to seven days. The AAN scale (table 4.2) rates the concussion based on loss of consciousness and duration of confusion. According to the AAN, any loss of consciousness or confusion lasting more than one hour warrants imaging, such as an X-ray, MRI, or CT scan.

Even without loss of consciousness, a concussed athlete should be assessed for confusion or amnesia (see table 4.3). Confusion is defined as any impairment in

CONCUSSION

(continued)

Table 4.1   Glasgow Coma Scale (GCS)

Eye opening response	
Spontaneous—open with blinking at baseline	4
To verbal stimuli, command, speech	3
To pain only (not applied to face)	2
No response	1
Verbal response	
Oriented	5
Confused conversation, but able to answer questions	4
Inappropriate words	3
Incomprehensible speech	2
No response	1
Motor response	
Obeys commands for movement	6
Purposeful movement to painful stimulus	5
Withdraws in response to pain	4
Flexion in response to pain (decorticate posturing)	3
Extension response in response to pain (decerebrate posturing)	2
No response	1
Head injury classification	
Severe head injury	Score of 8 or less
Moderate head injury	Score of 9 to 12
Mild head injury	Score of 13 to 15

From the Centers for Disease Control and Prevention, a division of the Department of Health and Human Services. Available: http://www.bt.cdc.gov/masscasualties/gscale.asp.

Table 4.2   American Academy of Neurology (AAN) Scale

Concussion grade	Loss of consciousness	Transient confusion
Grade 1	None	<15 minutes
Grade 2	None	>15 minutes
Grade 3	Any	

Data from The Quality Standards Subcommittee of the American Academy of Neurology, 1997, "Practice parameter: The management of concussion in sports (summary statement)," *Neurology* 48(3): 581-585.

awareness or orientation to surroundings. Amnesia is defined as the loss of recall of events just before, at the time of, or just after the injury occurred. Retrograde amnesia is the inability to recall events immediately preceding the trauma. Posttraumatic amnesia (also called anterograde) is further differentiated according to the length of time between trauma and the point of regaining normal continuous memory.

Sometimes athletes suddenly lose consciousness without trauma, such as when they are engaged in an aerobic activity and suddenly collapse. In such cases, the loss of consciousness is not related to a concussion. Instead, it may be secondary

CONCUSSION

Table 4.3 Confusion and Amnesia Assessments

Awareness or orientation to surroundings
What is your name?
Where are we playing? What's the stadium or field name?
Who are we playing? Who is the opposing team?
What day is it? Month? Year?
Retrograde amnesia
Do you remember getting hit?
What is the score of the game?
What happened earlier in the game?
Posttraumatic amnesia
Coach or trainer should repeat three words such as ball, chair, and car.
Ask athlete to repeat these words at one minute and then five minute intervals.
Posttraumatic amnesia is no longer present when athlete can recall the words.

to cardiac irregularities. If the athlete has neither a pulse nor spontaneous voluntary breathing, an ambulance should be called and cardiopulmonary resuscitation should begin.

Postconcussion Syndrome

Concussions sometimes cause a decrease of blood flow to the brain, which can result in postconcussion syndrome. The symptoms of postconcussion syndrome include headache, nausea, dizziness, balance deficits, visual deficits, attention deficits, and memory loss. Common visual deficits are blurriness and photosensitivity. These can occur immediately or over time. The athlete might feel fatigued or irritable and have unusual emotions or changes in personality. A sleep disturbance might occur, and the athlete might become depressed. The severity and duration of the symptoms can vary from days to weeks, depending on the severity of the concussion. Headache occurs in approximately 70 percent of those afflicted and is the most common symptom of postconcussion syndrome. The athlete might experience a headache during the initial sideline evaluation, which may become more intense over the ensuing hours or get worse with exertion. If a headache becomes severe or if the athlete is vomiting or experiencing a decline in mental status, he or she should be taken to an emergency room immediately so that a subdural hematoma (p. 62) or an intracranial bleed can be ruled out. Either of these conditions can be life threatening.

More postinjury difficulties involve amnesia than a loss of consciousness (Collins et al. 2003). A loss of consciousness does not necessarily signal deficits. The more symptoms the athlete has, the longer the symptoms last, and the greater the neurocognitive impairment, the more likely he or she will have long-term memory deficits.

Second-Impact Syndrome

If an athlete who is recovering from a concussion receives a second blow to the head, the consequences can be fatal. Second-impact syndrome is defined as massive cerebral edema, which is swelling of the brain. Clinically, the athlete demonstrates a rapidly decreasing level of consciousness.

(continued)

Treatment

If the cervical spine is determined not to be affected (see chapter 5), the conscious athlete with a head injury should be positioned upright to decrease intracranial pressure. Once the athlete is stable sitting, he or she can then stand and be helped off the field. If you suspect a cervical spine injury, do not remove protective equipment (shoulder pads, helmet) or articles of clothing if removal might cause motion in the cervical spine area, and protect the neck and spine with a stabilization collar, if available, or by placing rolled-up clothing alongside the neck to secure it from motion. If the athlete is unconscious, stabilize him or her and protect the airway. If the athlete is not breathing and has no pulse, call an ambulance and resuscitate with rescue breaths and cardiac life support. If obvious bleeding is noted, place a pressure dressing (or any dressing available) directly over the bleeding site. If bleeding is profuse, lie the athlete down and raise the legs slightly to help return blood to the heart.

Once the athlete is stable, he or she should be transported to a hospital's emergency room for further evaluation. He or she will be admitted if imaging results (X-ray, MRI, or CT scan) or neurological status remains abnormal. If the results of the neurological exam and imaging studies are normal, the athlete may be released. Once the athlete is home, family members should perform regular neurological checks, which include asking the athlete the day and date, the year, or the name of the president. They should also ask the injured athlete whether he or she has any headache, nausea, or weakness. If the responses to these checks worsen, the athlete should be transported to the physician or emergency room. Concussed athletes who suffer a second impact typically require a neuropsychological evaluation and cognitive retraining.

Return to Action

When determining return to play postconcussion, appropriate guidelines should be followed based on the grade of the concussion. Both Cantu and the AAN have published return-to-play guidelines based on their respective scales. The two agree that athletes with a grade 1 concussion should be removed from play. Neurological exams should be done every five minutes, and, according to AAN guidelines, the athlete may return to play the day of a grade 1 concussion if he or she is symptom free within 15 minutes of the injury. Cantu guidelines allow a return to sport the day of a grade 1 concussion only if there are no symptoms at rest or upon exertion.

An athlete with concussion symptoms who returns to play during the resolution period is at risk for serious injury or even death. If a second grade 1 concussion occurs during the resolution period, the athlete is removed from the contest or competition. According to the Cantu guidelines, he or she may return in two weeks once no symptoms appear for one full week at rest or with exertion. According to AAN guidelines, the athlete may return in one week if he or she continues to be asymptomatic for one week after the second grade 1 injury.

Athletes with grade 2 concussions are removed from play with no return that day. Neurological exams are performed every 15 minutes for 24 hours to rule out any intracranial abnormality. If cognition remains impaired for longer than 60 minutes, or if any weakness or numbness is observed, the athlete should be sent to the emer-

CONCUSSION

gency room. According to the Cantu guidelines, an athlete with a grade 2 concussion may return to play in two weeks if no symptoms appear for seven full days at either rest or with exertion. The AAN again allows return to play in one week if the athlete is asymptomatic for the week. If a second grade 2 concussion occurs, the athlete is removed from play and may return in one month once asymptomatic for a week per Cantu. The AAN allows a return to play in two weeks in this case as long as the athlete has been asymptomatic for that time period. If any abnormalities, such as persistent confusion, memory impairment, or headaches, are discovered in an athlete with a grade 2 concussion, the athlete is out for the remainder of the season.

Athletes with a grade 3 concussion are immediately transported to the emergency room. The Cantu guidelines allow return to play in 30 days when asymptomatic for one week at both rest and exertion as long as imaging is negative. The AAN again allows return to play in two weeks if asymptomatic. Cantu and AAN agree that if a second grade 3 concussion occurs, the athlete is out for the season, even if imaging is negative. If a third grade 1 or 2 concussion occurs, the athlete is also out for the season and should consider restricting participation in contact sports.

In 2001, a group of experts met in Austria for the Vienna Concussion Conference. They reinforced the practice of removing athletes from a contest if they exhibit any signs or symptoms of concussion. They reinforced the following return-to-play guidelines but noted that decisions for any athlete should be individualized*:

1. Removal from game with any sign or symptoms of concussion
2. No return to play in game that day
3. Medical evaluation following injury including neuropsychological testing and radiographs to rule out more serious intracranial pathology
4. Adherence to stepwise return-to-play process:
   1. No activity until asymptomatic at rest and during exertion
   2. Light aerobic exercises
   3. Sport-specific exercises
   4. Noncontact drills
   5. Contact drills
   6. Game play

The two most important factors in making an individualized decision are the athlete's age and concussion history. Children have more prolonged and diffuse cerebral swelling and are at an increased risk for a second head injury (Pickles 1950). It is important to note that the speed of recovery is, overall, the same for all age groups, thus negating the theory that "kids heal faster." Knowing if the athlete has a history of concussions at the time of a new injury is important. Cumulative neuropsychological and subtle neurocognitive deficits can be seen after multiple concussions. After three or more concussions, the athlete becomes more vulnerable to subsequent injuries (Collins et al. 2002). There is no data on time between injuries and cumulative deficits or cause of subsequent injuries.

*Adapted, by permission, from P. McCrory et al., 2005, "Summary and agreement statement of the 2nd International Conference on Concussion in Sport, Prague 2004," *Clin J Sport Med* 15(2): 48-55.

SUBDURAL AND EPIDURAL HEMATOMA

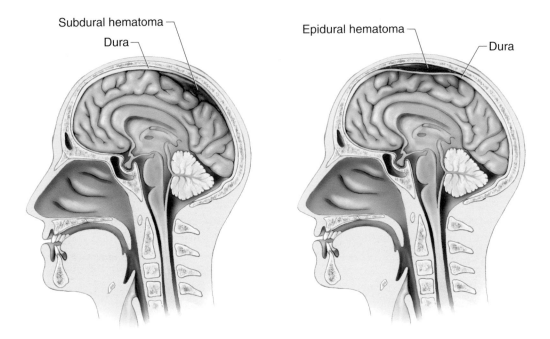

Common Causes

Subdural and epidural hematomas are caused by a direct blow to the head and occur primarily in contact sports. A subdural hematoma is bleeding between the outer layer (dura) and middle layer (arachnoid) of the membrane covering of the brain, and an epidural hematoma is bleeding between the outer membrane of the brain (dura) and the skull.

Identification

An athlete with an epidural hematoma typically experiences a decreased level of consciousness and a severe headache. A variable lucid period is followed by a rapidly declining level of consciousness. A subdural hematoma or intracranial bleed results in loss of consciousness with little to no lucidity. Vomiting, seizure activity, and hemiparesis may be evident. Eye pupils are often unequal and dilated.

Treatment

The athlete with symptoms of either an epidural or subdural hematoma should be immediately removed from the game and transported to a hospital emergency room. Note that the initial blow to the head causing the bleed or traumatic brain injury does not always appear to be severe.

Return to Action

Because symptoms vary so much depending on the degree of the injury, there is no set standard for return to play for subdural and epidural hematomas. Each case must be evaluated individually. That said, many athletes with relatively mild hematomas return within weeks of the injury. Others take much longer.

SKULL FRACTURE

Common Causes

An athlete with a skull fracture exhibits different symptoms depending on the type and degree of the fracture. A skull fracture may be caused by a blunt blow to the head, a fall onto the head, or other trauma to the head. Skull fractures typically occur in contact sports such as American football but can also result from a direct hit by a baseball or hockey puck or a fall as might occur during gymnatics or horseback riding.

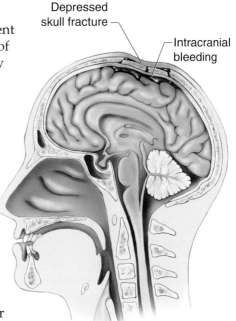

Depressed skull fracture

Intracranial bleeding

Identification

A deep bruise or laceration with accompanying pain and headache signals a possible skull fracture. Other indications include sunken black eyes, bleeding from ears or nose, and swelling or discoloration behind the ear. Clear fluid draining from the nose or ears is indicative of a cerebral spinal fluid leak associated with a severe skull fracture or head injury. Unconsciousness and unequal pupils are signs of serious underlying intracranial bleeding associated with a skull fracture.

There are several types of skull fractures. A linear fracture is a simple crack in the cranium. A comminuted fracture is a crack that radiates from a center point. A depressed fracture, one of the more serious fractures, is when bone fragments are separated and driven inward. A basal fracture involves the cranial floor.

Treatment

If the fractured pieces of skull are aligned, no treatment is generally needed; the fracture must be allowed time to heal before the athlete returns to play. A depressed skull fracture generally requires neurosurgery. Athletes with this fracture typically need oxygen, anticonvulsants, and osmotic diuretics (such as Mannitol) to reduce brain swelling. After the athlete is treated and becomes stable, extensive rehabilitation, including physical, occupational, and speech therapy, follows.

Return to Action

With any significant head injury, a full neuropsychological evaluation should be performed before clearing the athlete to return to play. Persistent cognitive or neurological impairment including weakness, numbness, or balance deficits disallows any return to contact sports.

NASAL AND MANDIBLE FRACTURES

Common Causes

Fractures to the nose and jaw are seen most often in contact sports. They are caused by a direct forceful blow to the face.

Identification

A nasal fracture can be identified by pain and tenderness, bleeding, and increased mobility of the nose. There is typically a displacement deformity of the nose. An athlete with a mandible (jaw) fracture has a painful and swollen jaw and difficulty opening the mouth. The athlete will have difficulty speaking and often have loose or knocked-out teeth. There might be significant facial distortion. Blunt trauma in contact sports can also result in other oral trauma, such as when lips and gums are forcefully compressed against teeth. If blunt trauma occurs to the oral region, a laceration and sometimes dislodged teeth could result.

Treatment

As initial treatment for a nasal fracture, maintain an open airway by suctioning, positioning, and controlling bleeding. If there is no associated skull or neck fracture, the athlete should be positioned forward to avoid blood draining into the throat. If the athlete is unconscious, immobilize the neck first because posterior head and cervical spine injuries are often associated with nasal fractures. Nostrils should be pinched to control bleeding unless the nose is draining clear fluid, which indicates a skull fracture. Apply a cold pack to decrease blood flow to the area.

As initial treatment for a mandible fracture, maintain an airway and dress the wound. The lower jaw should be supported and immobilized with a cravat or strap placed under the jaw and wrapped around the top of the head and tied in a knot above the ear. The athlete should then be transported to the emergency room for evaluation by an oral surgeon. If teeth are dislodged, they should be carefully removed to avoid airway obstruction.

Return to Action

For a nasal fracture, once the nasal bones are healed and the airway passage has been opened with or without surgical intervention, the athlete may return to play in approximately six weeks. The athlete should wear a protective face mask for the remainder of the season. For a jaw fracture, once the jaw has healed and the athlete is cleared by an oral surgeon to return to play, he or she should wear a mouth guard to prevent a recurrent injury. A mouth guard should also be worn by athletes who have experienced other oral trauma.

EAR TRAUMA

Common Causes

Blunt trauma to or pulling on the ear can result in what is known as a "cauliflower" ear caused by a hematoma or collection of blood in the outer ear. This injury is most common in wrestling and is sometimes called wrestler's ear.

Identification

The injury shows up as a shapeless, purplish mass on the outer ear caused by a calcified hematoma. It may cause mild to moderate local discomfort.

Treatment

The mass, or clot, must be removed by an incision to remove the clot. This can be done in an office setting with local anesthesia.

Return to Action

Once the incision has healed, in approximately four to six weeks, the athlete can return to play.

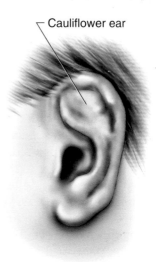
Cauliflower ear

EYE INJURIES

Common Causes

Eye injuries are generally associated with direct trauma to the eye, such as getting poked in the eye by an opponent's finger while going for a rebound in basketball.

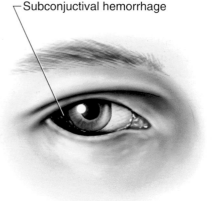

Subconjuctival hemorrhage

Identification

An athlete may sustain any of a variety of eye injuries. With a subconjunctival hemorrhage, the athlete has a red or bloodshot eye, equivalent to a bruise to the eye. More serious eye injuries include foreign bodies and puncture wounds to the eye. A foreign body in the eye usually results directly from major or minor contact to the eye. The athlete may experience a burning, pain, or discomfort in the eye. Generally, the foreign body is identified with fluorescein staining of the eye.

Treatment

A subconjunctival hemorrhage will generally resolve without treatment within two weeks. If a foreign body is identified in the eye, the eye should be shut and the athlete evaluated by an ophthalmologist (eye doctor). The foreign body should never be removed or the cornea of the eye touched by an untrained professional. If the foreign body is chemical in nature, immediately and extensively irrigate the eye for 15 to 20 minutes with water or a saline solution that is flushed into the eye. Antibiotic ointment and a patch should then be applied. The athlete should be evaluated by an ophthalmologist to rule out further damage to the eye.

If the eye injury is traumatic, a medical professional will need to check for eyelid perforations or corneal abrasions. These injuries are extremely painful, and initial treatment is often aimed at pain control. A cup or loose protective dressing should be placed over the injured eye and the athlete transported to an emergency room for evaluation by an eye doctor. The pupils are then dilated with atropine and antibiotic eye drops applied.

Return to Action

A subconjunctival hemorrhage will generally not keep an athlete from returning to play. Once the foreign body has been removed, the cornea healed, and normal vision is restored the athlete may return. Return time depends on the extent of the corneal abrasion. Direct penetrating trauma, usually with a sharp object, results in a puncture injury to the eye. Return to play after a puncture, chemical, or blunt injury requires full healing and clearance by an eye doctor.

CHAPTER 5

Neck and Cervical Spine Injuries

Greg Rowdon, MD; Hank Sherman, MD

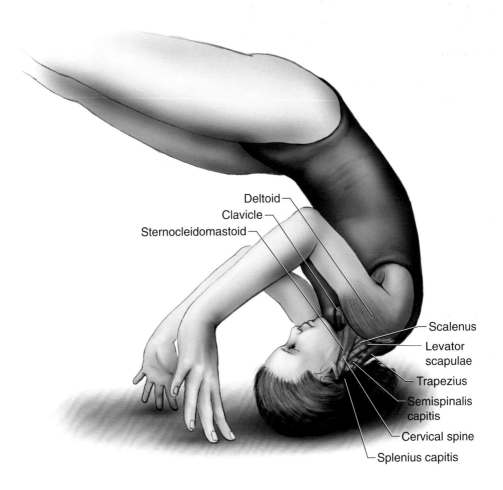

Deltoid

Clavicle

Sternocleidomastoid

Scalenus

Levator scapulae

Trapezius

Semispinalis capitis

Cervical spine

Splenius capitis

Athletes at any level of competition are at risk for injuries to the neck and spine. These injuries—whether soft tissue injuries or neck or spinal fractures—can occur as acute events or as flare-ups of a chronic, degenerative process. Such injuries might cause mild, transient limitations in function or might be catastrophic and life changing.

A big part of preventing neck and spinal injuries involves educating athletes in contact sports on proper hitting and tackling of an opponent. An athlete should always maintain eye contact on the opposing player and avoid putting his or her head down and dropping the shoulders during contact. Proper contact prevents the head and neck from being driven into hyperextension, which causes most cervical spine injuries. Protective equipment, such as shoulder pads and neck rolls, helps absorb the shock at impact and prevent hyperextension and excessive lateral flexion. Pads should fit well, feeling comfortable but stiff at the base, to protect the neck. Preparation should also include ensuring that necessary first-aid equipment, such as a backboard, rigid cervical collar, and resuscitation equipment, is available in case of injury. For helmet sports such as American football, a Phillips screwdriver should always be on hand for face-mask removal.

In this chapter we review several kinds of neck and spinal injuries, including an example case of each injury and the immediate and long-term management of each condition. Regardless of the type of injury, the injured athlete should be examined by medical personnel before resuming activity.

Neck and Spine Injuries

WHIPLASH

Common Causes

Common athletic causes of this injury include falling on the neck after making a tackle in football or rugby. The most common cause outside athletics is a rear-end motor vehicle collision.

Identification

Whiplash, or cervical strain, injuries are generally stable injuries of the soft tissues of the neck caused by acute trauma when the neck is violently jammed or forcibly flexed, extended, or rotated. Athletes might have diffuse neck pain anywhere from the base of the skull to the shoulder region (deltoid and trapezius muscles). They will generally complain of neck pain throughout the various ranges of motion of the neck, and often have accompanying cervical muscle spasm, but they usually have complete range of motion of the neck. Athletes should not have tingling, numbness, or weakness of the arms, and the pain should not radiate into one or both arms.

Treatment

Customize treatment of cervical strains to the severity of the injury and to the athlete's symptoms. Most cervical strains are self-limited conditions that resolve spontaneously over several days. Manage pain with analgesics and anti-inflammatory medications, when appropriate, until full, pain-free range of motion is reestablished. Muscle relaxant medications might also be prescribed by a physician. Physical therapy such as massage, hot packs, electrical stimulation, and ultrasound aimed at reducing muscle spasms in the area to reestablish pain-free range of motion and strengthen cervical muscles can be helpful. X-rays, a CT scan, or MRI should be considered if the athlete has point tenderness over the bony prominences of the neck, persistent pain, marked limitation of cervical range of motion, or neurological symptoms such as pain, numbness, or tingling that travels down the arm.

Return to Action

The athlete should be able to resume full athletic participation once comfortable and free of pain. Some athletes might choose to wear a neck roll, cowboy collar, or another soft cervical collar to prevent neck extension and lateral bending so they can return more quickly to activity and avoid future cervical strain. These devices are most commonly used in American football. Teaching proper tackling techniques reduces the incidence of cervical strain.

BURNERS

Common Causes

Also known as transient neuropraxia or "stingers," this injury is almost always related to American football. The injury occurs during tackling or blocking when the neck is either pinched toward the side of injury or stretched to the opposite side.

Identification

A burner is a cervical nerve root contusion outside the spinal cord. The nerve root is the start of the nerve, where it exits the spinal cord. Burners occur during neck extension combined with same-side lateral neck flexion. The athlete's symptoms include a burning sensation that begins in the neck and radiates down the arm on the affected side. These injuries are not typically bilateral in nature. Athletes might also have associated numbness or tingling of the upper extremity on the affected side and possibly weakness of the deltoid or biceps muscles. The symptoms of burners are transient, usually lasting seconds to minutes. There is usually no neck pain or reduced cervical range of motion.

Treatment

Rule out more serious pathology of the neck and arm by taking a thorough history and physical examination. The symptoms of burners subside spontaneously and do not require further treatment. Recurrent burners or prolonged symptoms lasting from hours to weeks require detailed evaluation by a physician. Recurrent burners or stingers may signify a spinal problem or entrapped nerve. Electromyography (EMG) is used when persistent neurological symptoms occur.

Return to Action

Athletes may return to play under three conditions: when all symptoms have subsided, when they have painless and complete cervical range of motion, and when they have full upper-extremity and shoulder girdle strength. Prevention of burners and stingers includes year-round regimens of cervical muscle and shoulder muscle strengthening and conditioning. Proper tackling techniques in contact sports and properly fitting equipment, specifically shoulder pads in American football, are also imperative. Protective devices such as neck rolls, cowboy collars, and high-riding shoulder pads have also been developed to help prevent these injuries.

General guidelines exist that help determine level of risk in returning to play after burners. One guideline that most practitioners agree on is that players with any persistent neurological deficits should not return to play that day. Another is that any athlete with tenderness over bony prominences or painful limited neck range of motion should get X-rays before returning to play. If the athlete's only symptoms are transient numbness and tingling, and these symptoms quickly resolve, he or she may return to play under three conditions: the neurological exam is normal, the range of cervical spine motion is normal, and the Spurling maneuver is negative. To perform the Spurling maneuver, an examiner first has the athlete extend the cervical spine (neck) and turn the head toward the affected side; the examiner then gently compresses the spine by placing his or her hand on top of the head and gently pushing down. In a positive test, the athlete notes pain radiating into the arm toward which the head is rotated. In a negative test, no such pain is noted by the athlete (local neck pain alone is considered a negative test).

CERVICAL OSTEOARTHRITIS

Common Causes

Cervical osteoarthritis is a chronic process most common in men and women over 60, unless history of a trauma exists. Cervical osteoarthritis is not caused at the time of an injury, but a prior injury might predispose athletes to future osteoarthritis.

Identification

Cervical osteoarthritis refers to degeneration of the cervical vertebrae and intervertebral discs (discs that sit between the bones and act as "shock absorbers"). This degeneration might have several effects on the cervical spine, including bone spurs, disruption or fusion of the facet joints (the joints that connect one block of the spine to the next), narrowing of the foramina (the openings in the bone through which the nerves pass), nerve root compression, and cervical stenosis (see p. 75).

Characteristic symptoms of cervical osteoarthritis include vague or generalized neck pain—often most noted in the early morning, popping or grinding sensations in the neck, and reduced cervical range of motion. Spasms in the muscles supporting the spine might occur following a change in posture. As the process advances, other damage along the spine could occur, including cervical strain (injury to the soft tissue in the neck), cervical radiculopathy ("pinched nerve"), cervical disc herniation (rupture), and cervical stenosis. The symptoms might then progress to numbness, tingling, burning, or decreased sensation in the arms. Athletes might become weaker as muscles of the shoulders, arms, and hands atrophy.

Treatment

Treatment of cervical osteoarthritis is both preventative and reactive (symptom guided). Osteoarthritis does not have a cure at this time. Preventative measures include proper posture and proper athletic techniques (especially tackling). Cervical muscle strengthening programs might also provide a benefit. Once an athlete has cervical osteoarthritis, treatment focuses on pain management, muscle strengthening, and prevention of further deterioration. Initially, analgesic and anti-inflammatory medications may be prescribed. Cervical X-rays should be taken to evaluate foraminal narrowing, cervical stenosis, bone spurs, and intervertebral disc space. Physical therapy may be prescribed to decrease pain, improve cervical muscle strength and range of motion, and teach improved cervical posture. Cervical traction might provide benefits depending on the type of cervical pathology. Corticosteroid injections (e.g., cortisone shots) into the epidural space (the area outside the tough membrane that covers the spinal cord) or the areas of the facet joints (the joints that provide spinal stability and allow the body to bend and twist) might also reduce inflammation and alleviate, or even eliminate, pain. Finally, surgical consultation might be warranted depending on the cervical damage present and its symptoms.

Return to Action

Future participation in sports and recreation is recommended for athletes with cervical osteoarthritis, as long as there is no evidence of existing or pending nerve injury or neck instability. Athletes may, however, need to modify activities depending on the severity of symptoms and type of injury. Cervical muscle strengthening programs and improved cervical posture could certainly be beneficial.

CERVICAL DISC INJURY

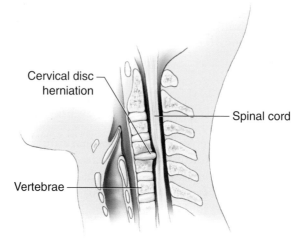

Cervical disc herniation

Spinal cord

Vertebrae

Common Causes

Cervical disc injuries occur when the cervical intervertebral disc ruptures or herniates and the bulging tissue entraps or irritates cervical nerve roots, either by direct mechanical irritation or via chemical irritation (the ruptured disc exudes various chemicals, which can irritate local nerves and muscles). Cervical disc injury can result from pure rupture of the intervertebral disc, deterioration of the intervertebral disc space, foraminal narrowing of the cervical spine, bony deterioration and osteophyte (bone spur) formation in the cervical spine, or any combination of these. Acute cervical disc rupture is rare in athletes; in most cases the rupture occurs gradually as a result of chronic injury and deterioration.

Identification

Athletes with a cervical disc injury often have chronic neck pain and commonly have progressively worsening numbness, tingling, and weakness in the arms associated with nerve irritation. Many times, the affected athlete can demonstrate specific movements that reproduce their symptoms. As the condition gets worse, symptoms might become constant.

Treatment

Treatment depends on the severity of symptoms. Cervical spine X-rays should be done at the outset to assess bone damage of the cervical spine. Anti-inflammatory medications or oral steroids may be prescribed to reduce inflammation around the irritated nerve. Physical therapy aimed at strengthening cervical musculature and improving cervical posture can alleviate symptoms. Cervical traction, which must be prescribed by a physician, might help reduce the pressure of the ruptured disc on the nerve root. If symptoms progress to cause constant, uncontrollable pain or muscle weakness and atrophy, surgery might be recommended. As an alternative or precursor to surgery, epidural steroid injections (an injection directly to the ruptured disc area) or a nerve block injection (an injection into the nerves directly alongside the cervical vertebrae) might be recommended by physicians to reduce the surrounding swelling and size of the ruptured cervical disc.

Return to Action

Management and return-to-play criteria for a cervical disc injury should be conservative and managed by a physician. Most athletes will be able to return to full activity after treatment. Athletes who require surgery should follow the return-to-activity guidelines outlined by their surgeons. If suspicions of spinal instability arise, contact sports may be prohibited.

CERVICAL STENOSIS

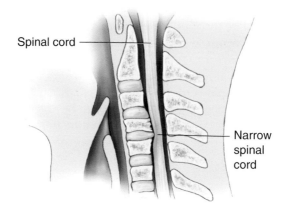

Spinal cord

Narrow spinal cord

Common Causes

Cervical stenosis, or transient quadriplegia, refers to a condition in which the spinal canal is abnormally narrow. This condition might be congenital or the result of degenerative conditions such as osteoarthritis, excessive cervical ligament laxity, or cervical disc ruptures.

Identification

Most athletes will be unaware of congenital cervical stenosis. Athletes with acquired degenerative cervical stenosis might know of their condition if they have seen a physician and had images taken (e.g., X-ray or MRI). In the acute setting, a forced hyperextension, hyperflexion, or axial load on the cervical spine and spinal column initiates symptoms. Signs of cervical stenosis range from no symptoms to transient quadriplegia (temporary loss of sensation and muscle function in arms and legs) after an acute injury. The athlete might have numbness, tingling, burning pain, or loss of sensation of any or all extremities. Neck pain need not be present. If the injury occurs in the middle to lower part of the neck (spinal cord) only, the upper extremities could be involved and the athlete might experience "burning hand syndrome" because the nerves in the middle to lower part of the neck are the ones that travel to and supply sensation and strength to the hands. Although transient quadriplegia and burning hand syndrome are caused by trauma, they are more likely in athletes with cervical stenosis. Episodes typically last from several minutes to hours and do not require treatment. Athletes should regain complete neurological function.

Treatment

Treatment of cervical stenosis is very limited. Individuals with congenital stenosis are generally unaware of the condition. Knowledge of the condition influences the athlete's future involvement in sports, particularly collision sports. Acquired cervical stenosis can be treated, depending on its cause. Initial cervical spine imaging (X-rays, CT scans, or MRI) will be ordered by a treating physician. Analgesic and anti-inflammatory medications are used for pain and symptomatic treatment. Physical therapy to strengthen cervical muscles might improve the athlete's function. Cervical traction is sometimes an option to alleviate symptoms. Corticosteroid injections (e.g., cortisone shots) might be prescribed by a physician, depending on the cause of the stenosis. In some cases, surgery is necessary.

Athletes with a history of transient quadriplegia (weakening that comes and goes) should be checked for underlying spinal abnormalities including fractures at all cervical levels. Anyone with symptoms of quadraparesis (a weakening of all four limbs), no matter how transient, should have MRI.

Return to Action

In general, athletes should not return to collision or contact sports unless the cause of the stenosis can be corrected (i.e., it is the acquired form). Once an athlete has no symptoms and no significant spinal stenosis, he or she can return to play without restriction. Congenital stenosis usually ends a collision-sport athlete's career. In some cases, year-round neck exercises can help prevent future symptoms. Noncontact sports and activities are encouraged.

Most athletes with stenosis and a history of transient quadriplegia do not progress to permanent neurological injury. Athletes with permanent quadriplegia generally have no history of transient neuropraxia or significant spinal stenosis (Torg et al. 1997). Based on these studies, Torg allows return to play in athletes with spinal stenosis as long as they have no symptoms. However, studies have shown that cervical stenosis is a factor in occurrence and severity of neurological injury after spine trauma. For these reasons, Cantu believes that athletes with functional spinal stenosis should not participate in contact sports but may participate in noncontact sports (Cantu 1998).

Some medical practitioners believe stricter criteria should be followed; they recommend absolutes regarding circumstances in which an athlete should not return to play:

- If initial symptoms in the limbs last longer than 36 hours
- If the cervical cord is affected or involved or if ligaments are unstable
- If the athlete has congenital abnormalities (structural defects) in this region of the body or has any vertebral fusion
- If the athlete has a loss of range of motion in the neck or neurological deficits or disorders (dizziness, lapses in consciousness) that last over time

CERVICAL FRACTURE

Common Causes

Cervical vertebral fractures occur when the bones of the cervical spine are crushed, chipped, or cleanly broken. Such fractures occur as a result of degenerative processes such as osteoporosis or as a result of direct trauma to the neck.

Identification

Athletes with neck fractures might have various complaints and symptoms depending on the type and severity of the fracture. Possible symptoms include neck pain; painful neck range of motion; inability to move the neck; upper-extremity numbness, tingling, or weakness; or inability to move the extremities. Because of the complexity and potential severity of neck fractures, all athletes with neck pain, especially those with any history of trauma, should be evaluated by appropriate medical personnel.

Treatment

Treatment of cervical fractures is extremely complicated. The main function of the spinal column is to protect the spinal cord. Any fracture to this protective structure might in turn lead to injury of the spinal cord, which could cause permanent loss of leg function (paraplegia) or leg and arm (quadriplegia) function or even death. Any athlete with a suspected catastrophic neck injury should be properly immobilized on a spine board and with a cervical collar. Only trained medical staff should attempt to immobilize the athlete. Once transported, the athlete should receive X-rays or other imaging to rule out a neck fracture.

For stable types of fractures—those without obvious potential for spinal cord injury—treatment begins with pain management. Physicians may use analgesics or anti-inflammatory medications. Physical therapy may be prescribed to strengthen cervical muscles and improve posture. Soft collar devices may also be used. For unstable cervical fractures—those with potential for spinal cord injury—neurosurgical consultation is recommended, with imminent surgery likely.

Return to Action

All return-to-play decisions should be determined by the treating physician. These decisions generally depend on the type of fracture and its stability. Fractures to the spinous process (the bone you feel when you run your hand down your back), chip fractures, and compression fractures tend to be stable. After symptoms and physical exam abnormalities have been resolved, athletes who have suffered these fractures might be able to return to play. Catastrophic or unstable fractures resulting in any ligament instability or disruption of the anterior or posterior vertebral elements make a return to play unlikely, especially in collision sports.

CHAPTER 6

Shoulder Injuries

Edmund S. Evangelista, MD

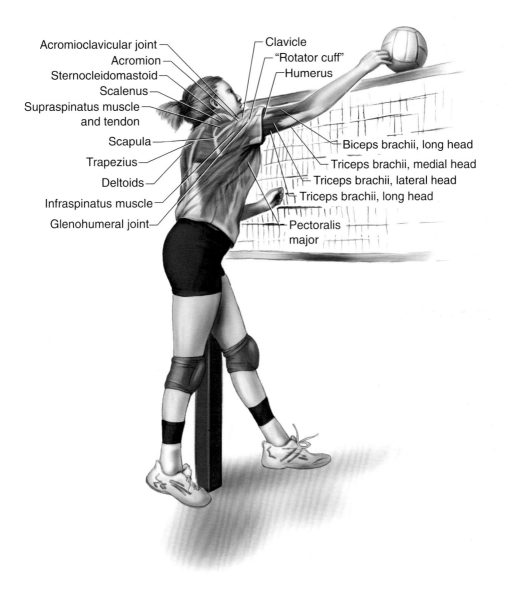

Acromioclavicular joint
Acromion
Sternocleidomastoid
Scalenus
Supraspinatus muscle and tendon
Scapula
Trapezius
Deltoids
Infraspinatus muscle
Glenohumeral joint

Clavicle
"Rotator cuff"
Humerus

Biceps brachii, long head
Triceps brachii, medial head
Triceps brachii, lateral head
Triceps brachii, long head
Pectoralis major

The shoulder is made up of two main joints: the *glenohumeral joint*, which is the "ball and socket," and the *acromioclavicular joint*, which is the smaller joint above the glenohumeral joint. All athletes are prone to shoulder injuries from both direct trauma and overuse. Throwing athletes and those performing repetitive overhead motions (e.g., swimmers, volleyball players) are especially prone to shoulder injuries caused by repetitive forces transmitted through the joint. In this chapter we review some of the common shoulder injuries encountered by athletes.

Most shoulder injuries can be treated conservatively. As described throughout the chapter, treatment principles for all shoulder injuries include relative rest and avoidance of the offending activity, decreasing pain and inflammation with ice and anti-inflammatory medications (if appropriate), restoring full pain-free range of motion, and strengthening of the shoulder, especially the rotator cuff muscles, which are the most important dynamic shoulder stabilizers. If an athlete experiences any of the following signs and symptoms after a shoulder injury, medical attention is required:

- Significant or persistent pain or deformity
- Persistent numbness or tingling
- Noticeable weakness or muscle wasting of the shoulder
- Inability to move the arm or shoulder
- Persistent or worsening pain despite conservative treatment

Shoulder Injuries

COLLAR BONE FRACTURE

Common Causes

Fractures of the collar bone, or clavicle, are among the most common fractures encountered in contact or collision sports such as American football, rugby, lacrosse, wrestling, and hockey. These injuries typically occur following a direct blow to the clavicle during contact or following a fall onto the top of the shoulder.

Identification

Following the injury, the athlete will complain of pain at the fracture site and might be unable to move the arm because of pain. Look for swelling and an obvious deformity at the fracture site. Tenting of the skin below the fracture might occur if the displacement is significant (that is, if one end of the fractured bone moves away from the other end).

Treatment

If a clavicle fracture is suspected on the field, keep the arm of the injured side against the body and immobilized until the athlete is evaluated by a physician. X-rays will confirm the diagnosis of a clavicle fracture. The majority of clavicle fractures are treated conservatively. Treatment includes immobilization with a figure-of-eight brace or a simple sling. Use ice and over-the-counter pain medications as needed for comfort. After three to four weeks, once healing is noted on a follow-up X-ray, the athlete may begin gentle range-of-motion exercises and eventually progress to light strengthening as pain allows. Most clavicle fractures heal uneventfully with conservative treatment. Even fractures with significant displacement heal surprisingly well. Most leave behind a visible deformity or bump at the healed fracture site.

Return to Action

Athletes may usually return to noncontact sports after six to eight weeks if the fracture shows healing on X-rays and if they have full pain-free range of motion and full strength about the shoulder. Avoid contact sports until after 12 weeks. Use donut padding over the healed fracture site for comfort and protection when returning to contact sports.

SHOULDER DISLOCATION

Common Causes

Most shoulder dislocations are caused by a forceful blow to the front of the shoulder when the arm is outstretched or overhead. Such a blow can occur during a fall to the ground, a collision with an object or another player, or during a tackle. Dislocation is common in sports such as American football, rugby, wrestling, and skiing.

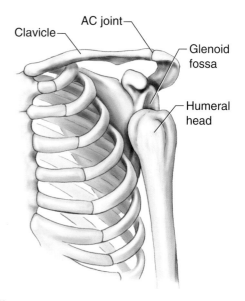

When the athlete's arm is stopped and the body continues to move forward, tremendous force is created across the shoulder joint. This force can result in the "ball" (humeral head or top of the humerus bone) slipping out of the "socket" (glenoid fossa, which is part of the scapula)—a shoulder dislocation. Athletes with a long history of participation in sports involving repetitive overhead motions or throwing, such as swimming, volleyball, or baseball, are more prone to suffering shoulder dislocations. The repetitive stretching of the shoulder capsule and ligaments that occurs over time causes the shoulder to become loose or unstable.

Identification

Following a shoulder dislocation, athletes usually complain of immediate pain with inability to move the shoulder or arm. They might report that the shoulder has "popped" out of place. A deformity might be visible, with prominence of the acromion (the upper part of the scapula that forms the roof of the shoulder, sometimes called the point of the shoulder) and a depression in the skin beneath it suggesting a dislocation.

During a shoulder dislocation, the shoulder capsule and glenohumeral ligaments, which hold the shoulder in place, are torn and stretched. There might also be detachment of the labrum (the anchor point for the shoulder capsule and ligaments) from the shoulder socket (glenoid fossa). Occasionally, other structures around the shoulder, such as the rotator cuff muscles or the surrounding nerves, are injured. Associated fractures can also occur during a shoulder dislocation, especially in older athletes. Greater tuberosity fractures have been reported to occur in up to a third of anterior shoulder dislocations. The vast majority of dislocations are anterior dislocations, in which the humeral head slips out through the front, but depending on the position of the arm at the time of trauma, the humeral head might slip from the socket through the back, producing a posterior dislocation.

SHOULDER DISLOCATION

Treatment

Initial management of an acute shoulder dislocation requires putting the shoulder back into place (placing the humeral head back into the socket), also known as a shoulder reduction. Shoulder reductions can often be done on the field (or court) by an experienced physician or athletic trainer. When the shoulder cannot be reduced on the field, the arm and shoulder must be immobilized while the athlete is transported to an emergency room, where X-rays can rule out an associated fracture and ensure that the shoulder is placed back into normal anatomic position. If you can't feel the pulse near the wrist on the side of the dislocated shoulder (and you can feel one near the other wrist), this is a medical emergency and the athlete must be transported immediately to a local emergency room.

Once the shoulder dislocation is reduced, all first-time dislocators should have their arm and shoulder immobilized in a sling or brace for three to four weeks to allow for adequate healing. A shorter period of immobilization (one to two weeks) is recommended for older athletes (over 40) to prevent joint stiffness and development of an adhesive capsulitis ("frozen shoulder"). For anterior dislocations, recent research suggests that immobilization in braces that keep the arm and shoulder rotated away from the body might lead to better healing of the shoulder structures and decrease the likelihood of future dislocations. Associated greater tuberosity fractures are usually treated conservatively with immobilization in a sling for four weeks. However, when a fracture shows significant displacement (greater than 5 mm, or .2 in.) from its normal anatomic position, surgery is usually recommended.

Following an appropriate period of immobilization, the athlete begins physical therapy to restore range of motion and strength in preparation for a return to play. Strengthening the rotator cuff muscles (supraspinatus, infrapinatus, teres minor, and subscapularis) is critically important in treating all shoulder disorders, and this is especially true for shoulder instability. These muscles are the dynamic stabilizers of the shoulder joint and help prevent recurrent dislocations by holding the humeral head in place within the socket. The muscles along the spine, the paraspinal muscles, play a role in shoulder function, and strengthening exercises geared toward these muscles—trunk rotations, sit-ups, reverse sit-ups, and so on—are also recommended.

Return to Action

Athletic arm activity should be restricted until the athlete has attained full pain-free range of motion and full strength in the muscles surrounding the shoulder. Depending on their sport, athletes may usually return to play within 8 to 12 weeks. When returning, they might wear a shoulder brace to protect the shoulder from another dislocation. Unfortunately, these braces work by restricting motion, so performance is affected.

RECURRENT SHOULDER DISLOCATION

Common Causes

Recurrent shoulder dislocations are caused by the same mechanisms as initial shoulder dislocations. However, athletes who have suffered previous dislocations might be prone to recurrent episodes with only minimal trauma.

Identification

A recurrent shoulder dislocation looks about the same as an initial dislocation, but the pain might be less severe, and in some cases athletes can reduce the shoulder back into place on their own. Many factors contribute to the risk for developing recurrent shoulder dislocations, including age, activity level, and structural abnormalities in the shoulder following an initial dislocation. A traumatic dislocation can lead to permanent stretching of the shoulder capsule and glenohumeral ligaments. There might also be permanent detachment of the glenoid labrum, which is the dense cartilage-like rim surrounding the outer edge of the shoulder socket (glenoid) that serves as the anchor point of the shoulder capsule and ligaments; this detachment is also known as a Bankart lesion. Athletes involved in repetitive overhead activities might develop stretching of shoulder capsule and ligaments over time, making the shoulder loose or unstable. These structural problems predispose an athlete to recurrent shoulder dislocations or shoulder instability.

Many studies have shown that the likelihood of recurrent dislocations is very high in young athletes, especially those involved in high-risk activities such as collision or contact sports. Researchers believe that failing to properly heal Bankart lesions, in addition to the high activity level in this population, contributes to the high incidence of recurrent dislocation. The inherent laxity or looseness of the shoulder capsule and ligaments, more common in young athletes, might also play a role.

Treatment

Initial treatment for a recurrent shoulder dislocation involves a period of relative rest, varying from a few days to four weeks, depending on the extent of the injury and the athlete's symptoms. A prolonged period of immobilization is typically not as necessary as for an acute first-time dislocation because athletes with recurring dislocations often have structural abnormalities that probably will not heal with additional immobilization.

In addition to restoring full pain-free range of motion, three options exist for managing recurrent shoulder instability. First, through diligent exercise, an athlete can try to optimize the strength and condition of the dynamic shoulder stabilizers (i.e., the rotator cuff muscles) to help prevent the shoulder from dislocating. This is especially important in "loose-jointed" athletes who have recurrent instability or dislocations not related to an initial traumatic event. These athletes have a better chance of responding to a prolonged rehabilitation and strengthening program that might take up to six months. Second, the athlete can avoid sports that carry a higher risk for dislocation (collision and contact sports). Doing so can dramatically decrease the risk of a recurrent dislocation.

RECURRENT SHOULDER DISLOCATION

However, if athletes continue to have dislocations despite conservative measures and still wish to participate in collision or contact sports, a third option is available. They can opt for surgical correction of the injured shoulder structures to prevent further dislocations. Surgery might include reattachment of the detached labrum and tightening of the shoulder capsule.

Return to Action

Following a recurrent shoulder dislocation, the athlete may return to play once he or she has attained full pain-free range of motion and full strength in the muscles surrounding the shoulder. This might take a few days to several weeks depending on the extent of the injury, the athlete's symptoms, and the sport. Prolonged immobilization is usually not necessary. As is the case for first-time dislocations, athletes might consider using special shoulder braces that prevent the arm from going overhead into a position that can lead to a dislocation. As noted previously, however, these braces might not be acceptable to the athlete. If an athlete opts for shoulder stabilization surgery, he or she will usually not return to play for about six months, depending on the sport.

Because of the risk of recurrent dislocations, especially in young athletes involved in high-risk sports, the decision to return to play should be seriously considered. Athletes who continue to suffer shoulder dislocations can do further injury to the structures of the shoulder, including the capsule, ligaments, rotator cuff, cartilage, and even nerves about the shoulder. Over time, repetitive injury to these structures can lead to persistent pain, stiffness, loss of motion, and early arthritis.

SHOULDER SUBLUXATION

Common Causes

A shoulder subluxation occurs when the humeral head slips *partially* out of the socket, but not completely out as in a shoulder dislocation. Shoulder sub-luxations are much more common in younger athletes, especially those who are loose jointed. Athletes with a long his-tory of participation in sports involving throwing or repetitive overhead motions such as baseball, softball, volleyball, water polo, or swimming are predisposed because of the repetitive stretching of the shoulder capsule and glenohumeral liga-ments that occurs over time. When the shoulder capsule and ligaments become stretched and loose, they can no longer adequately stabilize the joint, especially during overhead sports, which transmit high amounts of forces across the joint. Thus, the humeral head has a higher likelihood of slipping out of the shoulder socket. Colli-sion and contact sports such as American football, rugby, hockey, or wrestling can also lead to shoulder subluxations.

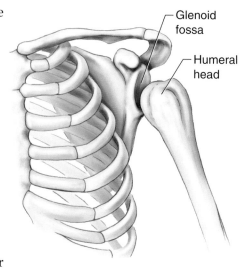

Glenoid fossa

Humeral head

Identification

Athletes with shoulder subluxations might have a variety of symptoms. Some might say their shoulder joint feels loose and briefly slips out of place during activity. Others might feel only pain during certain activities. Some have a transient numbness or tingling sensation down the arm ("dead arm syndrome"). Some develop symptoms following an initial traumatic event, but many develop symptoms gradually without any trauma.

Whereas some athletes might have mild instability and subluxations with only minimal or no pain, other athletes can develop pain that inhibits them from playing. Pain results from the repetitive subluxation that leads to irritation and inflamma-tion of the shoulder structures, including the capsule, labrum, bursa, and rotator cuff tendons. As the humeral head slips out of the glenoid, the shoulder structures (especially the bursa and rotator cuff tendons) can get impinged underneath the roof of the shoulder (the acromion), leading to further inflammation and pain.

Treatment

In cases of an acute first-time shoulder subluxation caused by a traumatic event, immobilization in a sling or brace for up to four weeks might be necessary to allow healing of the injured shoulder structures (shoulder capsule and ligaments). In non-traumatic cases related to repetitive overhead activities or throwing, immobilization is usually not required. In these cases, the athlete should rest and avoid throwing and overhead activities until pain and inflammation subside. Icing, anti-inflammatory medications, and physical therapy can help reduce pain and inflammation and restore full pain-free range of motion.

The next step in managing the injury is a structured rehabilitation program that focuses on correcting muscle imbalances and strengthening the dynamic shoulder stabilizing muscles, specifically the rotator cuff muscles. Optimizing the strength of these muscles can stabilize the joint by helping to hold the humeral head within the glenoid, thus compensating for the loose, stretched shoulder capsule and ligaments commonly found in athletes with subluxations. Many athletes develop muscle imbalances about the shoulder because of repetitive stresses placed across the joint, which allow certain areas to get overly stretched or strong while other areas get tight or weak. Correcting these imbalances can lead to better stabilization across the shoulder joint and decrease the risk of recurrent subluxations. A structured rehabilitation program, which may last up to six months, is often successful in athletes with subluxations, especially those not related to trauma.

Along with focusing on strengthening the shoulder, technique should also be addressed (see Return to Action below), as should the condition of other areas of the body that might affect the stress and forces transmitted through the shoulder. By correcting technique and correcting deficiencies in other areas of the body used in the sport, the athlete might be able to reduce undue stress across the shoulder.

Athletes who continue to suffer from recurrent shoulder subluxation despite extensive conservative management might need to consider giving up their sport or consider surgery to tighten the ligaments of the shoulder capsule.

Return to Action

Time required before returning to play varies from a few days up to several weeks, depending on the athlete's symptoms, the extent of injury, and the sport. Because acute first-time shoulder subluxations caused by trauma are usually treated with a period of immobilization followed by gradual range of motion and strengthening exercises, it might take 6 to 12 weeks to return to action.

However, athletes who have recurrent nontraumatic subluxations might be able to gradually return to sport sooner once they have attained full pain-free range of motion and full strength in the muscles surrounding the shoulder. Athletes should stop participating if symptoms recur. In some cases, they will need to modify their participation to prevent recurrence of symptoms. For example, a swimmer might eliminate certain strokes or events, a pitcher might limit the number of pitches thrown, and a volleyball player might move to the back line to avoid the repetitive overhead motion. Athletes might also benefit from modifying technique once they return to play. For example, a baseball pitcher obtains much of the power in his throw from his hips and trunk. If he loses power in his throw because of deficiencies in his technique or an underreliance on his hips and trunk, he might try to compensate by overloading the shoulder. Improving technique and throwing mechanics can help reduce undue stress across the shoulder joint.

LABRAL INJURY

Common Causes

The glenoid labrum is the dense cartilage-like rim that surrounds the shoulder socket (glenoid) and serves as the anchor point for the shoulder capsule and ligaments that help stabilize the shoulder. Injuries to the labrum are common in sports in which the athlete sustains shoulder subluxations and dislocations, such as collision or contact sports (American football or rugby), throwing sports (baseball or softball), sports involving repetitive overhead motions (swimming or volleyball), or sports in which athletes might fall to the ground onto the shoulder or arm. A traction-type injury to the shoulder and arm, such as can occur when holding the rope while water skiing, can also produce an injury to the labrum.

When the humeral head slips partially or completely out of the glenoid, a tearing or detaching of the labrum can result. The long head of the biceps tendon attaches to the superior part of the labrum, and repetitive traction to this area from the throwing motion can cause a strain or detachment of the superior labrum, also known as a SLAP (superior labrum, anterior to posterior) lesion. Detachment of the anterior–inferior portion of the labrum is known as a Bankart lesion and commonly occurs after an anterior shoulder dislocation.

Identification

Athletes with labral injuries or tears might complain of deep, ill-defined shoulder pain with an associated painful clicking, popping, or catching sensation. Some might have symptoms that start after an initial traumatic event, but many symptoms occur gradually and might be chronic by the time the athlete seeks professional advice. Pain might be reproduced with the throwing motion or when reaching overhead, which can make a labral tear difficult to distinguish from shoulder impingement symptoms. Many times the diagnosis of a labral tear is made by MRI or during surgery. The symptoms from a labral tear are usually caused by the labrum getting caught in the glenohumeral joint during motion. In addition to pain, the athlete might have recurrent subluxations or dislocations caused by more significant labral injuries, such as a Bankart lesion that has not healed.

Treatment

The management of labral injuries caused by shoulder dislocations, recurrent dislocations, or subluxations follows the same guidelines as prescribed for those injuries (see pp. 80-85). Because pain from a labral injury can be difficult to distinguish from the pain of shoulder impingement, treatment for a possible underlying shoulder impingement should also be considered, including a trial of physical therapy and a possible cortisone injection. An athlete with persistent pain or instability symptoms related to a labral injury or detachment that has been unresponsive to conservative treatment might consider surgery. If a labral tear has not healed initially, it is unlikely to heal over time. If the athlete is unable to live with the symptoms, surgical debridement or repair of the torn labrum should be considered.

LABRAL INJURY

Return to Action

For labral injuries resulting from shoulder dislocations, recurrent shoulder dislocations, or shoulder subluxations, see the return-to-action guidelines for these injuries on pages 80-85. For painful labral injuries treated conservatively, gradual return to sports may be initiated once the athlete has attained full pain-free range of motion and full strength about the injured shoulder. Depending on the severity of the strain, degree of symptoms, and the sport, a full return might take anywhere from a few days to several weeks. Taping or bracing is usually not helpful for painful labral injuries. Participation in sport might need to be modified to avoid painful motions. For example, a tennis player might avoid a painful overhead serve, or a weightlifter might steer clear of certain exercises at the gym. If a labral tear is continually aggravated or stressed through participation in sports or activities, the injury could become worse, resulting in more painful symptoms.

ACROMIOCLAVICULAR JOINT INJURY

Common Causes

Acromioclavicular (AC) joint injuries are common in contact or collision sports such as American football, rugby, hockey, or lacrosse. The injury typically occurs during a fall directly onto the acromion, or the point of the shoulder. It can also occur when an athlete sustains a direct blow on top of the shoulder when trying to tackle or hit another player.

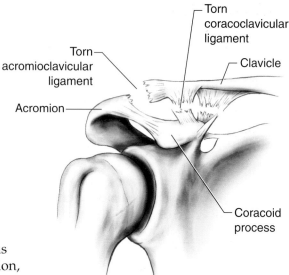

Torn acromioclavicular ligament

Torn coracoclavicular ligament

Clavicle

Acromion

Coracoid process

Identification

An AC joint injury is also known as an AC joint sprain, AC joint separation, or shoulder separation. This type of injury involves a disruption to the joint formed between the end of the clavicle (collar bone) and the acromion. Athletes with this injury usually have pain and swelling directly over the AC joint and difficulty raising the arm overhead. An obvious deformity might also be present caused by the separation of the acromion and clavicle. This separation is known as a "step-off deformity."

After AC joint separations, a deformity with a bump at the AC joint often persists even after healing. This deformity is usually cosmetic with no related pain or symptoms. In rare cases when the athlete has persistent pain and symptoms following an AC joint separation, surgery might be an option. Athletes who have recurring injuries to the AC joint might develop early arthritis in the joint.

Treatment

Most AC joint injuries are treated conservatively. When a step-off deformity is present, X-rays can assess the degree of separation and rule out an underlying collar bone fracture. Only injuries with significant separation or displacement of the clavicle from the acromion might require surgery. Ice and anti-inflammatory medications can help reduce pain and inflammation. Short-term immobilization in a sling can be used for comfort, followed by gentle range-of-motion exercises as pain allows.

Return to Action

Following mild sprains of the AC joint without any deformity or separation, athletes can usually return to sports quickly. Depending on the degree of pain, return to play may be immediate or take up to one to two weeks. The athlete should have full pain-free range of motion and full strength in the muscles surrounding the shoulder before attempting a return. Following more significant injuries with obvious deformity and separation, athletes should usually avoid contact sports for a minimum of three weeks to allow for healing of the injured ligaments. Use foam padding or a donut cushion over the AC joint for extra protection and comfort when returning to contact sports.

ROTATOR CUFF TEAR

Common Causes

Rotator cuff tears usually occur in athletes over 40 who have a long history of involvement in repetitive overhead sports such as swimming, surfing, volleyball, or throwing sports. A fall or a direct blow to the shoulder during any sport can cause acute tearing or straining of the rotator cuff in such athletes. Several factors are thought to contribute to the development of rotator cuff tears. Many believe they result from repeated episodes of impingement (see p. 90). Over time, repeated inflammation and irritation of the rotator cuff can cause the cuff to tear. Other factors possibly contributing to tearing include repetitive microtrauma and overuse, degeneration of the cuff from aging, poor circulation to the rotator cuff tendon, and acute injury superimposed on chronic cuff degeneration. Rotator cuff tears typically occur in the outer aspect of the tendon near its attachment to the humerus. The supraspinatus tendon of the rotator cuff is the tendon most commonly torn.

Identification

Rotator cuff tear symptoms are similar to symptoms of impingement, rotator cuff tendinitis, or bursitis. Athletes have pain in the front or side of the shoulder that is aggravated by reaching or overhead activities. With smaller tears, weakness might not be apparent. With larger tears, weakness can be prominent. With massive tears, the athlete might be unable to hold the arm up at the side. Athletes with rotator cuff tears are typically over age 40 and might have a past history of recurrent episodes of rotator cuff tendinitis or bursitis. Pain might start suddenly after a precipitating event or occur gradually with no obvious cause. Severity of pain varies from minimal to severe. Studies show that some people may have no symptoms whatsoever.

Treatment

Treat most athletes with rotator cuff tears conservatively. Treatment varies depending on the athlete's age, level of function, size of the tear, weakness, and pain. Larger tears in younger athletes who are very active might require early surgery. Conservative treatment is identical to the treatment of athletes with shoulder impingement, rotator cuff tendinitis, and bursitis: relative rest, reducing pain and inflammation, restoring full pain-free range of motion, and progressing the athlete to a strengthening program for the rotator cuff and surrounding shoulder muscles.

If symptoms persist after conservative treatment, surgery might be necessary. MRI will usually show the location and extent of the tear. Surgery might include repair of the torn rotator cuff tendon and a subacromial decompression to shave off arthritic bone and spurs to allow more room for the rotator cuff to travel.

Return to Action

After treatment, athletes may gradually return to their sport once they have full pain-free range of motion and full strength in the injured shoulder. Return time depends on the size of the tear, the athlete's symptoms, degree of weakness, and the sport. A full return often takes up to three months. If symptoms recur, stop participation. Taping or bracing is usually unnecessary on return. Athletes might need to adjust their participation or technique to avoid recurring symptoms. Athletes who undergo surgical repair of a torn rotator cuff usually cannot return for at least six months.

SHOULDER IMPINGEMENT

Common Causes

Shoulder impingement is common in sports that involve repetitive overhead motions or throwing, such as swimming, surfing, baseball, softball, water polo, and volleyball. During normal shoulder motion, the rotator cuff and subacromial bursa travel smoothly beneath the acromion in the subacromial space (the space between the acromion and humeral head). Additionally, the subacromial bursa, a small fluid-filled sac, helps the rotator cuff travel smoothly beneath the acromion and AC joint. In shoulder impingement, however, the rotator cuff and bursa get pinched or impinged underneath the acromion during overhead activities, resulting in pain.

Several factors can contribute to shoulder impingement. Structural or anatomic abnormalities might result in a narrower subacromial space. For example, some people are born with a curved or hook-shaped acromion that narrows the subacromial space. With aging, development of AC joint arthritis and bony spurs underneath the acromion can also narrow

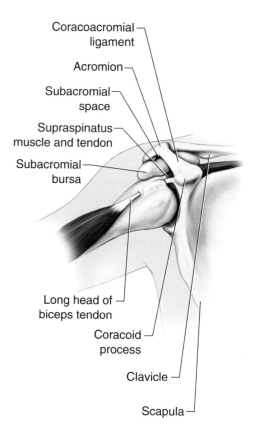

Coracoacromial ligament

Acromion

Subacromial space

Supraspinatus muscle and tendon

Subacromial bursa

Long head of biceps tendon

Coracoid process

Clavicle

Scapula

the subacromial space. The less room there is for the rotator cuff and bursa to travel, the more likely it is that these structures get pinched during shoulder motion.

A second factor is inflammation. Overuse or repetitive irritation of the rotator cuff underneath the acromion can lead to inflammation and swelling of the rotator cuff tendons and overlying bursa (tendinitis and bursitis). Not only are the inflamed tendons and bursa painful, but pain is aggravated when these inflamed and swollen structures get pinched or impinged underneath the acromion during overhead motions.

A third factor is shoulder instability, especially in young athletes. If the structures of the shoulder are ineffective in stabilizing the humeral head within the socket (glenoid fossa) during overhead motions, the humeral head might migrate upward out of the socket, causing impingement. Underlying shoulder instability is likely a primary cause of impingement symptoms in young athletes.

Identification

Shoulder impingement is an extremely common condition that affects athletes of all ages. Athletes typically experience gradual pain in the front or side of the shoulder that is aggravated by reaching or overhead activities. Sometimes the pain radiates down into the upper arm. They might have decreased range of motion and subjective weakness with difficulty raising the arm overhead or behind the back. Night pain and difficulty sleeping on the affected shoulder are also common.

Repeated impingement usually leads to rotator cuff tendinitis (inflammation of the rotator cuff tendons) and bursitis (inflammation of the subacromial bursa that overlies the rotator cuff). Again, these two conditions can aggravate the impingement symptoms.

Treatment

Athletes can begin treating shoulder impingement at home. They should avoid repetitive overhead activities and other aggravating activities until pain and inflammation subside. Anti-inflammatory medications (e.g., ibuprofen) and ice might also be helpful in reducing pain and inflammation. Early in treatment, athletes should begin range-of-motion exercises to help restore normal pain-free motion; progress exercise as pain allows.

If symptoms persist despite initial treatment, formal physical therapy might be needed to assist in decreasing inflammation and pain through electrical stimulation, ultrasound, or other modalities. A cortisone injection into the subacromial bursa can be a quick, effective way to reduce pain and inflammation. Eventually, all athletes should begin a shoulder-strengthening program with particular attention to the rotator cuff muscles. This is especially important for younger athletes, in whom impingement symptoms usually involve underlying instability.

Athletes who continue to have disabling symptoms may require surgery to correct underlying structural or anatomic abnormalities causing the impingement. In older athletes, this might involve a subacromial decompression in which arthritic bone and spurs are shaved off the acromion to allow more room for the rotator cuff to travel. In younger athletes, shoulder stabilization surgery might be required to prevent impingement related to underlying instability. If shoulder impingement continues over time, the repeated inflammation and irritation of the rotator cuff might eventually cause the cuff to wear down, degenerate, and tear.

Return to Action

Most athletes improve with conservative treatment and gradually return to sport after attaining full pain-free range of motion and full strength in the muscles surrounding the affected shoulder. Return time varies from a few weeks to a few months, depending on the degree of symptoms, extent of injury, and the sport. Taping or bracing is usually not necessary when returning to play. If symptoms recur, the athlete should stop the sport or painful activity until the sport or activity is no longer painful.

To prevent recurrence of symptoms, athletes might need to limit or avoid certain movements in their sport. They might also benefit from modifying their technique. For example, a thrower might choose to throw sidearm instead of overhead, which might prevent the rotator cuff and bursa from getting impinged underneath the acromion.

BICEPS TENDON RUPTURE

Common Causes

The biceps muscle has two proximal tendons and one distal tendon. By far the most common tendon to be ruptured is the proximal long head of the biceps tendon. This tendon travels up and around the humeral head, through the shoulder joint, and underneath the acromion to attach onto the top of the glenoid (shoulder socket). Rupture of this tendon tends to occur in athletes over 40. It is more common in athletes with a prior history of shoulder impingement or bicipital tendinitis (see pp. 90 and 94) who are involved in repetitive overhead sports such as swimming, surfing, and volleyball or in throwing sports. Ruptures of the proximal biceps tendon usually occur because of a weakening and degeneration of the tendon over time. Because of its location beneath the acromion (roof of the shoulder), this tendon is predisposed to getting pinched during overhead activities, similar to the rotator cuff. Over time, the tendon can get frayed and weak and might eventually tear or rupture.

A biceps tendon can also rupture at its more distal attachment onto the radial tuberosity on the radius of the forearm. But a rupture at this location is far less common than a proximal rupture. Distal biceps tendon ruptures tend to occur in middle-aged weekend warrior athletes who are lifting heavy weights.

Short head of biceps tendon

Rupture of proximal biceps tendon

Long head of biceps tendon

Rupture of distal biceps tendon

Identification

Typically, athletes with a proximal biceps tendon rupture describe a sudden pain in the shoulder often accompanied by an audible snap or tearing sensation. Within a few days, bruising develops in the biceps area, and a bulge in the lower biceps is readily apparent. This bulge is accentuated when flexing the biceps muscle (think of Popeye after eating some spinach). The bulge occurs because the torn biceps tendon and muscle get bunched up into the lower aspect of the upper arm. Sometimes when a proximal biceps tendon rupture occurs acutely, very little pain results, and the injury might even go undetected. Because the other proximal biceps tendon remains attached to the coracoid process in the shoulder, significant weakness is rarely a complaint.

Athletes with a distal biceps tendon rupture might describe a sudden pain in their distal arm and over their elbow. They often say the injury occurred while they were trying to lift a heavy load; they might mention hearing or feeling a snap or pop in their arm. They might also note swelling and bruising at the elbow. Unlike a proximal tendon rupture, a distal rupture is likely to result in arm weakness.

BICEPS TENDON RUPTURE

Treatment

For most proximal biceps tendon ruptures, treatment is conservative. Because of the intact remaining proximal biceps tendon, and because other muscles assist in flexing the elbow, little loss of function or strength occurs. The cosmetic deformity (loss of the normal biceps muscle contour and the bulge in the lower biceps area) is usually acceptable to most athletes. As needed, over-the-counter anti-inflammatory medications and ice may be used for pain. Range-of-motion exercises followed by gradual strengthening exercises for the shoulder and upper arm may be done as tolerated. Surgical repair of the torn tendon might be considered in younger athletes with high activity levels. Any surgery should be done within a few weeks to prevent retraction of the tendon, making the repair more difficult.

Distal tendon ruptures cause functional impairment. A full-thickness distal tendon biceps rupture almost invariably leads to significant weakness. In active people and athletes wishing to return to sport, surgical repair of the tendon is usually required. If the rupture is incomplete, or if the patient is older and does not need to be physically active, conservative care, including rest, ice, and immobilization, followed by structured physical therapy, is an alternative to surgery.

Return to Action

If treated conservatively, a proximal biceps tendon rupture might allow a return to play within four to six weeks. Before considering a return, athletes should have full pain-free range of motion and close to full strength about the injured shoulder. Taping and bracing is usually not necessary. After a surgically repaired proximal biceps tendon rupture, a return takes at least three to six months.

A full-thickness distal biceps tendon rupture, when treated conservatively, makes a return to sport unlikely. If treated surgically, a return can take up to six months. Following surgery, the elbow is typically immobilized for one to two months, followed by two to three months of physical therapy. The athlete should have full pain-free range of motion and close to full strength with elbow flexion and supination before attempting a return to sport.

BICIPITAL TENDINITIS

Common Causes

Bicipital tendinitis (also called biceps tendinitis) is an inflammation of the long head of the biceps tendon as it passes up through the bicipital groove of the humerus (upper-arm bone). Because of its location, the tendon is prone to irritation and inflammation by the same mechanisms that cause shoulder impingement. During overhead motions, the biceps tendon can get pinched or impinged between the humeral head and the acromion, leading

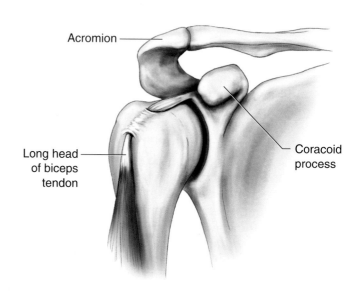

to inflammation and pain. This injury is common in sports that involve repetitive overhead motions or throwing, such as swimming, surfing, baseball, softball, water polo, and volleyball. Although most cases of bicipital tendinitis are related to impingement, the inflammation might occasionally be related to primary overuse from repetitive stress placed on the tendon caused by repetitive throwing, overhead hitting, racket sports, or doing arm curls with weights using improper technique.

Identification

Athletes with bicipital tendinitis typically complain of gradual pain over the front of the shoulder that might radiate down the biceps muscle. They mention pain with overhead activities and throwing, and they might have pain at night. Activities that stress the biceps tendon might be painful, such as biceps muscle contraction when doing arm curls, lifting objects in front of the body with a straight arm, or turning a door knob or screw driver in a way that the palm faces up (supination). Because bicipital tendinitis most commonly occurs with shoulder impingement, it is common in athletes over 40. However, younger athletes who perform repetitive motions such as throwing can also develop bicipital tendinitis.

Treatment

Initial treatment includes relative rest and avoiding activities or motions that elicit pain. Use icing and anti-inflammatory medications (e.g., ibuprofin) to reduce pain and inflammation. Range-of-motion exercises should be started early in the treatment course and progressed as tolerated to restore normal pain-free range of motion. Formal physical therapy may be considered to assist in reducing pain and inflammation through the use of electrical stimulation, ultrasound, or other methods. In refractory cases, a steroid injection (cortisone shot) into the biceps tendon sheath may be considered to eliminate persistent pain and inflammation.

BICIPITAL TENDINITIS

Once pain and inflammation subside, begin strengthening exercises to restore full strength about the shoulder with particular attention to the rotator cuff muscles. This is especially important for younger athletes, who might have impingement and irritation of the bicipital tendon caused by underlying instability.

If the athlete continues to have disabling symptoms despite conservative measures, surgery may be considered. For older athletes, surgery may involve a biceps tenodesis, in which the tendon is transferred to the upper humerus to relieve the repetitive mechanical irritation. A subacromial decompression may also be performed in which arthritic bone and spurs are shaved off the acromion to address the impingement anatomy. In younger athletes, a shoulder-stabilization surgery could be required to prevent impingement and irritation of the biceps tendon that might be related to underlying instability. If bicipital tendinitis continues over time, the repeated inflammation and irritation of the tendon might eventually cause it to wear down, degenerate, and tear (proximal biceps tendon rupture).

Return to Action

In general, athletes may gradually return to sport once they have attained full pain-free range of motion and full strength in the muscles surrounding the affected shoulder. Return time might vary from a few weeks up to a few months depending on the degree of symptoms, extent of injury, and the sport. Taping or bracing is usually not necessary when returning to play. If symptoms recur, athletes should stop the sport or painful activity. They might need to modify their sport participation to prevent recurrence of symptoms.

SUPRASCAPULAR NERVE INJURY

Common Causes

Suprascapular nerve injury, also known as suprascapular neuropathy, suprascapular nerve entrapment, or suprascapular nerve palsy, is a relatively less common cause of shoulder pain in athletes. The injury tends to occur most often in volleyball players or overhead throwing athletes. The suprascapular nerve might be damaged because of a traction or stretch injury to the nerve caused by the repetitive overhead or throwing motion. The nerve might also be damaged because of compression by a ganglion cyst. Tears of the glenoid labrum are sometimes associated with formation of ganglion cysts that can compress the suprascapular nerve. Sometimes a direct trauma or fracture to the scapula can cause an injury to the suprascapular nerve.

Identification

An athlete with a suprascapular nerve injury typically complains of shoulder pain that is deep and poorly localized but often felt more in the back or side of the shoulder. The athlete might describe a feeling of weakness. Eventually, athletes might have wasting (atrophy) of the supraspinatus and infraspinatus muscles, which are the rotator cuff muscles behind the shoulder blade (scapula) that are innervated by the suprascapular nerve. The suprascapular nerve can be damaged at a few points along its course to innervate the supraspinatus and infraspinatus muscles. Depending on where the nerve is damaged, it can affect one or both of these muscles.

With weakening of the rotator cuff muscles, some athletes might develop instability and secondary impingement pain because these muscles can no longer hold the humeral head in its socket (glenoid). In many cases, the athlete might continue to play and function despite the injury and without seeking medical attention. The weakness might be detected incidentally on a preseason physical exam, or sometimes a family member or friend will notice the athlete's muscle wasting with prominence of the shoulder blade, prompting a visit to the doctor.

The diagnosis of a suprascapular neuropathy is usually made by a physician or other medical professional. Strength testing reveals weakness with shoulder abduction or external rotation. An electromyograph (EMG)/nerve conduction study (test of the muscles and nerves) is usually ordered to confirm the diagnosis and determine the extent of nerve injury. An MRI of the shoulder can help to identify a ganglion cyst compressing the suprascapular nerve.

Treatment

Treatment for suprascapular neuropathies depends on the cause of the nerve injury. If an obvious ganglion cyst has formed or another lesion is compressing the nerve, surgery might be necessary to remove the compressive lesion and relieve pressure on the nerve. If the injury is caused by a traction or stretch injury from repetitive throwing or overhead activities, athletes must rest and avoid these activities. Over-the-counter anti-inflammatory or pain medications may be used as needed. Strengthening exercises (especially shoulder abduction and external rotation) are performed to strengthen the weak rotator cuff muscles as well as the surrounding shoulder muscles. In cases in which the athlete fails to improve within three to six months of conservative treatment, surgical exploration may be considered. In severe cases, the athlete might be left with some chronic wasting (atrophy) and mild weakness of the affected muscles.

Return to Action

Return time ranges anywhere from six weeks to several months, depending on the severity of the nerve injury. In general, once the athlete's pain resolves and strength improves to approximately 80 percent of normal, the athlete can initiate gradual return to play. The athlete should be monitored for any recurrence of weakness and should stop play if weakness or pain recur. Taping and bracing is usually not necessary when returning to play. In some cases, if weakness and symptoms fail to improve, the athlete might need to consider modifying or changing sport participation to avoid the repetitive overhead motion.

DEEP VEIN THROMBOSIS

Common Causes

Damage to the blood vessels in the arm (as in other parts of the body) may trigger the formation of thrombi (clots) in the blood vessels. When these thrombi form in the deep veins, the condition is known as deep vein thrombosis (DVT). There is a risk that the thrombi will break away from the vessel wall and travel to the lungs or brain, causing serious injury and, in rare cases, death.

Identification

When an athlete develops vague shoulder or neck discomfort, swelling of the limb, and possibly a low grade fever, DVT must be considered. If this condition is suspected, the athlete must be referred to a physician immediately.

Treatment

Depending on the underlying cause, DVTs are generally treated for at least three to six months with anticoagulation therapy. Often, the athlete with a DVT will initially receive an anticoagulating medicine such as heparin, which is given via an IV, or low-molecular-weight (LMW) heparin, which is given subcutaneously once or twice daily. He or she is then transferred over to warfarin (Coumadin), which is given orally. It is important that the athlete's blood be monitored while he or she is taking warfarin because the levels of this medication in the blood may fluctuate and dosages may need to be adjusted. Until adequate anticoagulation is reached (typically in three to seven days), the patient should not use the affected extremity.

Return to Action

Athletes should not return to *contact* sports until they are finished with anticoagulant therapy. During therapy, there is a significant risk of bleeding from contact. Athletes may return to *noncontact* sports (e.g., running) once their blood is fully anticoagulated (typically within three to seven days of treatment initiation) and they have pain-free range of motion. Until adequate anticoagulation is reached, the affected extremity should not be used to reduce the risk of dislodging the clot and sending it to the lung or brain.

Robert S. Gotlin, DO, and Grant Cooper, MD, contributed this injury text.

CHAPTER 7

Arm and Elbow Injuries

Andrew L. Sherman, MD, MS

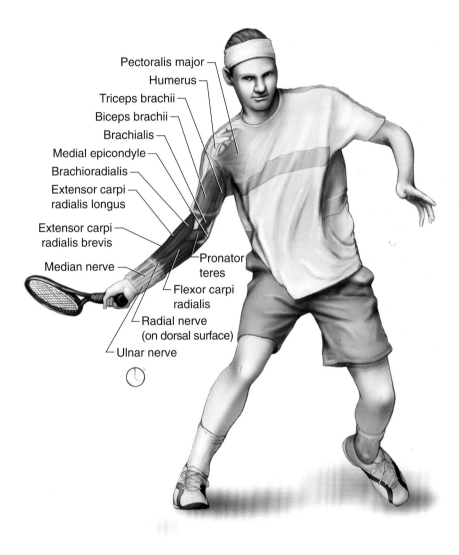

Pectoralis major

Humerus

Triceps brachii

Biceps brachii

Brachialis

Medial epicondyle

Brachioradialis

Extensor carpi radialis longus

Extensor carpi radialis brevis

Median nerve

Pronator teres

Flexor carpi radialis

Radial nerve (on dorsal surface)

Ulnar nerve

Elbow injuries in young throwing athletes are surprisingly common and most often caused by repetitive stress on an immature skeleton. The overhand throwing motion of most baseball pitchers exposes the medial, lateral, and posterior elbow to forces of tension, compression, shear, and torsion. One recent survey of 172 pitchers found an injury incidence of 40 percent in 9- to 14-year-old pitchers who were followed for one full year. Additional sports that expose the elbow to repetitive strain and injuries include golf, tennis, squash, racquetball, and volleyball. Certain sports, such as American football, skiing, hockey, and soccer, are associated with traumatic arm and elbow injuries such as fractures and dislocations. Although most traumatic and nontraumatic arm and elbow injuries are minor and respond well to a short period of rest and rehabilitation, some of these injuries progress over time, threaten the growth plate, and can lead to permanent loss of function and lost future athletic opportunities.

Arm and Elbow Injuries

TENNIS ELBOW

Common Causes

Tennis elbow is a common sports malady that affects more than just tennis pros and weekend tennis warriors. Tennis elbow, or lateral epicondylitis, occurs as a result of repetitive twisting and torquing of the forearm and elbow from activities such as tennis, golf, baseball throwing, racquetball, bowling, and squash. Laborers such as carpenters are also often afflicted with tennis elbow.

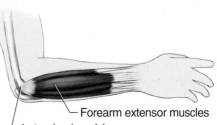

Forearm extensor muscles
Lateral epicondyle

Tennis elbow occurs in female athletes more often than male athletes by a 2 to 1 margin. The injury is common in athletes between the ages of 30 and 49 years but also occurs in younger or older athletes. Tennis elbow is caused by an overuse of the extensor or supinator muscles of the forearm and wrist (the muscles that turn the palm upward and that straighten the elbow). Many activities can cause tennis elbow, but it is the backhand motion of the tennis swing that has the most direct impact on tennis players and gives the condition its name.

Certain risk factors make getting tennis elbow more likely. Studies find the incidence of tennis elbow increases in athletes over 40 who play more than two hours per week of tennis. Improper equipment might also be a culprit. A racket grip that is too small or too large can cause poor mechanics that lead to tennis elbow. A wet and heavy ball, a racket that is strung too tight, or a stiff racket head can increase stress on the elbow. Finally, athletes who are improperly conditioned are at higher risk for injury because their muscles are not strong or limber enough to handle the stress of competition.

Identification

Athletes who develop tennis elbow often complain of pinpoint, knifelike pain over the (outer) lateral surface of the elbow. The pain is felt most during wrist extension (when the wrist is in a position used for a push-up) and forearm supination (when the palm is facing upward)—motions used in the tennis backhand. A physical exam will often confirm the pinpoint tenderness and even swelling on the outside of the elbow. The pain can be reproduced by forcibly resisting wrist or finger extension. X-rays and MRI usually show no abnormalities, though they might reveal a bone spur or calcium deposit outside the lateral elbow joint. If the condition is significant, MRI may reveal a partial or complete tear of the muscles involved, most commonly the extensor carpi radialis brevis (ECRB). If the athlete complains of pain radiating down the forearm, this pain must be distinguished from nerve entrapment and radial nerve pain (see radial tunnel syndrome on p. 106).

Treatment

Treatment of tennis elbow is typically nonsurgical. About 95 percent of athletes who develop this injury should achieve excellent functional recovery with conservative treatment. Tennis elbow can be separated into three distinct categories in terms of

(continued)

healing. The most benign cases of tennis elbow behave much like any typical sprain or strain. Relative rest, refraining from sports participation, and over the counter medications are all that's needed in this scenario. In approximately three to six weeks, the condition resolves and the athlete returns to his or her preinjury state.

Injuries in the second category can take three to six months to heal. Treatments here include those previously noted as well as physical therapy, counterforce bracing, cortisone injections, prolotherapy, and extracorporal shock wave therapy. Counterforce braces reduce the muscle tension on the elbow. A tennis elbow brace is a thin strap with an air bubble centered on one area of the strap. The air bubble is placed directly over the muscles just below the elbow to gently compress the area. A wrist splint can also be used to reduce the motion at the wrist so there is less pull on the muscles at the elbow. Cortisone injections may reduce local inflammation, allowing the body's natural healing process to take over. In prolotherapy, a controversial but increasingly popular treatment for tennis elbow, a mixture of dextrose and normal saline is injected repeatedly into ligaments of the lateral elbow to stimulate healing. Physicians who advocate this procedure report promising results when it is used as an alternative treatment after traditional treatment fails. Extracorporal shock wave therapy, another controversial treatment option, uses sound waves to induce so-called microtrauma to tissues. Some researchers believe that microtrauma initiates a healing response and helps decrease inflammation, but study results have been mixed.

Injuries in the third category fail to respond to the treatments mentioned previously. Typically MRI reveals an abnormality. In this scenario, surgery is a consideration. Surgery is considered only after six to nine months of failed conservative management. Surgeons can remove a portion of the damaged tendon or release the attachment of the affected tendon. Postoperatively, the athlete usually wears a 90-degree elbow brace. Early motion in a brace may start after three to five days, and strengthening exercises may begin within three weeks. About 85 percent of people who fail conservative treatment and undergo the surgery report some degree of pain relief.

Return to Action

When full pain-free range of motion is achieved, the athlete may begin strengthening. Initial strengthening should focus on the muscles that can stabilize the upper body and reduce strain on the elbow. For example, strengthening the latissimus dorsi (the muscle covering the lumbar region of the back), shoulder rotators, and upper-back muscles helps create a more balanced upper body, which can support the weight of the racket better, thereby reducing stress on the lateral elbow. As the athlete's condition improves, the wrist and forearm may be strengthened. Finally, sport- or activity-specific training can be implemented to complete the rehabilitation.

Only when the athlete has pain-free range of motion in the elbow, has normal wrist extensor strength, and can apply this strength to a normal swing can he or she return to competitive tennis play. If the athlete has had surgery, a return to tennis or other racket sports can be expected after four to six months. As in the case of other musculoskeletal injuries, athletes who have been treated for tennis elbow should return to play only after normal strength, endurance, and flexibility are restored.

TENNIS ELBOW

Those who return too early risk reinjury and an inability to play the sport at a high level. Athletes who are not adequately recovered might compensate for continued pain in the elbow by putting too much stress on another part of the body, such as the shoulder or lumbar spine, causing an injury there.

Because tennis elbow does not usually result in fractures or permanent disability, some recreational athletes may gradually return to play at below full physical capacity. Taking steps to change swing technique, training habits, and equipment or wearing an elbow counterforce brace can speed up a return to competitive or recreational sports.

To maintain a healthy wrist, tennis players must make sure their racket grip is the proper size for their hand. Correct grip size can be obtained by measuring the distance from the bottom lateral crease in the palm to the tip of the ring finger (figure 7.1). If your hand measures between grip sizes, use the smaller size and add an overgrip or heat-shrink sleeve to attain the right size. For an Eastern forehand grip (in which the palm is placed against the same bevel as the string face), you should be able to fit the index finger of the nonhitting hand in the space between the ring finger and palm.

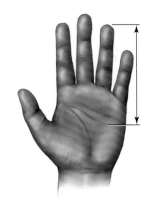

Figure 7.1 Grip measurement.

Common Causes

Similar to tennis elbow, golfer's elbow (or medial epicondylitis) occurs as a result of overuse stress placed on the musculotendinous junction of the inner aspect of the elbow. Golfer's elbow is seen most commonly in males 20 to 49 years of age. The injury also occurs frequently in tennis players, weightlifters, and baseball pitchers who throw too many breaking balls. The most common cause of golfer's elbow is repetitive stress on the tendons that originate on the medial epicondyle (inside of the elbow). The pain originates in the forearm tendons where they attach to the elbow. In the acute form (occurring suddenly), a true tendinitis with inflammation of the tendon can occur. In the chronic form (occurring over time), a failure to fully heal microtears of the tendon leads to tendinosis with chronic pain and dysfunction.

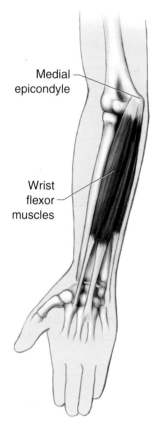

Medial epicondyle

Wrist flexor muscles

Similar to tennis elbow, golfer's elbow can progress due to poor swing mechanics and equipment issues. The medial elbow pain occurs most commonly in the trailing, or dominant elbow. Too strong a grip can cause increased stress on the wrist flexor muscles, increasing stress on the tendon at the elbow. Many clinicians believe that smaller golf club grips elicit the greater wrist tension that causes golfer's elbow. Finally, an incorrect plane in the backswing and downswing might cause abnormal stress on the elbows and wrists.

Identification

The athlete who develops golfer's elbow most often complains of pain along the inner side of the elbow. The pain is worse with wrist flexion (palm bent back as when you wave to someone) and pronation (the motion used to turn a dial counterclockwise). Some athletes also complain of tingling or numbness in the fourth or fifth fingers. This suggests either irritation or entrapment of the ulnar nerve (the forearm nerve that supplies the fourth and fifth digits of the hand) as it travels through the ulnar groove in the elbow. This injury, called cubital tunnel syndrome (see p. 116), must be suspected when an athlete's hand or grip strength has decreased to the point that he or she is dropping the ball or even simple household objects. You may know the affected area as the "funny bone." When you inadvertently strike this area, you feel the sensation of electricity traveling down the arm.

You can reproduce the pain of golfer's elbow by touching the inside of the elbow or the bony protuberance just below the inner elbow. The range of motion of the elbow is usually normal, and discoloration or swelling in the joint is unusual.

Golfer's elbow tends not to show up on X-rays or MRI. An X-ray might rule out any loose bodies or bone spurs. MRI scanning can investigate the condition of the ligaments, particularly the ulnar collateral ligament, for tearing or inflammation. In the case of neurological abnormalities, a nerve condition velocity study (NCV) and needle EMG study might be done to investigate the function of the ulnar nerve as it courses through the elbow and wrist.

Treatment

Initial treatment of acute golfer's elbow focuses on the PRICE principles (protection, rest, ice, compression, elevation) or on relative rest, medial counterforce bracing, icing, and anti-inflammatory medications. Rarely, a cortisone injection may be warranted. Once the acute phase has resolved or the pain is reduced, treatment should focus on rehabilitation, including forearm muscle strengthening, and preventing recurrence.

Return to Action

Athletes may return to action when they have full pain-free range of motion of the elbow. Grip strength should be nearly symmetric. Before considering a return, remember that many athletes with golfer's elbow, particularly baseball pitchers and golfers, also suffer from weak upper-back, neck, and thoracic muscles. Coupled with tight latissimus dorsi (back) and pectoralis (chest) muscles, these muscular deficiencies often lead to poor posture and altered sport mechanics that produce abnormal stress on the inadequately supported elbow, shoulder, and wrist joints. Thus, the rehabilitation program must focus on recreating proper body posture, improving upper-body muscular strength to better support the distal extremities and the weight they bear, and teaching improved sport mechanics to prevent future symptoms. Once that program is complete, the athlete can focus on strengthening the hand, wrist, and forearm.

RADIAL TUNNEL SYNDROME

Common Causes

Radial tunnel syndrome is most often caused by repetitive twisting and torquing of the elbow, especially the repetitive motion of the throwing arm. Repeated pronation and supination of the elbow, seen often in pitchers, can aggravate the radial nerve. Eventually scarring or an extra ligament traps the radial nerve in the proximal elbow. The most common sports in which this injury occurs are tennis, racquetball, golf, baseball, and other throwing sports.

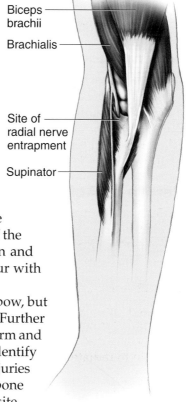

Biceps brachii

Brachialis

Site of radial nerve entrapment

Supinator

Identification

In radial tunnel syndrome, the motor branch (the part of the nerve that causes the muscles to move) of the radial nerve becomes entrapped. Symptoms of pain and numbness in the back of the hand and forearm occur with weakness in extending to the wrist and fingers.

The athlete might at first appear to have tennis elbow, but the injury does not improve with usual treatment. Further examination reveals neurological deficits in the forearm and back of the hand. X-rays or MRI typically cannot identify the nerve injury or entrapment but can reveal other injuries to the bone or tendons, such as a stress fracture or bone avulsion. Electrodiagnostic testing can identify the site of nerve entrapment and confirm the severity of any nerve damage. Neuromusculoskeletal ultrasound can also identify injuries to the nerve and tendons.

Treatment

In the short term, alternating ice and heat to the elbow can reduce inflammation and pain. Anti-inflammatory medication can be prescribed. Initially, stretching can increase the flexibility of the overlying tendons and improve the symptoms. For a more severe or chronic problem, the athlete should see a professional, who will prescribe rehab specific to the athlete's needs and goals. If conservative treatment fails and pain or neurological symptoms become even more severe, surgery to decompress the nerve might be required.

Return to Action

The throwing athlete can return to action when the pain has improved to the point at which a full pain-free throwing range of motion is achieved. Most athletes can achieve this through exercise, stretching, and rehabilitation. Rehabilitation should be guided by an experienced clinician. A gradually progressing throwing program can prevent reoccurrence of the injury. If, however, surgery is performed, the athlete is looking at a longer road to recovery. Some markers such as equal grip strength, wrist extensor strength, and finger extensor strength should be achieved before returning to throwing, golf, or racket sports.

POSTERIOR INTEROSSEOUS NERVE SYNDROME

Common Causes

Posterior interosseous nerve (PIN) syndrome, in which a branch of the radial nerve is impinged or irritated, occurs most often in tennis players and results in weakness of the muscles used in finger extension. Symptoms of PIN syndrome mimic radial tunnel syndrome in that the finger extensors are weak but differ in that PIN does not produce wrist extension weakness. The cause is repetitive rotation of the forearm.

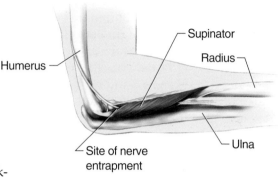

Humerus

Supinator

Radius

Ulna

Site of nerve entrapment

Identification

Athletes with PIN often complain of pain in the lateral elbow. They notice difficulty in extending their fingers. Numbness is unusual. Examination typically reveals local tenderness on the outside of the elbow. Tapping on the elbow usually causes "electrical" pain to radiate down the outside of the elbow.

Treatment

Initially, control the inflammation at the elbow. Rest, ice, anti-inflammatory medication, and sometimes splinting should reduce pain and inflammation. Severe cases that include weakness or numbness likely require physician input. Electrodiagnostic testing is often necessary to identify the severity of the injury. Although conservative treatment usually resolves PIN, surgery might be necessary to free the nerve in the elbow and forearm.

Return to Action

Athletes may return to sport when they have a normal grip and when strength is restored to the upper limb. The elbow must be pain free throughout the throwing motion. A period of rehabilitation supervised by a trainer or physical therapist will be needed to restore that strength.

PRONATOR SYNDROME

Common Causes

Pronator syndrome, often termed "anterior interosse-ous syndrome," occurs when the median nerve (one of the two main nerves that supply function to the hand and sensation to the thumb and first finger) is compressed near the crease of the bent elbow. The most common cause of the injury is hypertrophy (an increase in mass) of the volar (front) forearm muscles caused by weightlifting or similar activi-ties. The injury is usually transient and benign. Most susceptible to this injury are weightlifters, who are often told they have "Popeye arms." They will notice a gradual weakening and asymmetry of their ability to perform wrist curls and grip-type exercises. Baseball pitchers with overdeveloped forearms can also acquire pronator syndrome. If the injury is left untreated, or in the case of severe ligament entrapment, pronator syndrome can result in permanent injury to a motor branch of the median nerve and result in forearm muscle atrophy and weakness of muscles in the lower forearm and hand.

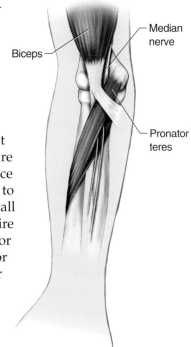

Biceps

Median nerve

Pronator teres

Identification

The compression of the median nerve most often occurs in the arm or forearm, com-monly between the two heads of the pronator teres in the area of the elbow crease. Usually, only the motor branch of the nerve is affected, resulting in motor but not sensory deficits (there may be muscle weakness but no loss of sensation).

Avid weightlifters with this injury might experience symptoms of performance decline in the affected extremity caused by painless muscular weakness. Alternatively, athletes can complain of pain described as a dull ache. The pain is localized to the flexor forearm (often in the belly of the pronator teres muscle) and is worsened with pronation movements (turning the palm down when the upper arm is straight out in front of you) or prolonged activity. In contrast to carpal tunnel syndrome (see p. 126), nocturnal pain is uncommon. A physical exam will reveal significant weakness in the finger flexor muscles, and especially in the thumb flexor muscles. Pronator strength is often preserved because the pronator teres muscle is not usually compressed.

Pronator syndrome is less common than other upper-limb entrapments, so other conditions that cause pain, weakness, or numbness, such as carpal tunnel syndrome, must be ruled out. Nerve-conduction studies and needle EMG are required to distin-guish these often overlapping and sometimes coexisting problems. MRI of the elbow can sometimes show ligament entrapments and abnormal signal within the median nerve but is more likely to be of value when performed in the cervical spine to rule out a herniated disc that might mimic pronator syndrome symptoms.

PRONATOR SYNDROME

Treatment

Treatment consists of initial rest to the affected upper limb and avoiding athletic activity. Although there is no clear evidence for its efficacy, you can try applying a wrist-immobilization splint in 15 degrees of flexion for the athlete to wear for four to six weeks. The athlete is taught to perform friction massage at the site of entrapment or muscular restriction. Quite often, the rest, forearm stretching, and possible antagonist strengthening of the wrist extensors resolve the symptoms. But if symptoms do not improve, and if a physician suspects the ligaments might be entrapped, surgical exploration might be necessary.

Return to Action

Weightlifters with this injury may return to exercises that stress the front of the forearm and wrist only when they feel no pain when performing the exercise. Gradually, they will need to strengthen the area again to attain symmetry with the uninvolved side. Throwing athletes with this problem on the dominant side should return to their sport only when the injured side is at least 80 percent back to normal and no pain occurs during the throwing motion.

ULNAR COLLATERAL LIGAMENT TEAR

Common Causes

Injuries to the ulnar collateral ligament (UCL), the ligament on the inner side of the elbow, are common in baseball pitchers. The UCL, about three-quarters of an inch (1.9 cm) away from the medial epicondyle (bone on the inside of the elbow), is a tremendously important structure stabilizing the inside of the elbow. When the elbow is flexed 90 degrees, as occurs during a wrestling match or American football tackle, the UCL distributes over 50 percent of the medial support of the elbow. After the initial windup during a baseball throw, and then during the transition between bringing the arm back and then forward, the UCL is at maximum stress. During the throwing motion, the UCL pulls the forearm forward with the rotating upper arm. The tremendous tension produced in the relatively small UCL during a properly executed throw is close to its limit. When an athlete uses improper mechanics or if arm muscles become fatigued, the load might be more than the UCL can withstand and may cause small microtears. If such microtears are not addressed with rest and therapy, a devastatingly large tear, or strain, can occur.

Identification

Pitchers with UCL injuries often describe feeling or hearing a pop in the elbow during a particular pitch. Many experts believe that the one particular pitch was just "the straw that broke the camel's back" and produced a final microtear that led to a large tear. A pitcher who tears the UCL loses a significant amount of support and strength in the elbow, thus limiting his ability to perform at the highest level. Acute and then chronic pain in the medial side of the elbow will persist if the pitcher tries to pitch through the injury. MRI scans are necessary to confirm and then determine the extent of the injury. Alternative injuries such as elbow stress fractures must be ruled out.

Treatment

Although nonoperative management of the tear might reduce the pain and swelling in a noncompetitive athlete, it will not enable a competitive athlete to recover completely. In most cases, the forces that high-level athletes place on the elbow are too strong for them to compete with a UCL tear. Surgery in which a tendon is woven back and forth between the bones of the elbow (ulna and humerus) to fabricate a new ligament is almost always recommended. The success rate of the surgery has been overwhelmingly positive; some pitchers even remark that they throw harder after the surgery than before they were injured. This procedure has been coined "Tommy John" surgery because one of its first applications was on then-famed Major League pitcher Tommy John.

Recovery is a long process if the athlete wishes to regain lost skills. During the first three weeks after surgery the goal of rehabilitation is to brace the elbow for support and restore lost elbow flexion, pronation, and supination motion. When athletes can touch their shoulder with their fingers, they may begin strengthening the wrist flexor and pronator muscles. Once full extension is achieved, the athlete can begin to strengthen the shoulder, elbow, and grip. Stressing the elbow should be avoided for four months.

ULNAR COLLATERAL LIGAMENT TEAR

After three months, the athlete can begin a throwing program with a foam ball for two weeks, a tennis ball for two more weeks, and then a hardball. Many physical therapists and sports medicine specialists recommend that no throwing take place until the athlete achieves what they consider to be a normal strength ratio of the external and internal rotator muscle groups. The ratio that they consider normal is when the external rotator strength is 65 percent of that of the internal rotators.

Return to Action

Only the athlete's physician, with input from the trainer and physical therapist, should give the athlete clearance to return to competitive play after a UCL tear. On return, the athlete must still adhere to a strict, slowly progressive throwing program to avoid a second injury or relapse. In all cases, progress depends on such factors as age, experience, injury status, and healing patterns. Address soreness with care, allowing an extra day of rest between workouts.

Before full return to competition, the athlete should be tested in a simulated game situation. For example, for a baseball pitcher, the simulation should be off a regulation mound with the same type of throwing as he would do during a game—same number and mix of pitches. If the simulation is successful, he may return to real games. After surgery and proper rehabilitation, athletes can expect to return to preinjury level. In some cases, they might be even stronger than they were preinjury.

Common Causes

Little League elbow (LLE) is an overload injury to the medial elbow that occurs as a result of repetitive throwing in the immature throwing athlete. During the throwing motion, the valgus stress on the elbow creates tension on the elbow's medial structures and compression of its lateral structures. Most injuries occur during the acceleration phase when the elbow is maximally flexed.

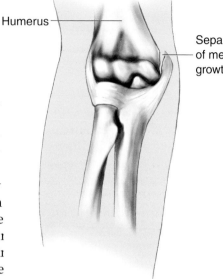

Humerus

Separation of medial growth plate

The acceleration phase of a throw subjects the elbow to valgus stress on the UCL, medial epicondyle (the bone on the inside of the elbow), and ulnar nerve. The proximal end of the UCL in skeletally immature athletes is attache outside the elbow joint itself to the unfused medial humeral apophysis (the area of a bone where tendons attach, near the area where bone growth occurs). In one type of LLE disorder, excessive overhand throwing can cause a subclinical medial elbow stress fracture and eventually a partial separation of the medial apophysis (growth plate) from the humerus. Such microtrauma can add up and cause the partial separation to become a complete avulsion (tearing away) of the growth plate off the humerus, a much more devastating injury.

The elbows of skeletally immature overhead-throwing athletes have secondary ossification centers at the radial head and olecranon (prominent bone on the upper end of the ulna behind the elbow joint). When subjected to the repetitive stress of overhand throwing, the growth plates of these unfused centers are more vulnerable to injury than the adjacent muscle–tendon units are. Thus another common LLE injury is avulsion of the posterior olecranon epiphysis. The chronic repetitive throwing in the young adolescent with lax joints can cause impingement of the medial tip of the olecranon during the terminal swing phase of throwing, resulting in similar pain.

Identification

With Little League elbow, the athlete will complain of medial elbow pain. Often the pain is associated with one of the following factors:

- Throwing too hard too often
- Increasing the number of pitches thrown per week too quickly
- Throwing too many curves or sliders at a young age
- Changing to a league in which the pitcher's mound is farther from home plate or the mound is elevated

LITTLE LEAGUE ELBOW

Most adolescent pitchers who experience severe disabling pain are still at a reversible stage. However, when elbow weakness is evident, a single hard throw might partially or completely tear the medial apophysis from the epicondyle.

Proper diagnosis is important in achieving a good outcome. The clinician must be able to identify stress fractures in the arm and elbow, nerve injuries, and muscle or ligament strains that might require surgery to repair. In most cases in which medial elbow pain does not improve quickly, X-rays or MRI are required.

Treatment

Initially, treatment should be conservative and focus on reduction of pain and inflammation with PRICE. Athletes *must* refrain from throwing. Once the elbow is completely pain free, rehabilitation and alteration of throwing mechanics can help make recurrence unlikely. Many young throwers are not taught to use the trunk and lower limb muscles properly to reduce stress on the elbow. Teaching youngsters to strengthen and properly use these muscles often prevents future recurrence of elbow injuries and could result in a few extra miles per hour and more movement on the fastball.

If initial efforts fail to reduce pain and inflammation, medical evaluation is needed. Treatment of elbow pain in the immature athlete starts with the proper diagnosis. X-ray of the elbow is of paramount importance to investigate for bony avulsions or fractures through the growth plates. If ambiguity exists, MRI is required to check for stress fractures and to look at the integrity of the UCL and other soft tissue structures.

Most elbow injuries are caused by repetitive stress, so it is important to eliminate as much stress on the elbow as possible. Modalities such as electrical stimulation and pulsed ultrasound may help. If an athlete's injury has progressed to stress fracture or avulsion, he or she should not throw at all for 6 to 12 weeks or until the condition resolves. Occasionally, surgery is required to reattach an avulsed fragment.

Return to Action

After an athlete returns to pitching, preventing reinjury takes on primary importance. Proper stretching exercises and warm-up throws are essential. The American Physical Therapy Association publishes a set of stretching exercises recommended for Little League pitchers. A therapist or trainer can also provide the team with exercises. After the game, applying ice to the elbow for 10 to 15 minutes should reduce inflammation and prevent the kind of soreness that can lead to further injury.

Not all arm injuries can be prevented, but they can be minimized by limiting the amount and type of throws in the skeletally immature athlete. Limiting pitch counts is better than limiting innings because you never know how many pitches will be thrown in an inning (see page 38 in chapter 2). Most authorities agree that athletes under 13 cannot throw breaking balls or curveballs without risking short-term or long-term injury.

OSTEOCHONDRITIS DISSECANS

Common Causes

Osteochondritis dissecans (OCD) is an inflammation of the bone and cartilage that most often affects adolescents and young adults. The area of the elbow most frequently affected is the anterolateral surface of the humeral capitellum (the outside of the elbow). The cause of the injury is repetitive throwing and strain on the elbow. As a consequence of repetitive strain, the medial or lateral elbow suffers a localized separation of a segment of articular cartilage and subchondral bone.

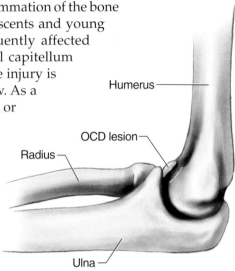

Identification

Elbow pain in young throwers is commonly known as Little League elbow; OCD is another less common elbow problem. Little League elbow typically produces pain along the medial (inner) side of the elbow while OCD usually produces pain along the lateral (outer) side of the elbow. However, the two injuries often occur simultaneously. Nearly 90 percent of those diagnosed with OCD have a history of elbow pain, and almost 55 percent report a loss of range of motion. Symptoms generally occur gradually. Pain is usually intermittent and occurs with activity, especially hard throwing or increased stress on the elbow. OCD of the capitellum is more often seen in adolescents ages 13 to 17 and is caused by repetitive lateral compression of the elbow during overhead motions. A radial head stress fracture can occur in similar fashion and might need to be ruled out by a physician.

Many athletes have symptoms similar to those with apophysitis or Little League elbow, and it is impossible to tell the difference between the two conditions without X-rays. X-rays might show loose bodies within the joint or secondary ossification (bone formation) centers within the joint that are abnormal. MRI of the elbow can rule out stress fractures and ligament tears. MRI should also reveal bone fragments and cartilage damage. Because a bone scan can detect such small changes in lesion (osteoblastic) activity, a scan provides a sensitive way to identify OCD lesions.

Treatment

Whether surgery is required depends on the size of the bony lesion and its location. The presence of loose bodies and the condition of the articular cartilage of the capitellum and radial head also help determine the need for surgery. The earlier OCD is detected, and the younger the age of the athlete, the greater the likelihood that no surgery will be needed. Conservative care consists of limiting throwing, using anti-inflammatory medications, and doing forearm strengthening exercises under the guidance of a skilled therapist or trainer. If conservative measures fail after 8 to 12 weeks, surgery may be considered. There are many surgical options, including arthroscopic debridement with curettage. In this procedure, a device called an arthroscope is placed through the skin and into the elbow joint. The arthroscope has a camera attached to it so that the surgeon can clearly see the joint space while operating. Once inside the joint, the surgeon may simply remove any loose bodies in the elbow or he or she may opt to drill the OCD lesion, which helps stimulate bone regrowth.

Because OCD occurs primarily as a result of overuse, both the injury and its reoccurrence can be prevented. As stated earlier, the number of pitches in both the skeletally immature *and* the mature athlete must be limited appropriately. Coaches, parents, and athletes must become thoroughly educated so they can recognize the injuries early. All baseball players and other at-risk athletes such as javelin throwers, shot-putters, and even tennis players must learn proper technique and conditioning.

Many throwing elbow injuries commonly occur when the throw involves a whipping or snapping motion with the arm in a relatively horizontal position during delivery. Thus, baseball pitchers should avoid opening their lead shoulder and lifting their back foot from the ground too soon. Preventive strengthening of forearm muscles, including flexors and extensors, scapular muscles, and supportive trunk and even pelvic and thigh muscles should begin long before the season starts and continue throughout the schedule.

Return to Action

As pain in the elbow subsides and full range of motion returns, athletes may start a gradual throwing program to increase endurance. Throwing technique must be evaluated by trainers and coaches familiar with the sport, and corrections must be made immediately. Serial MRI tests might be of some value, but the athlete's description of symptoms is the best signal of when to return. If the athlete is pain free, the elbow has full range of motion, and proper grip strength is fully returned (equal to the nonaffected side), the athlete may be cleared for full throwing activities.

CUBITAL TUNNEL SYNDROME

Common Causes

Cubital tunnel syndrome is caused by repeated throwing motions that result in excessive bending and twisting of the inner elbow. This injury is seen most often in baseball pitchers who throw curveballs, other throwing athletes, and golfers. Racket athletes can also suffer from this problem.

Identification

This injury is the result of irritation or entrapment of the ulnar nerve (the forearm nerve that supplies the fourth and fifth digits of the hand) as it travels through the ulnar groove on the inner elbow. If the ulnar nerve is entrapped such that nerve conduction is blocked or actual nerve fibers (axons) are damaged, the athlete might have numbness in the pinky finger and outside half of the ring finger. The athlete will also have atrophy and weakness of the inner hand muscles.

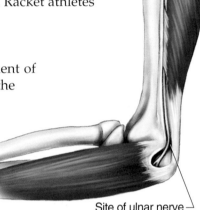

Site of ulnar nerve compression

Often athletes with an entrapped ulnar nerve in the cubital tunnel have a valgus deformity to the elbow (a lateral bend of the extended elbow). Athletes with weak intrinsic muscles of the hand cannot make a tight thumb–pinky finger pinch.

Treatment

Short-term treatment involves reducing inflammation, rest, and splinting. Anti-inflammatory medication might be prescribed. The elbow is splinted in a natural 45-degree bend to reduce stress on the nerve. The therapist can provide forearm and wrist stretching to mobilize the nerve and significantly reduce symptoms. Once elbow pain and hand numbness subside, the hand and grip should be strengthened by a professional hand therapist or occupational therapist.

If the symptoms do not improve, or if the hand weakness gets worse, surgery might be required to decompress the nerve. After surgery, a period of immobilization is necessary. Following this period, a professional therapist spends many weeks or even months helping the athlete regain wrist and forearm strength. Many different techniques are employed using hand weights and resistive straps to regain strength.

Return to Action

Throwing athletes may return to sport only when they can demonstrate pain-free range of motion of the elbow and grip and forearm strength equal to the opposite side or close to preinjury levels (if the dominant hand was injured). Athletes require sport-specific training before being able to safely return to sport.

HUMERAL STRESS FRACTURE

Common Causes

A throwing athlete who develops pain in the arm above the elbow after repetitive throwing might have a stress fracture in the mid-arm or humerus bone. A stress fracture differs from a true fracture in that the bones are not displaced, so no resetting is necessary. However, if a stress fracture is not recognized, and the athlete continues to throw competitively, the stress fracture can destabilize into a full fracture. Also, a thorough medical investigation sometimes reveals that what seemed to be a routine arm fracture is in fact bone cancer, which if treated early can prevent its spread throughout the body. Stress fractures can also occur at the radial head, shoulder, wrist, and lower extremities. Wheelchair athletes, who use their upper limbs to bear weight, are at particular risk for upper limb and elbow stress fractures.

Identification

The athlete with a stress fracture often has chronic, increasing pain in the arm or elbow after throwing a certain number of pitches or after a certain amount of time. The symptoms usually vanish with rest but then recur when activity resumes. Examination by the trainer or physician will often identify areas of local tenderness in the arm or, in the case of radial (arm bone) head fracture, the distal elbow. X-rays might not show the abnormality, which makes MRI or bone scan necessary to reveal the stress fracture.

Stress fractures in a non-weight-bearing bone are rare, so other causes, such as benign lesions, cancer, or infection (osteomyelitis), must be considered. In the unfortunate case of bone cancer, a biopsy will need to be ordered by the treating physician if the MRI is suspicious.

Treatment

The athlete should abstain from activity that stresses the affected area. For stress fractures in the upper extremity, throwing and activities in which the arms bear weight (such as poling in cross-country skiing) should be avoided. Typically, recovery time is about six weeks but will vary depending on the severity of the fracture. MRI and bone scan will remain abnormal for a prolonged period of time (a few months for MRI and up to two years for a bone scan) after the fracture has healed, so these are not usually repeated unless symptoms return.

Return to Action

After about six weeks, reassess the athlete; if pain free, he or she can start throwing again and begin to train for a return to play. A gradual return makes it less likely for the fracture to recur, but if it does, it will need to be rested again. Muscle strengthening around the injured arm might also prevent recurrence and should be supervised by the trainer or physical therapist.

ELBOW DISLOCATION

Common Causes

Elbow dislocation is the most common dislocation in children and second most common in adults (shoulder dislocation is number one). Sports injuries account for at least 50 percent of dislocations in children and adolescents. Ninety percent of dislocations occur posteriorly (with the bone moving out or away from the arm) and 10 percent anteriorly (with the bone moving in toward the arm). Most posterior dislocations occur when athletes fall on an outstretched hand with the elbow only slightly flexed. Anterior dislocations usually occur secondary to a direct blow to the back of the elbow, thrusting it forward (anterior). The major risk with elbow dislocation is its potential to compromise the nerves and blood vessels in the area. While the obvious concern may seem to be the pain and possible fracture(s) associated with a dislocated elbow, the urgent need is to ensure that the athlete has sensation, strength, and a pulse in the lower forearm and hand. If the skin appears pale (cyanotic) or there is little voluntary wrist-hand motion and a lack of feeling on the skin of the hand, this is a medical emergency, and the athlete must be transported to the local ER immediately.

Identification

The athlete will feel immediate pain. If the median or ulnar nerve is injured or stretched, the athlete will feel numbness and tingling in the hand on the injured side. If the brachial artery is injured, the hand may become pale or bluish (cyanotic) due to lack of blood supply. In young athletes, elbow subluxations of the radial head (in which the head of the elbow is moved out of position) can occur with a pull on the elbow. The child will hold the elbow close to the body and refuse to allow movement of the elbow.

Dislocations are typically diagnosed on plain X-rays of the elbow, which are also needed to rule out associated fractures. For younger athletes, the clinician should be aware of the six ossification (bone forming) centers of the elbow joint as well as the annular ligament (a strong band of fibers in the arm). Ossification can be mistaken for fractures on X-ray.

Treatment

Immediate treatment is to reduce the dislocation (relocate the elbow), but before that can happen, the athlete needs analgesia and sedation, not only for comfort but to allow adequate relaxation in the arm. Relocation can be accomplished in the prone or supine position but should occur in a controlled environment in the emergency room or be supervised by trained medical personnel. The prone position with the arm hanging over the bed and applying downward traction is usually preferred for relocation.

A complete examination of surrounding nerves and blood vessels is essential both before and after the reduction. Any vascular (blood flow) compromise requires immediate attention and might even require immediate action to reduce the dislocation. However, avoid on-the-field reduction in most cases because unrecognized fractures might be associated with the dislocation. If there is any question of vascular compromise, the athlete should be admitted into a hospital for 24 hours of observation. Follow-up X-rays will be required to rule out fractures.

ELBOW DISLOCATION

After the dislocation is reduced and the elbow stabilized, a period of immobilization is required. How long the elbow remains immobilized depends on the presence or absence of fractures (which occur in up to 15 percent of cases). An injury to the ulnar nerve (the nerve running from the shoulder to the hand) also occurs in up to 15 percent of cases and might need a period of immobilization to heal. As soon as the athlete is cleared by the surgeon, rehabilitation should begin as soon as possible.

During the acute phase of rehabilitation, the therapist will control any excessive accumulation of fluid (edema) and restore the athlete's elbow range of motion. Once adequate range of motion has been achieved, the athlete may begin strengthening of the forearm and arm muscles. Once adequate muscle strength has been restored, sport-specific training will optimize recovery and help prevent reinjury to the elbow.

Return to Action

Athletes involved in nonthrowing sports, such as soccer or American football, who suffered trauma to the elbow that caused the dislocation may return to sport in six weeks if adequate elbow range of motion and arm strength has returned. Throwing athletes might need to wait as long as three months or more to recover well enough to return to sport. The throwing athlete will require full pain-free elbow range of motion, restoration of arm strength, and participation in a gradually increasing throwing program before resuming full participation.

OLECRANON BURSITIS

Common Causes

Mild but repeated trauma to the elbow is probably the most common cause of olecranon (tip of the elbow) bursitis. For example, people who lean on their elbows a lot cause friction and repeated mild injury over the olecranon. Informal names have been given to olecranon bursitis when the cause is obvious, such as "student's elbow," caused by studying while leaning on elbows placed on a

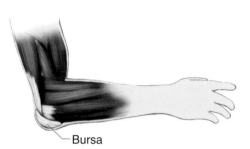

Bursa

desk. Alternatively, a one-time injury such as a blow to the back of the elbow can also set off inflammation. This injury often occurs in American football, hockey, soccer, basketball, and other contact sports. An infection to the olecranon bursa might occur if the skin over a bursa is cut and allows in bacteria; the infection can become dangerous if not treated right away with antibiotics or surgery. In the end, many cases of olecranon bursitis are idiopathic, meaning that no cause is ever found. Some are likely caused by old injuries that have been long forgotten.

Identification

Olecranon bursitis is not an extremely common injury. But once bursitis occurs, the superficial nature of the elbow creates a situation in which repeated trauma leads to a recurrent injury that can be frustrating to treat. Symptoms of bursitis include all the components of an inflammatory problem: pain, redness, heat, and swelling. A large amount of redness and heat along with systemic fevers might indicate an infection, so a physician should be consulted immediately. In the inflammatory form of bursitis, the swelling might not be painful but might lead to a reduced range of motion that impairs athletic performance.

Treatment

Treat immediately with anti-inflammatory measures such as ice to the elbow, nonsteroidal anti-inflammatory medications, wrapping of the joint, and rest. The athlete should see a physician to rule out more serious pathology, such as infection or systemic arthritis.

The swelling should subside once the athlete avoids trauma to the tip of the elbow. A padded brace might be helpful in this regard. In cases in which the amount of fluid is extremely large, or when fluid is not receding despite treatment, needle aspiration and a cortisone shot might be required. If so, maintain sterile conditions so an infection is not introduced into the bursa and joint.

Return to Action

Athletes with olecranon bursitis may return to sport when the pain subsides and full range of motion to the elbow is restored. If a rest was required, rehabilitation of the surrounding arm and forearm muscles might be necessary. Athletes with recurring bursitis should consider wearing an elbow pad.

CHAPTER 8

Wrist and Hand Injuries

Frank C. McCue III, MD; Susan Saliba, PhD, ATC, MPT

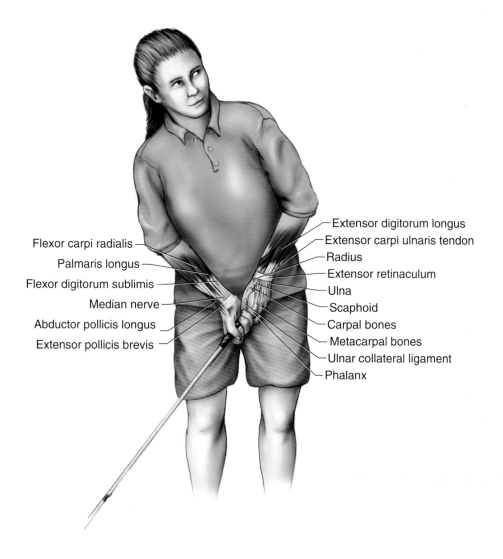

Flexor carpi radialis

Palmaris longus

Flexor digitorum sublimis

Median nerve

Abductor pollicis longus

Extensor pollicis brevis

Extensor digitorum longus

Extensor carpi ulnaris tendon

Radius

Extensor retinaculum

Ulna

Scaphoid

Carpal bones

Metacarpal bones

Ulnar collateral ligament

Phalanx

Injuries to the wrist and hand are very common in recreational and competitive athletics. The small joints of the fingers get twisted and jammed, and the wrist is vulnerable in falls. Most athletes disregard a sprained finger or swollen wrist when the injury does not prevent continued participation. But improper attention to a swollen finger or a sore wrist can lead to malalignment, further injury, or permanent dysfunction. This chapter focuses on the common injuries of the wrist and hand and how to identify when these injuries should be referred to a physician for further evaluation and treatment.

Wrist and Hand Injuries

WRIST FRACTURE

Common Causes

Wrist fractures are caused by trauma, such as when athletes fall and catch themselves with their hands. Wrist fractures are common in in-line skating or skateboarding.

Identification

The most common wrist fracture is of the distal radius, one of the forearm bones. The radius is broad at the wrist and cups the proximal row of carpal or wrist bones. When the wrist is forced back, the carpal bones are jammed against the radius and can cause a break in the bone. This injury causes immediate pain and swelling at the back of the wrist. The athlete feels pain with any wrist movement, and the pain can be localized to one location at the site of the fracture. Deformity or an angulation of the wrist might occur with a fracture of the radius.

A common wrist fracture that can cause serious problems is a fracture of the scaphoid bone at the base of the thumb side of the wrist. A scaphoid fracture causes point tenderness at the anatomical snuffbox (p. 124), pain with wrist motion, and decreased grip strength. This injury can be difficult to differentiate from a sprain because initial X-rays might not reveal a fracture line. Often, special X-ray views or MRI must be done to identify this fracture.

Treatment

If you suspect a fracture, protect the wrist from motion; the athlete should see a physician for further evaluation. Apply ice for swelling and pain. The physician who evaluates the injury dictates the time required for immobilization with a cast and whether the thumb or elbow should be included in the cast. A distal radial fracture heals well with cast immobilization, but the scaphoid has a poor blood supply and does not heal well, even when the wrist and thumb are placed in a cast. One part of the bone might deteriorate from lack of blood circulation and cause prolonged disability and pain. This can happen even with proper treatment.

When a concomitant rupture of a ligament causes instability or when the scaphoid bone is fractured at a dangerous location, surgery by a hand specialist might be necessary. Surgery commonly involves placing pins into the fractured site to stabilize the wrist and might include a bone graft to initiate healing of the bone. Surgery might occur soon after an acute fracture or after several weeks of conservative treatment.

Return to Action

Return to play should be decided by the athlete's physician. In most cases, athletes can return soon after the immobilization phase with a protective device or athletic tape or after adequate post-operative healing, as determined by the surgeon. Braces should be used to stabilize the wrist during normal activities or athletics or both. The athlete should work on strengthening the wrist by working on grip and weight bearing, exercising the muscles of the forearm and hand, and improving range of motion. If pain and lack of function persist, seek additional medical care.

WRIST SPRAIN

Common Causes

Sprains usually occur when athletes fall onto their hand(s). Sprains are also caused by repetitive overuse, as in gymnastics or even basketball shooting.

Identification

As you might recall from chapter 3, a sprain is the common term for an injury to a ligament or group of ligaments. A mild sprain is a stretching of the ligaments that usually heals with a few days to two weeks of rest. A severe sprain is tearing or rupturing of the ligaments and can lead to instability because the bones are no longer held together tightly. Eight carpal bones are in the wrist, arranged in two rows. These bones move together to allow the positioning of the wrist in any direction on the forearm. A sprain can cause excessive motion of one or more of the bones, causing pain with movement.

After a traumatic event, such as a fall, examine the wrist for swelling and tenderness specific to one site. If there is good alignment of the carpal bones and no deformity or localized swelling, the wrist might be fine, but have another look over the next few hours. If after the fall the athlete is in extreme pain with movement, or if numbness or deformity develops, splint the wrist and take the athlete to the emergency room for evaluation.

Once local trauma has subsided, observe the wrist and hand again for swelling. Compare the injured hand to the athlete's other hand. The athlete should move the wrist up and down and side to side to see if any motion causes consistent pain. Even if only mild pain occurs with movement, the joint should be protected against that motion until it heals completely; otherwise, the pain and injury may persist. Check for grip strength and for pain in the anatomical snuffbox (the area on the thumb side of the wrist demarcated by the long tendons of the wrist and thumb). If the athlete feels localized and sharp pain in this region, along with pain with movement and poor grip strength, the wrist should be evaluated by a physician to rule out a fracture of the scaphoid bone. If the athlete feels only generalized pain across the wrist and shows only minimal swelling, there is no need to seek immediate evaluation by a physician.

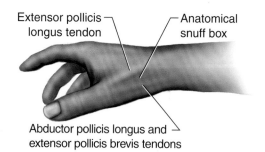

Extensor pollicis longus tendon

Anatomical snuff box

Abductor pollicis longus and extensor pollicis brevis tendons

Treatment

Treat a wrist sprain with ice until pain and swelling subside. The joints in the wrist are superficial and can be adequately cooled with a five- to seven-minute ice treatment. Apply cold therapy two or three times a day, gradually reducing frequency as pain decreases. Heat therapy is not necessary unless stiffness occurs (caused by extensive immobilization). If the athlete feels no pain with movement, or if the injury has been caused by repetitive microtrauma, apply a resting splint (which can be purchased at a drugstore) for daily activities. If the sprain does not heal within two weeks of rest, a physician should evaluate the injury.

WRIST SPRAIN

Return to Action

Most sprains heal quickly, but they are likely to persist if too much stress is placed on the injured extremity. An athlete can return to play sooner if joints are protected with athletic tape or a custom or commercial brace. Tape circumferentially around the wrist, as high on the hand as comfortable to provide stability and restrict motion (see p. 35 in chapter 2). If needed, a brace can restrict motion of the wrist, hand, or thumb to further protect the joints. These braces can be an encumbrance for play, especially in baseball and basketball, and are often discarded after a short time. The braces should be used, however, or else the athlete should choose not to participate until the injury has healed substantially, which might take six to eight weeks.

CARPAL TUNNEL SYNDROME

Common Causes

Carpal tunnel syndrome results from microtrauma sustained over a significant period of time. Rowers who sustain tension in the wrist or finger flexors are susceptible to this injury. Carpal tunnel syndrome might also occur after a sprain because small amounts of swelling can increase compression.

Identification

Carpal tunnel occurs when the median nerve is compressed in the palm side of the wrist. The median nerve is one of the two main nerves that supply function to the hand and sensation to the thumb and first finger. This nerve runs through a tight space, and any inflammatory condition can put pressure on it. In the initial stages of carpal tunnel syndrome, pain, aching, and numbness occur in the hand, usually in the thumb, pointer, and middle fingers. Certain positions and activities may increase discomfort, such as gripping an object tightly and flexing or extending the wrist. Repetitious movement of the wrist can also increase pain. If tapping gently over the wrist (on the palm side) produces a feeling of electrical shock radiating into the finger tips, this may be

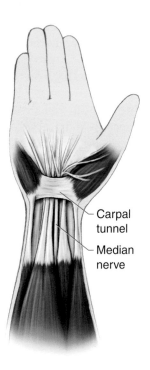

Carpal tunnel

Median nerve

an indication of carpal tunnel syndrome. Numbness often occurs at night when the wrist is flexed or placed in an awkward position for an extended time during sleep. In more advanced stages of carpal tunnel syndrome, the athlete might drop things, have weakness in the thumb, and experience greater pain.

Treatment

In the initial stages of carpal tunnel syndrome, use a resting splint (see p. \bb\ in chapter 2) to prevent excessive motion of the wrist and to minimize the extremes of flexion and extension. Because of the sensitivity of the nerves in this location, do not apply ice. Night splints are effective in minimizing extreme ranges of motion. Once the inflammation around the nerve has subsided, the pain might go away.

If a resting splint does not eradicate the symptoms, the wrist should be evaluated by a physician. An injection of steroid anti-inflammatory drug may be prescribed, which should gradually reduce symptoms over the next few days. Some athletes benefit from consuming vitamin B_6 (about 50 to 100 mg per day for one month), which acts as a diuretic and helps reduce inflammation in the area of the carpal tunnel. Rest and splinting are used to assist healing.

Electrodiagnostic testing (EMG) can assess how well the median nerve is working and is an excellent means of quantifying damage to the median nerve and the muscles it supplies. Even if the electrodiagnostic test is negative, carpal tunnel syndrome could still be the problem; the test may just not have revealed it. If the electrodiagnostic test is positive, the problem is definitely carpal tunnel syndrome. If the condition is in advanced stages, or if the injection does not help, surgery may be required to create a larger space for the nerve to travel in. After surgery, the hand should be splinted and protected while the incision heals for two weeks; then gradual motion is allowed.

Return to Action

Rehabilitation focuses on return of range of motion and grip strength. Thumb exercise should also be incorporated when the condition involves weakness of the thumb. Either preoperatively or postoperatively, athletes should avoid participating in their sport until their symptoms subside. If symptoms continue while playing sports, the median nerve could be damaged, which might cause permanent weakness and atrophy of the affected muscles. Generally, the longer the symptoms persist, the longer the rest period necessary to resolve the inflammatory process.

Once symptoms have subsided, circumferential wrapping of the wrist with athletic tape might stabilize the wrist, but this puts additional pressure on the carpal tunnel. Instead of taping, use commercial or custom braces for support.

Common Causes

Many of the tendons in the wrist can become inflamed, resulting in tendinitis. The back of the wrist has six separate compartments, each with its own synovial sheath. We can number these compartments one through six, starting on the thumb (radial) side. The synovial sheath provides lubrication against friction from bones and other tendons. The synovial sheath also contains fluid that accumulates in the case of an inflammation—much like a blister fills with fluid. Repetitive action of the wrist, such as shooting basketballs or hitting golf balls, can cause enough friction within the tendon to accumulate fluid, resulting in tendinitis (involving just the tendon) or tenosynovitis (involving the tendon and the synovial sheath). Some wrist tendons, such as the sixth tendon (called the extensor carpi ulnaris, or ECU) can become inflamed after a fall onto the hand.

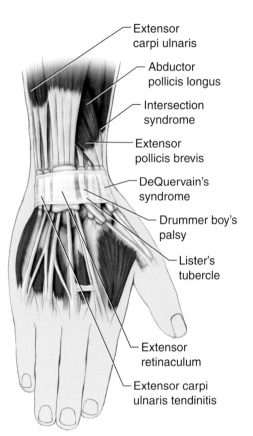

Extensor carpi ulnaris

Abductor pollicis longus

Intersection syndrome

Extensor pollicis brevis

DeQuervain's syndrome

Drummer boy's palsy

Lister's tubercle

Extensor retinaculum

Extensor carpi ulnaris tendinitis

Identification

Tendinitis is exemplified by swelling within the tendon. A crunching feeling (crepitus) is felt or heard when the tendon is pressed or the wrist moved. The wrist is very painful, and any stress to the involved tendon causes discomfort. The types of wrist tendinitis are grouped according to the affected tendon. Tendinitis in the fourth and fifth dorsal compartments is rare in athletics and is not addressed.

DeQuervain's Syndrome

When tenosynovitis is present in the first dorsal compartment, the condition is called DeQuervain's syndrome (also known as washerwoman's sprain). The involved tendons (the abductor pollicis longus and the extensor pollicis brevis) are held in a groove in the radius by a thickened portion of the extensor retinaculum. Discomfort is noted over the base of the thumb near the bump on the thumb side of the wrist. This syndrome is caused by repetitive motion that requires a forceful grasp.

Intersection Syndrome

Intersection syndrome is an inflammatory condition at the crossing point of the first and second compartments. These compartments cross at a 60-degree angle, and excessive wrist extension and bending the wrist toward the thumb side create the tenosynovitis in the second compartment. The inflammatory reaction places pressure on the first compartment, so patients may have stress on either site. Whereas DeQuervain's syndrome causes pain in the tendon near the thumb as it crosses the wrist, intersection syndrome occurs where the muscle bellies cross.

WRIST TENDINITIS

Drummer Boy's Palsy

The third dorsal compartment contains the extensor pollicis longus, which can rub on Lister's tubercle, a projection from the radius. Tendinitis, or even rupture, of this tendon is called "drummer boy's palsy" because of the prevalence of the pathology in drummers. In athletics, racket sports can produce the symptoms because of the firm grasp and the repetitive motion.

Extensor Carpi Ulnaris Tendinitis

The sixth compartment in the dorsal aspect of the wrist contains the extensor carpi ulnaris (ECU) tendon. This area is the second to DeQuervain's syndrome as the most common site of tenosynovitis in the wrist. The tendon might snap continuously with repetitive activities or dislocate traumatically and cause continued disability and pain. A snapping ECU commonly occurs when a baseball player swings a bat vigorously and misses, causing the bottom hand to turn forcefully. Pain is localized on the outside of the dorsal side of the wrist. There might be swelling and generalized pain. Athletes might not be able to reproduce the snapping of the tendon, but they will often report an immediate sensation of weakness when the wrist is stressed.

Treatment

Treat tendinitis with rest to prevent excessive motion in the wrist and anti-inflammatory agents (if appropriate) to reduce swelling. A splint helps to protect the wrist from further stress, but it is equally important to move the wrist to prevent stiffness and a recurrence of symptoms. The athlete should use a splint during daily activities to protect the wrist from further stress but remove it for gentle range-of-motion exercise at least twice a day to reduce the accumulation of fluid. Ice and self-massage can also help minimize swelling.

A thumb splint might be necessary for DeQuervain's syndrome and drummer boy's palsy. Corticosteroids can be injected to attempt to reduce the inflammatory process in DeQuervain's syndrome but should be discouraged in the case of drummer boy's palsy because of the possibility of tendon rupture.

When conservative management fails for intersection syndrome, surgery can decompress the first dorsal compartment, and then the second compartment as well if the retinaculum is constricted.

Stabilization of the wrist is necessary when the ECU is involved. This tendon is held in place by a ligamentous structure that has been compromised. The wrist should be protected while the ligament heals. Use athletic tape and commercial bracing. If the wrist continues to cause dysfunction and pain, consult a physician. On rare occasions, the tendon might need surgical stabilization.

Return to Action

Tendinitis is exacerbated by excessive stress, so until pain subsides the athlete should avoid activity that involves the wrist tendons. Playing through pain will cause a longer course of disability and might lead to a chronic disability. Once the wrist can be stabilized with taping or bracing and participation is pain free, a return to play is safe.

HAND FRACTURE

Common Causes

The long bones in the hand can be injured while punching; by a blunt, forceful contact; or as result of stress transferred through the fingers.

Identification

The metacarpals are numbered one through five, starting with the thumb and ending with the little finger. When a metacarpal is fractured, immediate and specific pain follows as well as swelling on the back of the hand. Once the initial pain has subsided, observe the hand for swelling and deformity. To differentiate between a bruise and a fracture, check for pain on both the back of the hand and in the palm. Apply force through each individual finger to check for tenderness in the hand. When the athlete makes a fist, each knuckle should be visible. Compare the hand to the athlete's other hand. Finally, check the fingers when making a fist. All fingers should point to the same location in the wrist. The rotation in a metacarpal fracture is amplified at the finger. If there is good alignment, poorly localized pain, and no deformity of the knuckle, the injury is probably a bruise and should subside quickly. Consult a physician if symptoms of a fracture are present or if there is uncertainty.

Treatment

The second through fourth metacarpals are relatively stable and usually require only cast immobilization with buddy taping of the fingers (taping fingers to each other) for good healing. The first metacarpal at the thumb has tendinous attachments that can pull the fracture out of line. These fractures often require surgical fixation. The fifth metacarpal is very mobile. This bone is often fractured with a punch, and is thus commonly called a "boxer's fracture." The mobility of the fifth metacarpal may also require surgical stabilization for good healing. Any hand fracture should be evaluated for rotation during the immobilization phase, which might indicate a need for surgical intervention.

To adequately immobilize the bones in the hand for healing from fracture, the hand and wrist should be put into a cast and the involved fingers splinted or taped together. The cast should allow good mobility of the metacarpophalangeal joints (knuckles) in the noninjured portion of the hand. Otherwise the hand will be stiff and require extensive mobility training to regain range of motion. Conversely, if fingers in the involved area are allowed to move freely, there is a potential for delayed healing or rotation at the fracture site. Buddy taping the fractured finger to an adjacent finger allows mobility of the metacarpophalangeal joint and prevents rotation.

Return to Action

Following immobilization, the hand is likely to be stiff and weak. Rehabilitation efforts should address these problems while protecting the hand from further injury. Strengthening exercises should be done for grip and wrist function as well as for the elbow and shoulder. Once X-ray indicates that the fracture is well-healed and mobility and strength are restored, the athlete may return to sports. If the injury requires surgery, the surgeon dictates the course of therapy and return to sports.

THUMB SPRAIN

Common Causes

The thumb, especially the ulnar collateral ligament (UCL), is vulnerable to sprains because of its mobility and unique abilities. It is located at the base of the thumb in the web space between the thumb and second digit. The UCL helps stabilize the metacarpophalangeal joint and is commonly injured when an athlete falls onto the hand or when the thumb is torqued by contact. The thumb can be injured from a fall, especially on a ski pole, and is often injured during contact from another player.

Identification

When the thumb is injured, immediate pain and swelling follow. Compare the appearance of the sprained thumb to the other thumb. Excessive swelling, point tenderness, and an inability to use the thumb are signs of more severe injury or fracture and should be evaluated by a physician. The integrity of the ligament is tested with a special test, and X-rays help to determine if a concomitant fracture has occurred.

Treatment

If the ligament is stretched or partially torn, splint the thumb so the ligament can heal. When the UCL is torn completely, the ruptured edge drops behind a muscle, and the ligament cannot heal without surgical repair.

Return to Action

During the healing phase, which generally requires six to eight weeks, the athlete should wear a splint or athletic tape during stressful activities. Commercially available splints can be used, but they tend to extend past the wrist, restricting the ability to play some sports. A custom brace can be made from a thermoplastic material to help prevent excessive stress to the thumb while allowing full mobility of the wrist. As long as there is no pain and the thumb is protected, the athlete may participate safely. When surgery is required to repair the ligament, the timing of a return is dictated by the surgeon.

FINGER SPRAIN

Common Causes

A sprained or jammed finger is probably the most common injury of the hand and is often caused by twisting with contact from another player. The finger can also be sprained by contact with a stick or ball. The injury is sometimes called "coach's finger" because it is often treated by the coach rather than by a health care professional.

Identification

There are two joints in each finger: the proximal (the joint after the knuckle) and the distal (the last joint of the finger) interphalangeal joints. When a finger is sprained, the ligaments are typically sprained in the proximal interphalangeal joint. The ligaments most commonly sprained are the ones running alongside the joint known as the collateral ligaments. In addition, the volar plate (a dense fibrous band) on the palm of the hand can be sprained. Volar plate strains often cause an inability to straighten the finger for several weeks.

A sprained joint in the finger can cause swelling, restricted mobility, and pain. Concomitant fractures in these small joints, when neglected, can cause permanent malalignment. Thus, any injury to the small joints of the fingers should be evaluated if swelling and decreased mobility do not subside within a few days.

Treatment

Remove any rings the athlete is wearing on the sprained finger. Because dislocations of finger joints are common, check that the finger is properly aligned with the other fingers. Friends who "pull out" a jammed finger rarely help the injury and can cause further damage if a dislocation has not been properly reduced (if the joint has not been put back into place). Once the initial pain has subsided, observe the finger for swelling and function of each joint. Also check the athlete's ability to move each joint independently. A physician should evaluate the injury if pain and swelling persist beyond a few days.

Return to Action

Finger sprains should be splinted for four to six weeks so that only the injured joint is protected during the day and during sports participation. Tape the injured finger to an adjacent finger for more support (this is especially helpful in the case of a collateral ligament injury). When the volar plate is injured, the finger should be splinted in a straight position, whereas a collateral ligament sprain should be splinted in 30 degrees of flexion.

FINGER OR THUMB DISLOCATION

Common Causes

The small joints of the fingers can be dislocated when the finger is torqued or hyper-extended. This type of force is common with contact from another player or contact from a ball. Basketball, football, baseball, and even soccer players often dislocate a finger. The injury rarely occurs in sports such as hockey or lacrosse, in which the fingers are protected by gloves.

Identification

Look for deformity of the finger. Dislocations of the finger usually occur at the bones on either side of the knuckle. After the dislocation, there will be an abnormal angle between these two bones. Fractures can occur along with this injury—either caused by the injury itself or by nonprofessional efforts to put the joint back in place. Any disruption in the architecture of the joint line can cause arthritis, poor mobility, and dysfunction.

Treatment

The dislocated finger should be evaluated by a physician for appropriate reduction (putting the joint back into place) and treatment. Some dislocations cause a permanent instability and become vulnerable to a repeat dislocation. This happens most often in the fifth finger because it is the least protected. Surgical reconstruction of the collateral ligaments might be necessary to provide stability when there are repeated dislocations.

Return to Action

Once the joint has been relocated, apply a splint to protect the finger. The splint might cover the entire finger for a few days and then be shortened to cover only the involved joint. Use buddy taping to help minimize forces while healing takes place. The finger should be protected from further injury during athletic participation for four to six weeks.

FINGER OR THUMB FRACTURE

Common Causes
Fractures in the fingers typically have the same causes as finger sprains and dislocations. Any contact with a ball or another player can cause a finger fracture.

Identification
Each phalanx (finger bone) can be fractured in a rotational or spiral manner, or it can be chipped at the joint. Damage to the fingernail might indicate a fracture to the distal phalanx. Any disruption in the integrity of the skin in the involved finger is treated as an open fracture. Take care to prevent infection in these cases.

Once initial pain has subsided, observe the finger for swelling, immobility, and deformity. Check each joint individually for mobility to make sure the tendons are functioning normally. A fracture causes pain when pressure is applied between the joints, so there should be one location that is much more tender than the others (unless there is more than one fracture). When the tip of the finger is tapped, pain occurs at the fracture site. If any of these signs are present, X-rays are needed. The finger should be splinted for protection and evaluated within one to three days.

Treatment
Treatment depends on the type of fracture. Chip or avulsion fractures are generally treated like sprains, with protective splinting for four to six weeks. Damage to the articular, or joint, surface, might require surgical repair to prevent arthritis. Spiral or rotational fractures might also require surgery for proper healing. Pins can be inserted through the skin. Small plates and screws may be required to stabilize some fractures.

If an injury occurs to the distal finger and the nail bed gets suddenly dark (blackness covering the majority of the nail bed), this may indicate a fracture of the nail matrix. This injury may require surgical repair to increase the likelihood of normal future nail growth.

Return to Action
If the injured finger is protected with a splint and buddy tape, the athlete can generally participate in his or her sport after four to six weeks. For fractures that require surgery, a physician should dictate return to play. Generally, the athlete may not participate when there are percutaneous pins (through the skin) in place or before any sutures have been removed. Focus is on protection from further injury.

MALLET FINGER

Common Causes

When the finger is struck at the tip, the phalanx at the fingertip (distal phalanx) is forced downward. This commonly happens in such sports as volleyball, basketball, or baseball in which the finger is held in extension and might be jammed into the ball. This force may rupture the extensor digitorum longus, which inserts onto the fingertip. The resulting condition is called mallet finger, in which the patient is unable to voluntarily extend the finger, although the joint can be moved into extension by the examiner or with the assistance of the athlete's other hand. The injury is sometimes termed "baseball finger" because it commonly occurs when the ball hits the fingertips. Mallet finger can also occur in American football or basketball when contact is directed to the fingertip.

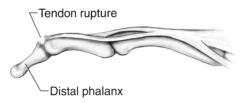

Tendon rupture

Distal phalanx

Identification

A mallet finger at first seems like a sprain to the distal interphalangeal joint. On examination, however, the athlete is unable to extend the distal phalanx actively. The fingertip droops downward and can cause a permanent extension lag if not treated properly. A mallet finger is categorized according to whether an avulsion fracture of the distal phalanx has occurred.

Treatment

The treatment for a mallet finger is continued splinting for eight to nine weeks. The fingertip must be held in extension so that the extensor tendon may heal. If the finger is allowed to drop into flexion, even for a brief time, time might be added to the healing process. A stack splint is used to immobilize the distal phalanx. This plastic splint allows mobility of the proximal interphalangeal joint while maintaining full extension of the fingertip. A stack splint is also perforated to help keep the skin dry.

You may also use metal splints with no padding to treat a mallet finger. Or a splint may even be applied to the dorsal side of the finger to allow perception of touch in the fingertip. The splint should ensure full extension or slight hyperextension and immobilize only the distal interphalangeal joint. When changing the splint, do not allow the finger to drop into flexion.

The care of the skin can become a concern because of the extensive splinting required. If the finger and splint get wet, either through washing or sweating, the skin might slough. This complication is exacerbated by a tight splint that restricts circulation. Teach the athlete to keep the finger dry and to move the splint if the skin becomes macerated.

Return to Action

The athlete might be able to participate in his or her sport with a splint in place. If the splint prevents participation, such as the inability to properly grip a bat, prohibit participation until the finger heals.

CHAPTER 9

Chest and Abdominal Injuries

Daniel A. Brzusek, DO, MSc

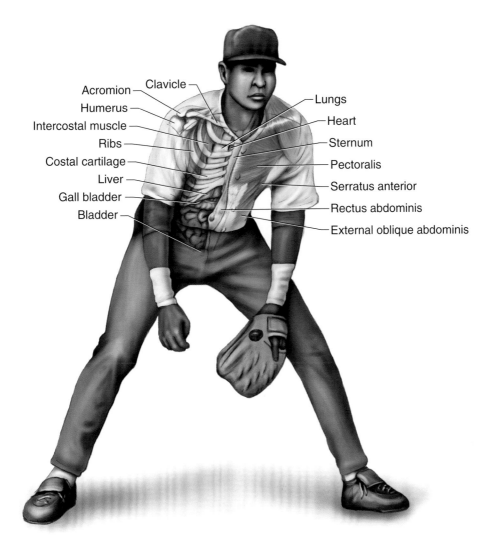

Chest and abdominal injuries in athletes are relatively rare, but when they do occur, they can be severe and gravely dangerous. All adults involved in sport should be able to recognize the warning signs of potentially life-threatening injury to the liver, spleen, or hollow abdominal viscera. Coaches or even team physicians cannot provide definitive treatment or diagnosis for many of these conditions on the field. However, they should be familiar with the usual clinical signs and symptoms of chest and abdominal trauma, and any athlete showing these signs should be transported to a medical facility for confirmation immediately. Referral to a sports medicine physician to seek diagnostic details and treatment options is also appropriate but should be made expediently for all chest and abdominal injuries.

On the field, decision making is extremely important because some chest and abdominal injuries can be life threatening. Coaches and trainers being aware of the symptoms and signs and reacting to them with all due efficiency might be the difference between life and death for an athlete.

Chest and Abdominal Injuries

HEMOTHORAX

Common Causes

A delayed hemothorax following blunt trauma is a rare but very serious, sometimes life-threatening injury. This injury is usually accompanied by displaced rib fractures and is most often seen in skiing, snowboarding, hockey, and baseball.

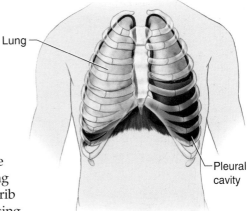

Identification

A hemothorax is a collection of blood in the space between the chest wall and the lung (the pleural cavity). In blunt chest trauma, a rib might lacerate the lung tissue or artery, causing blood to collect in the pleural space. Hemothorax can also be associated with pneumothorax, which is air trapped in the pleural cavity. Depending on the amount of blood or air in the pleural cavity, a collapsed lung can lead to shock and cardiac arrest.

Hemothorax or pneumothorax is usually one-sided. The athlete with one of these conditions usually has pain in the chest; signs of respiratory distress, such as shortness of breath or an inability to take in deep breaths; a sense of impending doom or anxiety; and hyperventilation or increased respiratory rate. If a stethoscope is available, listen for decreased or absent breath sounds on the affected side. The athlete might also have a very rapid heart rate and appear to be quite restless.

Treatment

If you suspect hemothorax or pneumothorax, keep the athlete calm on the field and then move him or her as quickly as possible to the nearest medical facility. An X-ray usually gives a quick diagnosis. The objective of treatment is to stabilize the athlete, stop the bleeding, and remove the blood or air in the pleural space. A chest tube is usually inserted through the chest wall to drain the blood and air. This tube is left in place for several days to reexpand the lung. The cause of the hemothorax, such as a broken rib, can then be treated. In most trauma patients, chest tube drainage is sufficient, and surgery is not required.

Return to Action

The athlete will probably not be able to return to action for six to eight weeks. It might be necessary to protect the affected area with a plastic shell, or flak jacket, to prevent further contact for several months following this type of traumatic event. Before returning to action, the athlete's lungs will need to be reconditioned, using exercises such as long-distance running and wind sprints. Complications are rare if the athlete is treated appropriately. Occasionally, the pleural space will become fibrotic or scar between the pleural membranes. Watch for athletes complaining of chest wall pain as they begin to run. Athletes should see a physician to determine if they have developed pleuritis (or pleurisy), an inflammation of the pleura, the lining of the pleural cavity surrounding the lungs. This condition might require surgery.

Common Causes

Commotio cordis refers to a circulatory arrest caused by a nonpenetrating blow to the chest. The condition can occur when an object, such as a baseball, hits the chest. It usually involves a high-speed (greater than 30 miles per hour) impact, but it can occur with a low-speed impact. There is usually no fracture to the ribs or sternum in commotio cordis. Blows directly over the center of the chest are more likely to cause this injury. In commotio cordis, the impact to the chest occurs at a critical time in the heart's cycle, when the normal rhythm is vulnerable. The impact sends the heart into a dysfunctional rhythm called ventricular fibrillation. Rather than

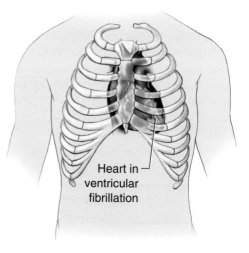

Heart in ventricular fibrillation

beating normally and pumping blood to the organs, the heart just quivers and fails to pump blood. In essence, the victim is in cardiac arrest.

Although such cases are relatively rare, an increasing number of deaths and a significant percentage of deaths on athletic fields are caused by chest wall impact. Commotio cordis is most frequently observed in young people from 14 to 18 but also occurs in adults. The most common activities during which this injury occurs include baseball, softball, hockey, and, to a lesser extent, karate, lacrosse, and American football. Rare cases have been reported in basketball, cricket, boxing, and martial arts other than boxing. In most instances (68 percent), the person is struck by a projectile—most commonly a pitched, thrown, or batted baseball or softball—estimated to be traveling 35 to 50 miles per hour. Other projectiles include hockey pucks and lacrosse balls. In 32 percent of instances, chest trauma resulted from bodily contact with another person or a stationary object. Examples include being hit by a player's helmet during a football tackle, being hit by the heel of a hockey stick, being struck by a karate kick, or receiving a body collision.

Identification

Individuals with commotio cordis are typically found to be unresponsive, apneic (not breathing), and without a pulse or audible heartbeat. Most are cyanotic (turning blue). Grand mal seizures occur with some cases of commotio cordis. Chest wall contusions and localized bruising that correspond to the site of chest impact are noted over the precordium (the front of the heart) in about a third of commotio cordis patients. Typically, the ribs or sternum are not broken or injured. Patients are often found in ventricular fibrillation (with an irregular heartbeat).

COMMOTIO CORDIS

Treatment

Given the generally young age and excellent health of the afflicted, resuscitation is more difficult than expected. The earlier treatment commences, the better the chance for successful resuscitation. Use of a precordial thump (a single very carefully aimed blow with the fist to the center of the sternum) during CPR is controversial, particularly in children. Expanded use of automatic external defibrillators (AEDs) may save the lives of some people who receive blunt trauma to the precordium and go into cardiac arrest. In such cases, the application of electric current, as delivered by an AED, may be the only chance to "jump start" the heart back into normal rhythm. Even when an AED is used by someone with minimal training, this device can recognize and automatically terminate arrhythmias.

The use of AEDs is not without controversy. There are people who shy away from using it due to liability concerns. However, using an AED is simple because the device guides the operator through its use. More and more youth leagues, public places, and industries have AEDs available in case of emergency, and most basic CPR courses now include AED training.

Until recently, AEDs were not approved for use in children younger than eight years of age who weigh less than 55 pounds. But the latest recommendations state that AEDs may be used in children from one to eight who have no signs of circulation. Ideally, if available, the device should be outfitted with a special pediatric pad and cable set, which attenuates the charge, delivering a more appropriate pediatric dose.

With more portable defibrillation units available, athletes who suffer commotio cordis can be greatly assisted in their survival rate. More modern, small, inexpensive, and efficient defibrillators are appearing in trainers' and sports physicians' on-the-field medical bags.

Return to Action

Return-to-action decisions should be left to a cardiologist. In all probability, the athlete will be out for at least two months. When people who suffer commotio cordis are treated successfully and survive, they are not necessarily susceptible to a recurrence. Nonetheless, a thorough cardiac evaluation before return to play is in order.

Baseball has one of the highest impact injury rates of all sports. These injuries are primarily attributed to impact by a ball after it has been hit, pitched, or thrown. Although the use of protective vests could decrease this condition, the incidence and severity of cardiothoracic trauma still appears to be in question. Studies have shown that safety baseballs (softer baseballs) do not prevent but do reduce the risk of sudden cardiac death. Soft baseballs should always be used with younger or less-skilled athletes.

RIB FRACTURE

Common Causes

The most obvious cause of rib fracture is a direct impact, such as when two bodies collide. Athletes' bodies might also be subjected to large indirect force from overuse. Rib fractures caused by overuse of remote portions of the body have been associated with golf and baseball pitching in particular. Direct impact fractures can occur during collisions in hockey, American football, soccer, lacrosse, and baseball.

Identification

The athlete with a rib fracture usually has pain over the affected area, particularly when taking a deep breath. Palpation shows tenderness. The athlete also breathes more shallow breaths. Interestingly enough, some mild compression over the fractured rib site while the athlete takes a deep breath might relieve the pain to some extent. Bruising is usually evident at the place of injury. Definitive diagnosis is made by X-ray, CT scan, and bone scan.

Serious rib fractures occasionally occur, the signs of which are rapid and shallow breathing, elevated heart rate, increased difficulty breathing, and coughing up blood. Place one hand on each side of the injured athlete's chest and observe the way the chest moves with inhalations. If one side of the chest rises during inhalation while the other falls, at least three ribs have been broken on the fallen side of the chest. This is called a "flail chest."

Treatment

When a rib fracture is suspected, the athlete should be taken immediately to a hospital. The injured athlete must be carried if there are any signs of respiratory distress but will be able to walk out with simple fractures. If you suspect the athlete has a flail chest, lay the athlete on the injured side and place a rolled piece of clothing under the fractured area to support it; this will help control the pain with breathing. Keep the athlete on his or her side and continue monitoring for difficulty breathing. The athlete might need to be rolled over to provide rescue breathing if he or she ceases to breathe.

Immediate treatment should be directed at alleviating pain. Ice packing the area will help. Until a definitive diagnosis is made and significant bleeding is ruled out, only acetaminophen should be administered for pain control; anti-inflammatories can promote bleeding. Once stabilized either at the site (for mild rib injuries) or at the local ER (for more significant injuries) further treatment can ensue. A newer, noninvasive and very effective method of treatment is the use of Lidoderm anesthetic patches, which help control pain by slightly numbing the area. A patch is applied for 12 hours at a time, followed by 12 hours off before another patch is used. These patches must be used with caution as prescribed by a physician. The use of these patches can lower the blood pressure of some people.

Rib fractures generally take three to eight weeks to heal. To speed the healing process, the athlete should avoid strenuous activities and take care not to bump the injured rib. The athlete should be encouraged to take deep breaths several times a day to keep the lungs free from infection. Rib belts or binders can be used for comfort but are not encouraged.

RIB FRACTURE

Return to Action

Healing usually takes a minimum of eight weeks. For displaced fractures, recovery may take longer, depending upon how the athlete responds and whether or not the fracture healing is delayed, as noted on X-ray, and the return to sports should be adjusted accordingly. Some athletes may require three months or more for healing to be sufficient to permit a return to play. Athletes who participate in contact sports and had displaced fractures or significant pain at the fracture site(s) should wear a Flak jacket for the remainder of the season. For athletes in noncontact sports, no binding or bracing is usually necessary unless they have local pain or breathing issues. Athletes who have been treated for a rib fracture should undergo a conditioning program to improve cardiorespiratory and pulmonary efficiency before returning to sports.

STERNAL FRACTURE

Common Causes

Most sternal fractures are caused by blunt trauma to the chest, although stress fractures have been noted in golfers, weightlifters, and other athletes engaged in noncontact sports. Direct impact sports such as hockey, American football, lacrosse, and soccer as well as falls from bicycles can also cause a sternal fracture. In the United States, motor vehicle collisions account for 60 to 90 percent of all sternal fractures.

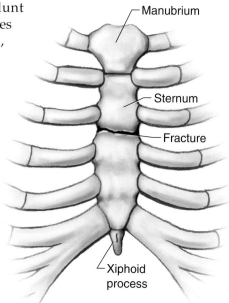

Manubrium

Sternum

Fracture

Xiphoid process

Sternal fractures are more common in mature athletes because of the elasticity of the mature chest wall. The mortality rate from isolated sternal fracture is extremely low. Death and morbidity are related almost entirely to associated injuries such as aortic disruption, cardiac contusion, pulmonary contusions, or unrelated injuries to the abdomen or head sustained in the incident. Children under 18 rarely have sternal fractures, but when they occur, they are often more severe.

Identification

Sternal fractures cause pain and tenderness over the sternum. A definitive diagnosis is made by bone scan or CT scan. Additionally, differentiating sternal fractures and rib fractures from sternocostal separation is difficult without an X-ray as both injuries produce significant pain.

Treatment

After a sternal fracture, the athlete should rest and avoid physical activity for four to six weeks. No particular rehabilitation program is required. The treatment for sternocostal separations is self-limited, although taping with elastic tape is used occasionally. Athletes may be left with a cosmetic deformity but no residual deficit, other than mild discomfort, is likely.

Return to Action

Prognosis is excellent for isolated sternal fractures. Most athletes recover completely over a period of four to six weeks and require no special treatment. The recovery timeline is similar for sternocostal separations. The athlete should be cleared by a physician prior to returning to athletic participation. A protective sternal pad may be used as a precaution but is usually not required once the fracture heals.

COSTOCHONDRITIS

Common Causes

Costochondritis is an inflammation of the junctions where the upper ribs join with the cartilage that holds them to the breastbone or sternum. The rib inserts into a cylindrical tube on the sternum. Usually this fit is very snug. However, direct trauma or unusual activity during sports such as weightlifting or swimming can loosen the fit, allowing the rib to rub against the sternal tubing, causing inflammation and discomfort. This injury occurs more often than is obvious and is usually disregarded as mild tendinitis.

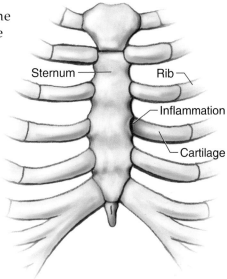

Identification

This condition is often misdiagnosed or undiagnosed. The athlete might have costochondritis for weeks or months before it is diagnosed. Athletes often note intermittent sharp, stabbing pain followed by a dull achy sensation that lasts for hours or days. Slipping and popping sensations are common in activities such as bending, coughing, deep breathing, lifting, reaching, or rising from a chair; stretching, turning, or twisting often exacerbates symptoms.

Costochondritis arises from hypermobility of the anterior ends of false rib costal cartilages. Hypermobility of the rib usually results from sports that require significant flailing motions of the upper extremities or from direct contact injuries. Hypermobility often causes the affected rib to slip under the superior adjacent rib. Slippage or movement can lead to irritation of the intercostal nerve, strain of the intercostal muscles, sprain of the lower costal cartilage, or general inflammation in the affected area. Costochondritis is also called Tietze's syndrome, clicking rib syndrome, displaced ribs, interchondral subluxation, nerve nipping, painful rib syndrome, rib tip syndrome, slipping rib cartilage syndrome, traumatic intercostal neuritis, and 12th rib syndrome.

Treatment

Treatment might include physical therapy and injection of the damaged cartilage with cortisone. Most often, it is treated conservatively with warm soaks and mild anti-inflammatory medications (if appropriate). If the cause of the pain is in question, consider transporting the athlete to the local ER to rule out possible cardiac causes for the pain. Surgery might be required in some cases.

Return to Action

Return time depends on how long it takes symptoms to subside. Surgical intervention is extremely rare. In most instances, the athlete may return to sports when relatively asymptomatic, but recovery may be protracted, and the decision should be based upon discussions between the athlete and physician. There is usually no need for special protective equipment upon returning to sports participation.

ABDOMINAL TRAUMA

Common Causes

In adolescents and children, the most common cause of abdominal injury is direct trauma. One study in the pediatric population of the incidents of recreational genitourinary and abdominal injuries found that kidney injuries were the most common at 44 percent, followed by spleen injuries at 36 percent, and liver injuries at 20 percent. Hockey, American football, snowboarding, sledding, and bicycling account for many incidents of abdominal trauma. Such injuries are quite rare in basketball or soccer. Kidneys are most at risk in American football. Spleen injuries can occur in all recreational sports.

Abdominal trauma injuries frequently occur in bicycling, often when child cyclists collide with handlebars, which can cause serious injury. Retractable bicycle handlebars, which consist of a spring-loaded damper system designed to retract and absorb the majority of energy at impact, reduces the risk of severe injury in young cyclists.

Identification

Look for abdominal pain in athletes after direct trauma. It may be vague or localized. In most cases of abdominal pain, the athlete should be immediately transported to an emergency facility that has the equipment required for ultrasounds and CT and MRI scans for diagnosis by a medical professional.

Treatment

In mild cases, when no particular organ damage is identified, treatment consists of rest until the athlete is pain free. Typically, this will take four to six weeks with ongoing close medical observation. General conditioning exercises are okay so long as abdominal discomfort is not increased. Occasionally, blunt abdominal trauma requires laparoscopic surgery for diagnosis or treatment. Surgery can be avoided in many cases if MRI rules out significant abdominal trauma or injury. On the other hand, if MRI reveals injured organs, internal bleeding, or other suspicious areas, surgery may be required.

Return to Action

Athletes may return to action after four to six weeks or when they are symptom free. Clearance to participate must be obtained from a physician. If surgery is done, clearance from the surgeon is required prior to participation, and recovery may take 12 weeks or more, depending upon the injury.

TESTICULAR INJURY

Common Causes

Despite the vulnerable position of the testicles, testicular trauma is relatively uncommon, perhaps partly because of the mobility of the scrotum. Still, traumatic injuries to the testicles deserve careful attention given the importance of preserving fertility.

Testicular injuries are divided into three broad categories based on whether cause of injury is blunt trauma, penetrating trauma, or degloving trauma, which involves shearing forces acting on the skin and is typically seen in males from 15 to 40.

Blunt injuries account for 85 percent of testicular injuries and penetrating injuries make up the majority of the rest. Most injuries are unilateral. In most cases, blunt trauma to the testicles is minor and requires only conservative treatment. Such injuries are reported in kick boxing, baseball, paintball, mountain biking, rugby, and hockey (usually when players are hit with a stick). Penetrating injuries are extremely rare in sports and are more common in auto accidents and work-related injuries. In athletics, testicular degloving injuries are rare due to the use of protective gear (such as a cup) but they can occur. In soccer, for example, a slide tackle gone wrong can catch the scrotum between the ahtlete's body and the turf, causing part of the scrotum to separate and tear.

Identification

The athlete typically has extreme pain in the scrotum, frequently associated with nausea and vomiting. Imaging tests such as MRI are required for specific diagnosis. Imaging determines the specific area of scrotal trauma, and evaluation by a urologist is essential.

Treatment

Treatment is either self-limited or surgical, with little range between.

Return to Action

If there is mild trauma without tissue tearing or functional loss, the athlete will be cleared to return to play by the urologist when symptom free. Following surgery, the athlete will be cleared by the surgeon for return to play after appropriate healing, which usually takes at least six weeks. Most players who sustain testicular injury are more susceptible to such injuries in the future. Use of an athletic protective cup is recommended.

BLADDER, KIDNEY, OR URETER INJURY

Common Causes

The most common cause is direct trauma during contact sports. Contact or collision sports are the usual culprits. However, falling from a bike, horseback riding, and simple jogging all can cause bladder or kidney damage.

Identification

Symptoms for these injuries include severe pain in the flank or lower back, nausea, vomiting, swelling of the abdomen, blood in the urine, fever, and shock. The kidney is the most commonly injured organ followed by the bladder, urethra, and ureter (tiny tubes that connect the kidneys to the bladder).

History is important in diagnosing this particular problem. Has the athlete previously experienced such problems? Did the athlete fall from a distance? Was there a direct blow to the flank region? These injuries may cause bleeding, either internally or in the urine. Specific diagnosis requires blood and urine tests, X-rays, CT scans, MRI, and other tests.

Treatment

Bladder injuries involve contusions and a small amount of blood in the urine, requiring no treatment. Most minor bladder and kidney injuries simply require healing time, usually a period of four to six weeks. There is no particular treatment required other than repeat blood and urine tests to assure medical stability. If the injury caused an internal laceration or tear, immediate surgery is required. Internal injury is diagnosed by imaging studies such as MRI or use of a cystoscope (a camera tube inserted through the urethra and into the bladder).

The severity of injury to the bladder, kidney, or urethra will be graded primarily on the findings of diagnostic tests. Most commonly, these injuries are low grade and include contusion, hematoma (collection of blood under the capsule of the kidney), or small laceration of the kidney, bladder, or uretal wall. Athletes with a low-grade injury usually manage with rest and observation. Athletes with more severe and less common injuries might require close observation in a hospital and surgery.

Return to Action

Due to the nature of these injuries, a prolonged healing time, typically a few months, is prudent. Return-to-play time is at least three months. No special rehabilitation program is required.

CHAPTER 10

Lower-Back Injuries

Stuart Kahn, MD; Arjang Abbasi, DO

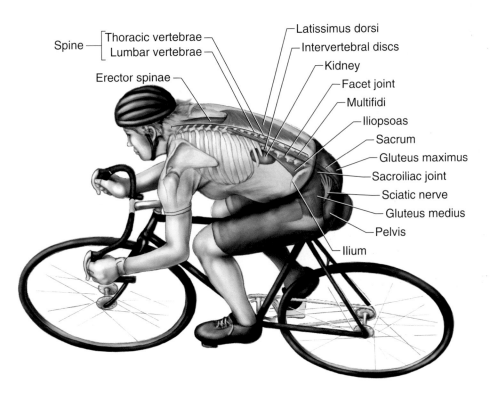

Injuries of the lumbar and thoracic spine are common in the athlete. It is estimated that 9 percent of all sport-related injuries involve lower-back pain. In the United States, 50 to 80 percent of the general population will have at least one episode of lower-back pain in their lifetime. In professional sports, lower-back pain is the most common reason that athletes miss a game, match, or contest. Over 90 percent of incidences of back pain are self-resolving (i.e., they heal themselves), so the exact incidence of thoracic (mid-back) and lumbar (lower-back) spine disorders in athletes cannot be determined.

Pain related to the middle to lower back can be generated by muscles, ligaments, discs, nerves, joints, or organs. There are 12 thoracic and 5 lumbar vertebrae. The vertebrae connect to one another through intervertebral discs and facet joints, allowing stability of the spinal column during motion. In this chapter we discuss the major causes of back pain related to common injuries in athletes. To maximize performance and minimize injury, athletes should understand the basic diagnostic criteria and preliminary treatment options.

Lower-Back Injuries

LUMBAR AND THORACIC AREA CONTUSION

Common Causes

Contusion, commonly called a bruise, occurs frequently in the lumbar and thoracic area, especially in contact sports or sports involving falls at high velocities. Muscle and soft tissue contusion occurs as a direct result of focal trauma to the tissues. This can occur in contact sports such as rugby, American football, boxing, or martial arts or during a fall or when accidentally running into a blunt object while playing a noncontact sport. The force of the blunt trauma, if great enough, causes injury to the soft tissue, stemming from the rupture of the cells.

Identification

While pain from a lumbar sprain or strain (see p. 152) peaks after about 24 hours, the localized pain from a contusion progressively worsens over the course of a few days. Pain is generally described as dull and nonradiating and is exacerbated by touching the area. Look for evidence of a bruise and tenderness in a specific area or signs of redness or black and blue discoloration (called ecchymosis).

Treatment

The treatment regimen is similar to the treatment for lumbar sprain or strain, including ice and anti-inflammatory medication initially. If the contusion or tenderness does not abate within a few days, consult a physician for further evaluation, including X-ray or other imaging, because serious injuries, such as organ damage, spleen rupture (p. 146), bone damage, and rib fracture (p. 142) can occur as a result of a contusion. Also, be aware that organ damage might mimic back pain. A collapsed lung and kidney contusion are prime examples; the athlete may feel discomfort in the flank area (in the lower back below the bottom of the rib cage) or in the chest. Physician consultation is critical if pain does not subside within a few days or in the case of accompanying abdominal pain.

Return to Action

Following a contusion affecting a ligament or muscle, the athlete may return to exercise or sports as soon as he or she has normal range of motion and is pain free. Typically, the return to play takes longer for an athlete involved in a contact sport than for an athlete in a noncontact sport. If there is no suspicion of flank injury, return to sport may occur in three to six weeks. If there is a significant flank injury and organ damage is suspected, the athlete may be out for several months as determined by the physician.

LUMBAR SPRAIN OR STRAIN

Common Causes

A sprain is a ligament injury caused by overstretching the ligament. A strain is a muscle injury involving a tear of the muscle fibers caused by overstretching. Pain from a sprain or strain is a result of the tissue being stressed beyond its pliable range. A sprain or strain can occur in almost any sport, from a contact sport such as rugby to a noncontact sport such as bowling. As previously mentioned, the lumbar and thoracic regions of the spine contain many layers of ligaments and muscles, so it is often difficult to determine the exact ligament or muscle in which the sprain or strain has occurred. Sprain/strain is the most common cause of mid- and lower-back pain in the athlete and is most commonly seen in individuals from ages 20 to 40.

Identification

Symptoms of a lumbar sprain or strain generally begin during an athletic event and grow worse over a 24-hour period. An increase in discomfort is often felt the day after the inciting injury. The most common symptoms are pain, stiffness, and spasm in the lower back accompanied by occasional radiating pain into the buttock. In this case, the pain radiating into the buttock is called referred pain and may or may not be caused by nerve irritation. Tenderness is usually felt in a small area of the lower back. Pain is exacerbated by certain activities, including bending or arching the back, and is typically improved by sitting or lying down.

The largest muscles of the back, the erector spinae, run longitudinally along the spinal column and aid with extension (leaning backward). Other major muscles, such as the multifidi group, sit more deeply and nearer to the vertebrae, run laterally, and aid mostly with rotation and stability of the lower back. The smallest and deepest muscles of the spine run within shorter lengths and, for the most part, provide stability to the region along with the ligaments. The muscles of the abdominal wall and iliopsoas are responsible for anterior stability and flexion.

Treatment

The initial treatment for any sprain or strain includes applying ice to the painful area three or four times daily. Each time, the ice should be applied in five-minute increments—five minutes on and five minutes off—for approximately 30 to 60 minutes. If the athlete has no allergies or previous gastrointestinal sensitivity to such medications, an over-the-counter anti-inflammatory such as ibuprofen and an analgesic such as acetaminophen might be useful to alleviate pain and discomfort. These steps will assist in reducing inflammation. In general, relative rest—that is, avoiding activities that exacerbate the pain—is preferred to bed rest. A physician should be consulted if pain does not improve within 48 hours or if there is loss in sensation in the buttocks area, sensory loss, weakness in the lower limbs, or loss of bowel or bladder control. In general, no X-rays are necessary for the first month if the injury is not traumatic or significant.

Once serious injuries are ruled out, other treatments such as a more potent prescription anti-inflammatory medication, muscle relaxants, physical therapy, osteopathic manipulation, chiropractic treatment, and acupuncture may be added to speed the recovery process. Physical therapy focuses on stretching exercises for the leg and lower-back muscles to restore a normal lumbar curvature and strengthen the abdominal and lumbar muscles. Ice, ultrasound, and electrical stimulation may be used as needed to reduce pain and inflammation. Exercises that focus on strengthening the core muscles and improving flexibility can further stabilize the spine and help prevent future injuries.

Return to Action

Once a full range of motion and simple activities of daily living can be accomplished without pain, the athlete may return to cross-training and sports activity, with pain as the limiting factor. Return to play typically occurs three to six weeks after the injury.

HERNIATED DISC

Common Causes

Lumbar herniated discs are rather common in athletes, particularly for those between the ages of 20 and 35. Sports that involve heavy lifting combined with bending and twisting pose the highest risk for herniated and injured discs. Athletes in throwing sports and twisting sports such as tennis, golf, American football (quarterback position), and baseball (pitcher) are also at risk. Sports with extreme forward bending such as yoga and gymnastics also pose a high risk for these injuries.

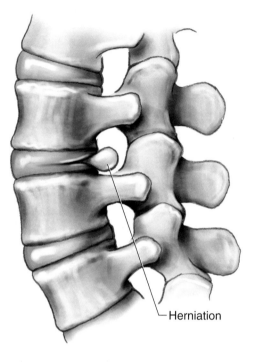
Herniation

The intervertebral discs are made of a fibrous band of material along the periphery called the annulus fibrosis and a central gelatinous material called the nucleus pulposus. These discs function as shock absorbers and prevent direct bone-on-bone contact of the vertebral bodies. A disc is herniated when a disruption of the annulus fibrosis allows the gelatinous material from the nucleus pulposus to either bulge into the annulus or to ooze out (like jelly from a jelly donut). The protrusion of the disc causes irritation of the nerve root, either from the disc directly pressing on the nerve or from inflammation of the nerve root caused by chemicals released in response to the herniated disc.

Identification

Typically, athletes with a herniated disc are more comfortable standing than sitting. Pain is often worse on one side and may radiate down the leg. Athletes tend to lean on the painless leg and favor the nonpainful side to reduce pressure on the disc. Pain is usually worse when sitting and improves when standing and walking (the opposite is true when the disc is herniated in the area known as the foramen). Complaints also include leg pain, weakness, and numbness. Physical exam maneuvers that duplicate radiation of pain into the affected leg are helpful in confirming the diagnosis.

Most discomfort related to a disc herniation is likely caused by inflammation rather than direct pressure of a disc on a nerve. Pain radiating into the lower extremity, numbness, or weakness is consistent with a herniated disc. If an athlete has back pain radiating into the legs with associated weakness, or if any of certain cardinal warning signs are present, a physician should evaluate the athlete as soon as possible as these symptoms indicate radicular pain or sciatica and may signify a significant disc problem. The cardinal warning signs are loss of bladder or bowel control, intractable pain, and progressive loss of neurologic function, i.e., rapidly progressing weakness.

HERNIATED DISC

If symptoms of lumbar disc herniation persist, the best method to evaluate the degree of herniation and the compression of the nerve root is via MRI. However, the appearance of the spine on MRI does not necessarily correlate with the degree of disability; people sometimes have herniated discs revealed via MRI yet are not symptomatic. MRI often is too sensitive and picks up things which are not clinically significant. But when symptoms *do* correlate with the findings on MRI, there is likely an association between disc herniation and symptoms.

Treatment

Various methods can treat an acute disc herniation with signs of sciatica (pain traveling from the lower back or buttocks region into the lower limb). If a short rest and mild analgesic or anti-inflammatory medications do not alleviate symptoms, a physician might place the athlete on oral steroids to reduce inflammation of the nerve root; the physician might also prescribe muscle relaxants and analgesics to control pain. The athlete is then reevaluated within a week, or sooner if pain or neurologic symptoms worsen. Symptoms of concern include the cardinal warning signs mentioned previously. If any of these occur, the athlete should immediately consult a spine surgeon or neurosurgeon.

If symptoms begin to improve and there are no special concerns, the athlete may begin exercising and start a course of physical therapy that focuses on extension-based exercises to reduce pressure on the disc. Abdominal and lower-back strengthening and stretching should help restore normal function. If symptoms fail to improve, if there is persistent pain and dysfunction, or if any signs of weakness in the legs occur, an epidural steroid or nerve block injection, under X-ray (flouroscopy), along with continued physical therapy might be attempted. If the athlete still shows no improvement with this conservative treatment, surgery might be considered to remove part of the disc.

In the rare event that an injured athlete has a sudden onset of bowel or bladder incontinence or saddle anesthesia (numbness in the buttock region), MRI, steroids, and possible emergency surgery might be indicated. This is a sign of a serious neurologic condition in which the herniated disc has compressed the nerves in the spinal canal that supply the lower parts of the body. The only treatment in this instance is rapid surgical decompression of the disc. Early surgery is advocated only with this condition or with progressive neurologic deficits.

Return to Action

Return to sport-related activity depends on the symptoms. The athlete should be pain free and should have undergone physical therapy including progressive cross-training, strengthening, and a return-to-sports program. The athlete needs to continue performing a home exercise program created by the physical therapist with the aim of strengthening the core muscles, maintaining flexibility, and relieving pressure from the spine to reduce the chance of recurrence of the symptoms. With conservative treatment for a herniated disc, the athlete can resume competition in approximately six to eight weeks. With surgical decompression, the athlete is usually out for the season or for at least three months.

ANNULAR TEAR

Common Causes

Annular tears are caused by disruption of the annulus fibrosis (the outer disc layer) without a frank disc herniation (see p. 154). Annular tears can occur in the same sports as herniated discs but are more common in twisting and torque injuries and nonviolent flexion injuries. You often seen annular tears in athletes involved in tennis, golf, yoga, or Pilates.

Identification

Athletes with annular tears generally experience axial (local), nonradiating lower-back pain. Pain is generally exacerbated by prolonged sitting, which causes pressure on the disc. Pain is generally worse when bending forward. No neurologic deficits (weakness, loss of sensation, or leg pain) are noted. A few tests to stress the discs might reproduce the symptoms. Any activity that takes the pressure off the disc, such as lying down, might improve symptoms. MRI is the most likely imaging mode to show an annular tear but is not foolproof. The gold standard for diagnosis is *discography*, in which a needle is inserted into the suspect disc and a mixture of fluid containing dye is injected into the disc. If the pain is reproduced by injection of fluid into the disc, and a tear is visible, a diagnosis of annular tear is confirmed.

In a less forceful disc injury, the outer disc layer (annulus fibrosis) might not be completely torn open but only the internal half. This creates a tear in part of the disc that contains a nerve that carries pain signals to the brain. In this case the pain is not from the nerves in the spinal canal or material causing pressure on the sciatic nerve roots but from the disc itself.

Treatment

First, treat the athlete to reduce pain. Medication, rest, and physical therapy, focusing first on pain reduction and afterward on nonpainful posture, is most beneficial. Follow up with core- and extension-based strengthening, stabilization of the lumbar spine, and long-term stretching. Medication may be prescribed to manage symptoms. If symptoms persist, more invasive approaches may be considered, such as a para-vertebral nerve block, epidural steroid injection (although this is not as effective as for a herniated disc), or minimally invasive intradiscal procedures. These injections are done by skilled clinicians who inject both an anesthetic agent and a cortisone preparation, under X-ray (flouroscopy), directly into or adjacent to the spinal canal; they are relatively minor procedures. Surgery is a last resort.

Return to Action

The criteria for returning to play and exercises prescribed to avoid recurrence of symptoms are similar to those for disc herniation (see p. 155) Annular tears can be more difficult to treat because they can be persistent, whereas the sciatica from a herniated disc tends to abate.

TRANSVERSE PROCESS FRACTURE

Common Causes

The transverse process (the bony protrusion on either side of the arch of a vertebra) is a part of the bony spinal column, which is a ridge of gray matter in each lateral half of the spinal cord—also called the dorsal column. Posterior column fractures are usually caused by direct trauma. These injuries are common in contact or collision sports especially those in which contact is made on the back (American football, rubgy, hockey and falls that occur in in-line skating and horseback riding).

Identification

Transverse process fractures are stable fractures that usually have no neurologic symptoms. The direct impact that caused the fracture, however, might have been sufficient to cause organ

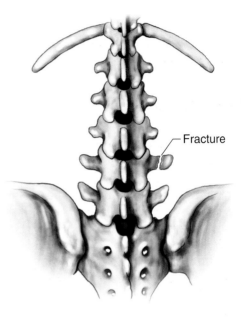

Fracture

damage. This depends on the level of the spine fracture. If it occurs in the upper spine area, the lungs, aorta, or pancreas may be affected. A fracture in the lower area may put the kidney or bladder at risk. Direct organ injury from transverse process fractures is rare. Nonetheless, it is crucial to assess any signs of abdominal discomfort. Ask the athlete if he or she has difficulties with urination (e.g., blood in the urine), which may be caused by kidney injury (see p. 146). Fractures are generally apparent on X-rays, but if the diagnosis is questionable, a CT scan might need to be performed. Physical examination reveals tenderness over the fractured area and sometimes a bruise is apparent. Pain may adversely affect spine motion. There typically is no neurologic damage.

Treatment

The treatment regimen consists of ice, analgesics, a soft brace, and physical therapy. The goals of physical therapy are to reduce pain, restore motion and strength, and improve flexibility.

Return to Action

Once pain is managed well enough that the athlete is able to move, begin gradual reconditioning. As pain subsides, the athlete can start sport-specific exercises with the goal of regaining complete range of motion and returning to participation once pain free. Clearance to resume participation is withheld if organ damage is present. The healing of the fracture takes approximately six to eight weeks for young athletes and three months for weekend warriors and older athletes.

COMPRESSION FRACTURE

Common Causes

Compression fracture is a fracture of the vertebral body in the anterior bony spinal column. It is caused in athletics by significant trauma that suddenly flexes the thoracic or lumbar spine. The flexion (forward bending) force is so great that the vertebral body collapses in upon itself. Fortunately, fractures of the spine are not common in sports. Sports in which you might see these injuries include tackling sports such as rugby and American football; falling sports such as horseback riding, gymnastics, and track and field; and sports that involve high-velocity crashes in which athletes might land in a flexed position (skiing or cycling).

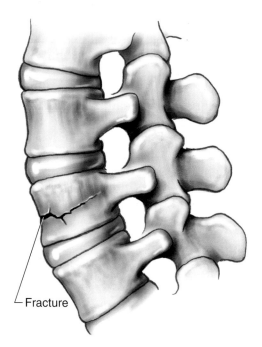

Fracture

Identification

The athlete with a compression fracture has constant severe pain that is made worse with nearly any motion but especially with extension. Usually, no neurologic deficits are seen after a compression fracture, unless there is a retropulsed bone fragment (a fragment that travels near the spinal cord). In the event of transient paralysis of the leg during the trauma or neurologic findings such as numbness, tingling, or weakness in the legs, consult a physician to rule out spinal cord injury. Diagnosis is made by X-ray.

Treatment

Thoracic compression fractures in which less than 50 percent of the height of the vertebra is lost are treated with analgesics for pain control and 6 to 12 weeks of bracing in an extension brace that does not allow the spine to bend forward. In some cases, compression fractures greater than 50 percent of the height of the vertebra might require surgery, kyphoplasty, or vertebroplasty; in the latter two techniques a balloon is inserted into the collapsed vertebra and is then inflated with material to increase the vertical height of the vertebrae.

Return to Action

Rehabilitation focuses on a return to a full range of motion without pain. Strengthening of the core muscles and reconditioning exercises should be included. For noncontact sports, athletes can probably return to play within 12 weeks if they have obtained full range of motion without pain. For contact sports, athletes should be advised of the risks of a repeat fracture and must weigh the risk-to-benefit ratio. Repeat fractures or further collapse of the vertebrae could cause postural changes and lead to painful conditions in the future.

BURST FRACTURE

Common Causes

Burst fractures are caused by a combination of axial (top to bottom) loading and flexion of the spine. In a burst fracture the force of the trauma causes the vertebrae to burst apart rather than to collapse upon itself, as happens in a compression fracture. Because of the type of fracture, a fragment of bone might lodge in the spinal canal, thus involving the anterior and middle columns of the spinal column. This is most severe when a bone fragment propels into the spinal canal and injures the spinal cord. Athletes at risk are those who play sports in which high-force blows to the spine occur. Rock climbers, horseback riders, American football players (especially those who might get thrown airborne), ski jumpers, and cliff divers are all at risk of burst fracture.

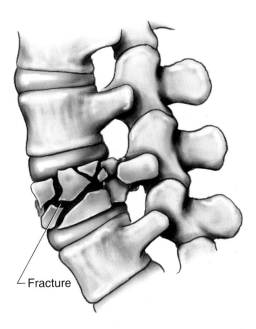

Fracture

Identification

Treat on-the-field spine injuries with great care and caution. These injuries should be viewed as emergencies. Any indication of weakness of the arms or legs or acute spine pain caused by trauma warrants immobilization on a spine board by trained professionals and immediate transfer to an emergency room. Athletes with a burst fracture that propels bone into the spinal canal will likely have spinal cord injury, which might leave them with paralysis of both legs and with bowel and bladder incontinence.

Treatment

Once at the emergency room, an athlete with a spinal cord injury will receive high-dose intravenous steroids, immediate MRI, and surgical evaluation. If a spinal cord injury has occurred and surgery is performed, the athlete will likely attend an intensive inpatient rehabilitation center to recover to the best functional level that neurologic impairment allows. When appropriate, a rehab counselor, physical therapist, or physiatrist can recommend a disabled athletic program; such programs are available in larger communities.

Return to Action

Recovery from surgery depends on the degree of nerve injury and can vary from full recovery to permanent paralysis. Healing requires a minimum of three to six months and most often is ongoing for several years or a lifetime. High-impact and high-risk sports are usually not permitted after these injuries.

SPONDYLOLYSIS AND SPONDYLOLISTHESIS

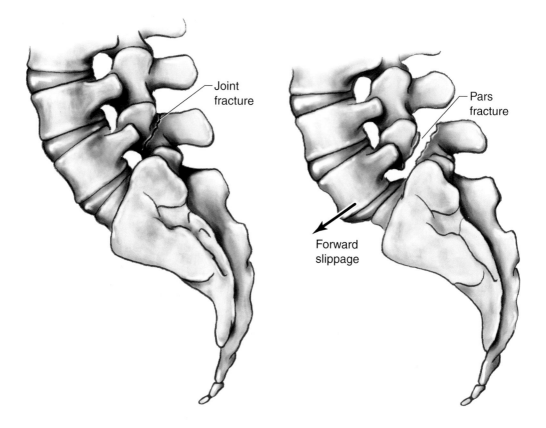

Joint fracture

Pars fracture

Forward slippage

Common Causes

Spondylolysis is a stress reaction or fracture of the joint between two adjacent vertebrae. The injury is caused by repeated hyperextension (bending backward) of the lumbar spine and is common in high-level athletes, especially gymnasts. It is more common in females than males. It most often occurs at the lowest lumbar segment (L5) or second-lowest lumbar segment (L4). Spondylolisthesis refers to forward (anterior) slippage of one vertebral body over the one below it. There are various types of spondylolisthesis, but in athletes the injury is usually caused by a fracture (specifically a pars fracture, and most likely a type of stress fracture) on both sides of a vertebral body.

Identification

Symptoms are generally described as a dull lower-back pain, occasionally radiating into the buttocks. Physical examination tends to reveal pain with extension with no evidence of neurologic deficits. Spondylolysis must be suspected in any athlete with extension-based pain who does not respond to conservative treatment, including analgesic and therapy, within a short time. Early evaluation of spondylolysis is crucial to prevent advancement of the stress reaction to a fracture. Because X-rays of the spine might not reveal findings early enough, a bone scan is often required if spondylolysis is suspected.

SPONDYLOLYSIS AND SPONDYLOLISTHESIS

Symptoms of spondylolisthesis are similar to spondylolysis, except in spondylolisthesis there is a history of occasional sharp radiating pain into the leg caused by irritation of the nerve because of the bony slippage. Spondylolisthesis can be detected on a plain X-ray. Flexion and extension X-rays are needed to assess if the degree of slippage changes with spinal motion, which is believed to be a much greater source of pain. Spondylolisthesis is categorized into grades I to V with each progressive number representing further anterior slippage of an upper vertebra onto the one directly below it. Surgical treatment is considered in grades III, IV, and V or if the athlete continues to experience pain radiating into the legs despite conservative treatment.

Treatment

Athletes with acute spondylolysis will be braced in an orthotic that prevents spinal extension until they are pain free for at least six weeks. The duration of treatment depends on whether symptoms are acute or chronic, the degree of pain, and whether there is a stress reaction or fracture.

Athletes for whom the problem is not caught early on might eventually develop chronic episodic recurring pain from spondylolysis or spondylolisthesis. These athletes will be treated with analgesics or anti-inflammation drugs (or both), muscle relaxants, and opioids, if needed. Physical therapy should focus on core stabilization, neutral spine pelvic floor strengthening, and biomechanics.

Return to Action

An athlete recovering from spondylolysis or spondylolisthesis is not allowed to participate in sports but may perform low-impact aerobic exercises such as bicycling with the brace. Physical therapy entails aerobic exercises as well as stretching of the lower-extremity muscles and core strengthening. Maintaining the routine core-strengthening exercises given by the physical therapist is important in preventing recurrent symptoms. Return to athletic participation after a diagnosis of acute spondylolysis or spondylolisthesis can range from 3 to 12 months, depending on the progress of healing and stability of the spine as assessed on follow-up X-rays. Return to sport is usually limited to a level of participation that does not exacerbate pain.

SACROILIAC JOINT DYSFUNCTION

Common Causes

The sacroiliac joint is formed by the articulation of the sacrum and ilium. Although the sacroiliac joint is not a part of the lumbar spine, pain from the sacroiliac joint can be very similar to lumbar spine pain syndromes. Sacroiliac joint dysfunction stems from a change in the position of sacrum on the ilium caused by an imbalance of the muscles attached to the pelvis, a ligamentous injury to the joint, a fracture of the sacrum or pelvis, or occurrences such as masses in the pelvis or pregnancy. Athletes, such as gymnasts and dancers, who jump, bend, stretch, and twist a lot are at risk for this type of injury.

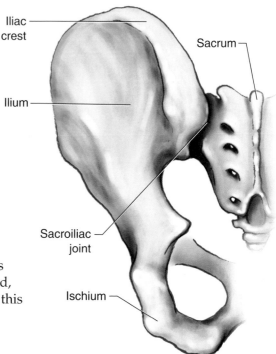

Identification

Athletes with sacroiliac joint dysfunction generally have pain and tenderness in the upper area of the buttocks. There is tenderness to touch at the sacroiliac joint. Pain might radiate into the lower buttocks, thigh, and down into the leg. Pain is worse with prolonged standing, sitting, turning on the side in bed, and stepping up on the painful side. Most often, an exam by a physician is sufficient for diagnosis. However, the gold standard test for diagnosis is performing a joint block. An anesthetic agent is injected into the sacroiliac joint. If pain subsides temporarily, a diagnosis of sacroiliac joint dysfunction is made.

Treatment

The initial treatment for sacroiliac joint dysfunction is rest and analgesics or anti-inflammatory medicine. Joint manipulation by a qualified practitioner such as an osteopathic physician, chiropractor, or physical therapist might help correct the muscle imbalance. Physical therapy that focuses on stretching of the muscles attaching to the pelvis, as well as strengthening the pelvic floor, abdominal, lumbar, and leg muscles, will also help. If symptoms do not improve, corticosteroids injections under X-ray guidance may be given. Some find relief with temporary use of a sacroiliac belt, which wraps around the hips to squeeze the sacroiliac joints.

Return to Action

The physical therapist should gradually increase activities and exercises during therapy sessions with the goal of preparing the athlete to return to sport-related activities. If no significant sacroiliac injury (fracture) has been identified and the athlete feels ready, he or she can return to sports as soon as one to two weeks after the injury. Stretching and strengthening exercises should continue long term.

FACET JOINT PAIN

Common Causes

Lumbar facet pain is caused by inflammation or arthritis of the facet joints (also known as zygapophaseal joints). Facet joints are located on the posterior aspect of the spine and they connect the posterior or rear portion of the adjacent vertebrae. The facet joint is a true synovial joint and when injured or inflamed can become swollen. This swelling can become large enough to cause pressure on the nerve root that passes through the joint. Athletes at risk for injuring facet joints are those involved in twisting activities, such as golfers, tennis players, and baseball pitchers.

Identification

Athletes generally complain of localized lower-back pain exacerbated by extension and rotation and relieved by flexion. Pain often radiates into the buttock on the same side. Diagnosis of facet joint pain is not always easy to determine. In such cases, diagnosis can be confirmed by a facet joint injection or blocking of the nerve that supplies sensation to the facet joint with an anesthetic agent.

Treatment

Initially treat facet joint pain with ice, analgesics, and anti-inflammatory medication. The athlete should avoid activities that cause pain. Spinal manipulation has been shown to help reduce facet mediated pain. These measures should be followed by physical therapy that focuses on strengthening the core muscles and stretching the leg muscles. Use ultrasound, ice, and moist heat to control pain. Avoid spinal extension at the early stages but introduce it as symptoms are controlled. The athlete needs to learn to use core muscles during activity to prevent hyperextension of the spine during motion and to avoid straining the facet joints. In cases in which these treatments do not resolve the pain, other procedures must be considered, including spinal-intervention procedures, such as fluoroscopic-guided facet injection or blocking and ablating the nerve that supplies the injured joint.

Return to Action

Athletes may return to sport once core muscles have improved to the point where there is no exacerbation of pain in practice and sport-specific training. This can occur in a relatively short period of time (two to three weeks) if only a synovitis is present but may take much longer (three months or more) if there are bony changes in the facet joint. Athletes with chronic facet pain may choose to continue to play sports but will need to modify their activity. If an athlete is willing to put up with a mild flare of pain for a day after sports and the condition is not deteriorating, there is no real health risk for continuing. Chronic patients sometimes preload with over-the-counter anti-inflammatory medications before an athletic contest.

LUMBAR DEGENERATIVE DISC DISEASE

Common Causes

Degenerative disc disease (DDD) occurs when one of the lumbar discs dries up and deteriorates so that the end plates or bones might rub against each other. This rubbing causes irritation to the remaining disc structures and can cause irritation of the bone. The pain is believed to emanate from inflamed fibers of the irritated disc. Although sports activities can aggravate the pain from DDD, they do not cause it. There is no specific cause. Clearly, people who have had a prior disc injury are at risk for having that disc deteriorate and become painful.

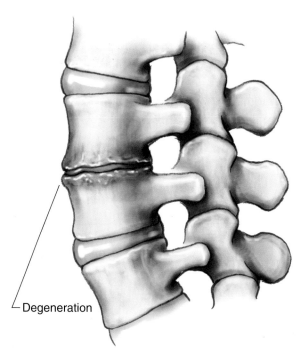

Degeneration

Identification

Athletes with degenerative disc disease experience tenderness in the lower lumbar spine. Pain is dull and might be located on one or both sides of the lower back; it may or may not radiate into the buttock. Pain is generally worse early in the morning, with stiffness and difficulty standing upright, and subsides as the day proceeds and returns at the end of the day. Spinal flexion might be limited by lower-back discomfort. Prolonged sitting is often uncomfortable. The pain is often not specific and difficult to describe. The condition can be confirmed by X-rays.

Treatment

Treatment of lumbar degenerative disease is similar to treatment for lumbar sprain or strain (p. 152). The most important factor in treating this condition is athlete education and maintenance of a core-strengthening and flexibility program.

Return to Action

The progression of therapy is guided by the athlete's pain and ability to tolerate activity. The athlete with lumbar DDD is prone to occasional bouts of severe back pain and thus needs to regularly perform core strengthening, lower-back and lower-extremity stretching, and extension-strengthening exercises to minimize recurrence of pain. All exercises for degenerative lumbar disease, including Pilates and yoga, need to be performed with caution. Avoid excesses of range of motion that might lead to aggravation. Modify yoga and Pilates to avoid forceful flexion exercises.

CHAPTER 11

Hip Injuries

Michael M. Weinik, DO; Ian B. Maitin, MD;
Ferdinand J. Formoso, DO

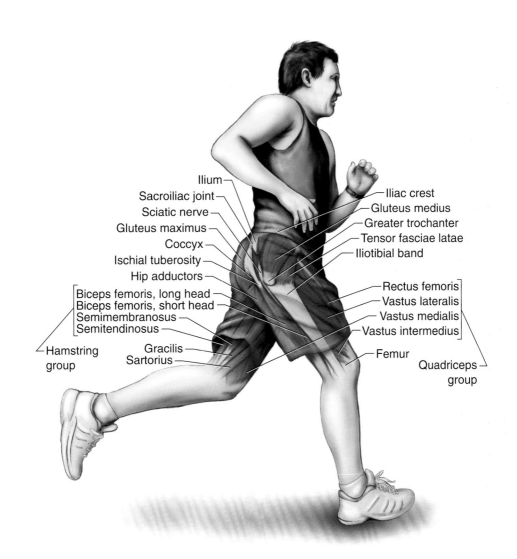

Ilium
Sacroiliac joint
Sciatic nerve
Gluteus maximus
Coccyx
Ischial tuberosity
Hip adductors
Biceps femoris, long head
Biceps femoris, short head
Semimembranosus
Semitendinosus
Hamstring group
Gracilis
Sartorius

Iliac crest
Gluteus medius
Greater trochanter
Tensor fasciae latae
Iliotibial band
Rectus femoris
Vastus lateralis
Vastus medialis
Vastus intermedius
Femur
Quadriceps group

The number of athletic injuries to the hip and pelvis in sports is low in general, ranging from 5 percent in the running athlete to 18 percent in hockey players. Amenorrhreic females may have a higher incidence of stress fractures, but males have higher percentages of injuries such as athletic pubalgia. As life expectancy increases for both sexes and the trend to remain physically active into later adulthood continues, it appears every athlete will have his or her fair chance of suffering a sports-related injury to the hip or pelvis. Nearly every competitive sport requires a strong contribution from the pelvis and hip.

Managing hip and pelvis injuries is difficult because the hip and pelvis are the coupling mechanism that transfers strength and power from the legs to the trunk and vice versa; they help absorb, dampen, and distribute the impact of running and jumping; and they provide the mobility to crawl, crouch, squat, bend, stand, and make every motion in between. Attached to the hips and pelvis are the largest and most powerful muscles in our bodies, which often act on the hip and pelvis with extremely long lever arms as created by the length of the legs and the height of the trunk. This fortunate anatomical arrangement allows the performance of amazing athletic feats but unfortunately places great physical demands on these structures, which sometimes leads to injury. In this chapter we discuss the more common injuries to the hip and pelvis in athletes and strategies to avoid and treat them.

Hip Injuries

ADDUCTOR TENDINOSIS

Common Causes

Tendinosis of the lower limb is quite common in athletes because of the elevated level of strain exerted on this limb during many sports. Although traditionally categorized as a tendinitis, which implies an inflammatory process, many clinicians now regard these injuries as resulting from a degenerative process. Adductor tendinosis is usually a chronic injury associated with repetitive strain of the muscular origin of the hip adductors. Microtears at the muscular origin might also occur that are not large enough to cause bleeding, and thus do not initiate healing, which chronically adds to the condition. Adductor tendinosis typically begins as a mild injury that is not properly rehabilitated or responds poorly to rehabilitation, and as the athlete continues to compete, the once-mild injury leads to loss of function. After a certain point, even minimal stress on the tendon origin produces pain. In an effort to minimize pain, the athlete adjusts his or her movements, which leads to localized weakness at the injury site, which ultimately ends in loss of endurance. Lower-limb tendinosis tends to be sport specific, with most hip injuries occurring in kicking athletes, hockey players, gymnasts, and horseback riders.

Identification

The diagnosis of adductor tendinosis is made primarily by the athlete's medical history and a physical examination in which tenderness is noted along the musculotendinous origin of the hip adductors, along the inferior edge of the pubic bone (in the upper thigh and groin). If the diagnosis is still in question, ultrasound or MRI might be useful in pinpointing the location and extent of injury.

Treatment

Traditional treatment for tendinosis includes physical therapy, analgesics, anti-inflammatory medications, and local injection of anesthetic and corticosteroid. If symptoms do not respond to this conservative approach after six months, surgery may be considered, which involves cutting through the principal tendon insertion and reattaching it into the pubis. Physical therapy typically consists of therapeutic massage, stretching, transcutaneous electrical nerve stimulation (TENS), and active strengthening of the hip musculature. Unfortunately, active physical therapy has been shown to be very helpful for only about one-third of athletes. The effectiveness of anti-inflammatory medication has not yet been proven. The injection of local anesthetic and corticosteroid usually gives only short-term relief of symptoms. As if treatment results were not grim enough already, another study (Akermark and Johansson 1992) showed that only 63 percent of athletes returned to their previous level of ability after surgery.

Although traditional treatments for this injury have been lackluster, the future holds promise that, with the help of physiatry, biomechanical abnormalities will continue to be identified and emerging modalities will prove to be more effective.

Return to Action

Athletes may return to action once symptoms have subsided, which might take up to six months. The rate of failure to return to previous level of ability can be as high as 25 percent. No significant bracing or taping options are available.

OSTEOARTHRITIS

Common Causes

Osteoarthritis (OA), sometimes called degenerative joint disease, is estimated to affect 12 percent of 25- to 75-year-olds in the United States. OA of the hip is typically a noninflammatory disease process characterized by destruction of the end of the femur bone as it attaches to the hip socket along with deterioration of the hip socket in which the femur bone rests. The loss of the articular hyaline cartilage surface of the bone as it wears down causes a narrowing of the joint space, subchondral cyst formation, and the development of marginal bone growth, otherwise known as osteophytes. The exact cause of these pathologic changes is uncertain, but physiologic and biomechanical factors such as age, obesity, genetics, joint alignment, joint laxity, and muscle weakness likely have a role in the disease process.

The condition is often aggravated by repetitive hip movements and strenuous prolonged physical activity involving standing, walking, running, climbing, and squatting. Athletes who participate in sport activity that requires single-limb support or pivoting of the hip joint, such as tennis, other racket sports, or track and field events, may have a particularly high incidence of OA-related pain. Episodes of single-limb support during sports can cause forces up to 14 times the body weight to be transferred through the lower limb. In a person with slowly developing hip OA that is asymptomatic during everyday activities, symptoms might be elicited in situations in which the hip is put under unusual stresses.

Identification

The typical symptoms of pain and stiffness most often occur after a period of inactivity, although OA of the hip usually has an insidious onset of symptoms, with a gradual escalation of pain that might become truly noticeable only during sports. Pain can be located in the groin, or laterally in the hip region, and might radiate down the thigh or even into the knee. Hip pain from OA is often relieved significantly with rest. Athletes with severe symptoms from OA might also report weakness in the hip muscles.

Diagnosis is typically made by a standard hip X-ray, which is ordered if the physician suspects OA based on physical examination findings such as limited passive hip range of motion and pain with movement, particularly internal rotation.

Treatment

Treatment begins with a conservative regimen consisting of some or all of the following: lifestyle modification, physical therapy, nutritional supplementation, and pharmaceuticals. In patients who are overweight, weight reduction can be one of the most important factors in relieving symptoms; in some patients, losing weight is enough by itself to relieve hip pain.

Physical therapy and an exercise regimen consisting of targeted muscle strengthening and improvement of coordination in conjunction with a stretching program can be quite effective in reducing symptoms. Use of heat and ultrasound at the affected region can also be helpful.

Analgesic medications, predominantly nonsteroidal anti-inflammatory medications (NSAIDs), are the mainstay of treatment for OA. Acetaminophen also works well for athletes with mild to moderate symptoms and athletes for whom NSAIDs are contraindicated or poorly tolerated.

If symptoms continue despite conservative treatment, intraarticular injection of cortisone (glucocorticoids) may be considered. According to the National Institutes of Health Consensus Conference, if moderate to severe symptoms or disability persist despite an extended course of nonsurgical management, total hip replacement is a reasonable option.

Return to Action

After treatment with conservative measures as described for three to four weeks, the athlete can slowly return to sport activity while being closely monitored for return of symptoms. If symptoms recur, the athlete should refrain from the inciting activity and return to the conservative regime of relative rest, physical therapy, and medications. Unfortunately, no significant taping or bracing options are available to treat hip OA, which underscores the importance of strengthening the hip muscles and stretching.

GREATER TROCHANTERIC BURSITIS

Common Causes

Trochanteric bursitis (bursitis of the hip) is relatively common, particularly in younger athletes. It includes inflammation of any or all of the bursae in the region.

Bursitis of the hip is often caused by changes in the attitude of the limb during activities such as adduction (movement of the lower limb toward the body) or internal rotation of the hip, which put the bursae under unusual stress, making them irritated and inflamed. Hip bursitis is commonly seen in long-distance runners. Bursitis is often associated with other pathologies of the lower limb, such as osteoarthritis (see p. 168), rheumatoid arthritis, iliotibial band tightness, and leg-length discrepancy. Tightness of the iliotibial band (ITB) also causes an increase in the compressive forces on the bursae against the greater trochanter, increasing the likelihood of irritation.

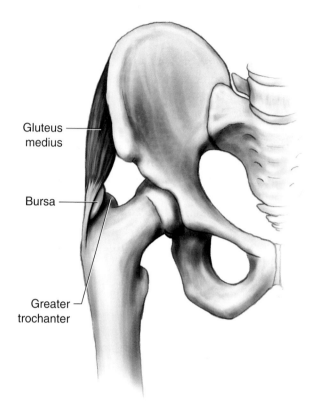

Gluteus medius

Bursa

Greater trochanter

Identification

The most common symptom of hip bursitis is lateral thigh pain that radiates down to the lateral knee. Night pain is common and individuals may not be able to lie on the affected side. Symptoms are exacerbated by activity such as walking, running, or climbing. This syndrome sometimes occurs acutely but most commonly progresses chronically.

No specific laboratory or imaging is needed to diagnose bursitis of the hip; typically, diagnosis is based on the athlete's history and a thorough neurological and musculoskeletal examination. An exam begins with an attempt to elicit tenderness with palpation over the greater trochanter; however, tender points might be present anywhere along the lateral aspect of the thigh. Forced passive adduction or active abduction (movement of the lower limb away from the body) and external rotation of the hip against resistance might make symptoms worse. The presence of iliotibial band tightness should be evaluated, as well as precise measurement of the leg lengths.

Treatment

Treatment options can be divided into musculoskeletal and pharmacological treatments. Musculoskeletal treatment includes relative rest, local heat, and therapeutic ultrasound for their analgesic properties and to facilitate stretching of the surrounding tissues; stretching exercises; correction of muscle strength imbalance; and correction of leg-length discrepancy (if present). Pharmacological treatment includes analgesic medications, anti-inflammatory medications, and corticosteroid injections (cortisone shots). For long-term success, both musculoskeletal and pharmacological treatments are usually needed. A plan that incorporates only pharmacological treatment ignores the structural pathology that caused the bursitis in the first place. That said, in some cases a correction of the musculoskeletal pathology is not possible, such as osteophytes (caused by osteoarthritis) irritating the bursae.

In the case of a mild hip bursitis, anti-inflammatory medications and rest might be all that are needed. In moderate to severe cases of hip bursitis, oral medication usually is not potent enough to take care of the inflammatory process. For these athletes it is necessary to perform a trochanteric bursa injection, which deposits a combination local anesthetic and cortisone directly to the involved bursa. When performed by a physician who can accurately access the inflamed bursa, this procedure is usually very effective.

Return to Action

The athlete may return to action once pain subsides, which typically occurs within a few weeks. Return should be slow and conservative. As is true of other hip injuries, there are no significant bracing or taping options.

ILIOPSOAS TENDINITIS

Common Causes

The iliopsoas muscle is the powerful thigh muscle that flexes the hip. It is one of the strongest muscles in the body. Iliopsoas tendinitis is an inflammation of the iliopsoas' tendon. Often, the inflammation spreads to the bursa, which rests next to the tendon, producing iliopsoas bursitis. Iliopsoas tendinitis is most common in runners, soccer players, gymnasts, and dancers who tend to perform repetitive hip flexion movements.

Identification

The most common symptom is pain in the front of the thigh, sometimes radiating down the thigh. A snapping sound or sensation may be noted as the tendon moves across the pelvis during hip flexion. Symptoms are exacerbated by activities that require repetitive hip flexion, including running uphill and kicking.

No specific laboratory test or imaging study is needed to diagnosis iliopsoas tendinitis, although ultrasound may be used to confirm the diagnosis. The diagnosis is typically made based on the athlete's history and a thorough neurological and musculoskeletal examination. Point tenderness over the iliopsoas tendon, and pain with resisted hip flexion is characteristic of the condition.

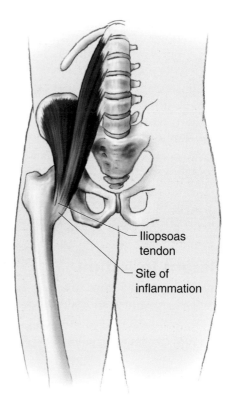

Iliopsoas tendon

Site of inflammation

Treatment

Intial treatment includes anti-inflammatory medication and avoidance of the offending repetitive motions. Ice may provide some relief, especially for very thin athletes as this tendon lies quite deep within the thigh. Physical therapy that incorporates a structured stretching and strengthening program can be helpful. In difficult cases, an injection of steroid and anesthetic can be performed under ultrasound guidance.

Return to Action

The athlete may return to action once pain subsides, which typically occurs within three to six weeks. Return to sport should be gradual. As with other hip injuries, no significant bracing or taping options are available.

ADDUCTOR STRAIN

Common Causes

The muscles of the medial thigh include the adductor muscle group and the gracilis. Adductor muscle strains are common in ice hockey and soccer but can be seen in all sports. Injury generally occurs following a sudden contraction of the adductor group with the thigh externally rotated and the hip abducted. Risk factors for adductor injuries include hip muscle weakness and imbalances (the adductors being weaker than the abductors), poor flexibility, and prior injury. These injuries are more likely to occur during the preseason and in athletes with less experience.

Identification

The athlete might experience the injury as a sudden painful event or a progressive, insidious development of pain. Pain is noted in the medial thigh or groin and is worse with adduction (pulling toward the midline of the body) against resistance. Tenderness at the musculotendinous junction generally occurs. Complete rupture results in a palpable defect or mass distal to the pubis. Avulsion injuries might occur, as might avulsion fracture of the origin of the adductor group. This is similar to a hamstring avulsion but involves a different muscle group with a different attachment site. Athletic pubalgia (see p. 182), osteitis pubis (p. 182), hernia (p. 186), and hip joint osteoarthritis (p. 168) should all be ruled out as possible sources of the groin pain. X-rays can rule out avulsion fractures and osteitis pubis. MRI can evaluate the possibility of other conditions and also localize and quantify the extent of muscle and other soft tissue injury.

Treatment

Treatment for adductor strains is similar to that for other muscle strains. The treatment starts with PRICE and the athlete using crutches if needed. Once pain subsides, the athlete can begin isometric exercises and then progress to isotonic exercises as tolerated. Ice and electrical stimulation are used throughout. Stretching is important and is done primarily to keep the muscle pliable and pain free, thus reducing risk of reinjury. Initiate jogging and sprinting as tolerated. If no pain occurs with straight running, begin pivoting and cutting activities. Surgical treatment (adductor tenotomy) may be considered if the athlete fails to improve after six months of physical therapy.

Return to Action

Athletes may return to play when flexibility and isokinetic testing of the injured leg is within 10 percent of the uninjured leg and when they can perform agility and sport-specific activities without difficulty. Return time can vary from one week for minor strains to six weeks or more for more severe strains.

Lisa M. Bartoli, DO, MS, contributed this injury text.

HIP LABRAL TEAR

Common Causes

The hip labrum is a cartilagenous extension of the bony acetabulum, adding depth and stability to the hip joint. Both nociceptive (pain) and propioceptive (position sense) free nerve endings exist in the labrum, accounting for the pain and perceived sense of hip instability when the labrum is injured. Labral tears often result from single traumatic events, such as a tackle in football or rugby, or a fall while skiing or cycling. They can also be caused by repetitive stress such as running or skating. Depending on the cause of injury, tears might develop along any area of the labrum.

Identification

Labral tears could cause pain in the lateral hip, anterior hip, medial groin, or even the buttocks, depending on the exact injury site. The anterolateral labrum is most commonly injured and should be suspected when the anterior labrum is stressed and produces either pain or a sense of instability when thrusting the hip forward, pivoting, or kicking. Suspect posterior labral tears when similar symptoms are elicited by pushing posteriorly through a flexed femur as when thrusting the hip backward. Active range of motion of the hip might produce a snapping sensation, which could be a result of a tight iliotibial band laterally or a hypermobile iliopsoas tendon anteromedially. Generally, if the hip is truly passively ranged (meaning the athletic trainer, physical therapist, or physician performs all the motion and the patient is at complete rest), these clicks are absent or less noticeable. However, should they persist or if range is restricted on passive motion, then an intraarticular injury such as a labral tear, chondral injury, or degenerative changes should be suspected.

Plain X-rays of the hip might prove helpful in identifying acetabular dysplasia, a condition in which the acetabulum, the cup-shaped portion of the hip joint, is irregular or abnormally shaped. Acetabular dysplasia allows abnormal and less constrained motion of the femoral head (the ball portion of the hip joint), which can stress the labrum and predispose an athlete to labral tears, osteitis pubis (p. 182), or osteoarthritis, which might mimic or accompany labral injuries. Magnetic resonance arthrogram, enhanced by a diluted contrast solution injected into the hip beforehand, has been shown to improve sensitivity of detection of labral tears over conventional MRI. Many labral tears fail to be detected and are found only on arthroscopic evaluation of the hip joint.

Treatment

Initial conservative treatments are often helpful in alleviating pain. Athletes should avoid activities that stress the labrum (e.g., pivoting and twisting on the hip) and excessive loading of the hip (e.g., squats and hip extensions). If pain is not relieved or range of motion not restored with these initial measures, a hip joint cortisone shot and use of a cane or crutches may be considered. A comprehensive course of six to eight weeks of rehabilitative therapies can help correct strength imbalances and flexibility deficits about the hip girdle, improve balance and proprioception, and identify errors in sport-specific activities or training programs that might have contributed to the labral injury.

Should the conservative measures fail to bring relief, surgical labral repair or debridement (the surgical removal of damaged tissues) must be considered. Pain relief is not the only reason to consider arthroscopic treatment of such tears. Some clinicians have postulated that hip labral injuries are similar to knee meniscal injuries in that the resulting incongruity of joint motion, subtle subluxation, and abnormal joint loading could predispose athletes to early arthritic changes of the joint.

Return to Action

Before athletes return to running or other fast-paced activities, they should have restored strength equal to the uninjured side. After surgical repair, depending on the demand of the sport and the degree of preoperative deconditioning, a return to competitive athletic activities could take up to six months.

ADDUCTOR CANAL SYNDROME

Common Causes

This syndrome involves compression of the superficial femoral artery at the level of the adductor canal (Hunter's canal). Compression of the artery occurs when an abnormal musculotendinous band arises from the adductor muscle mass. This might be either congenital or acquired as a result of training or an injury such as a kick to the inner thigh in soccer. This syndrome is very rare but is more common in young and athletic people than in other populations.

Identification

Athletes with this syndrome report worsening lower leg claudication (leg pain or fatigue from poor circulation), which is exacerbated by activity and relieved by rest. During physical exam, pulses are diminished or absent in the involved extremity. Arteriography is used to diagnose the occlusion of the superficial femoral artery at the Hunter's canal.

Treatment

Treatment involves surgical excision of the musculotendinous band compressing the femoral artery. If damage to the arterial wall has occurred, vascular repair might also be required. Following surgery, a rehab program is established that includes stretching, strengthening, and exercises to build endurance.

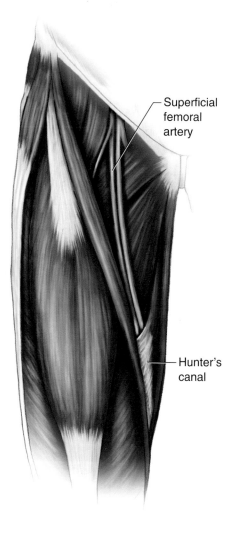

Superficial femoral artery

Hunter's canal

Return to Action

Return to sport depends on which and how much surgery has been done. Retraining can begin anywhere from two weeks to three months postsurgery and is overseen by the surgeon and a physical therapist.

Lisa M. Bartoli, DO, MS, contributed this injury text.

PELVIC STRESS FRACTURE

Common Causes

Because of the design and strength of the pelvis, it takes a great deal of force for a fracture to occur. Adolescents and amenorrheic women are most vulnerable to bony pathology of the pelvis. Stress fractures of the pelvis usually occur in the pubic rami (a group of four bones in the front of the pelvis) and are associated with long-distance running. Anorexic and amenorrheic female athletes are most vulnerable to pelvic stress fractures. The cause of injury is believed to be the repetitive pounding of forces transferred through the legs to the pelvis, making long-distance runners particularly susceptible.

Identification

Many stress fractures go undetected when athletes opt not to seek treatment for nonspecific pain. Most conditions improve with rest and analgesics. Complaints include pelvic and groin pain that gets worse with activity. Symptoms improve with rest. Many times exacerbations are associated with an increase in training activity. X-ray can detect stress fractures occasionally, but bone scan or MRI is more reliable. Stress fractures are most likely localized to the pubic rami but can occur elsewhere, including the neck of the femur.

Treatment

Treatment includes rest, analgesics as needed, and addressing the underlying cause of the injury. Nutritional and hormonal deficiencies should be corrected. If stress fractures recur, a thorough metabolic work-up is necessary. In females, bone density studies are recommended to check for underlying osteoporosis. Female athletes with stress fractures should be screened for the female athlete triad as an underlying cause; the triad includes amenorrhea, osteopenia or osteoporosis, and poor diet or disordered eating. If the triad is suspected, the athlete should be referred for counseling.

Return to Action

Athletes can usually return to action in four to six weeks. Activity should be ramped up gradually with modification of the regimen responsible for the damage. Preparation for return to sports should focus first on strengthening exercises and then on progressive increases in weight-bearing activities. Running mileage should start at 20 percent of the preinjury total and gradually increase over the course of the recovery period, usually several months.

PELVIC AVULSION FRACTURES

Common Causes

An avulsion is a tearing away. Avulsion fractures of the pelvis are seen primarily in adolescents and occur in three locations. Jumping sports such as basketball or volleyball can cause strong contraction of the sartorius muscle with an avulsion of the anterior superior iliac spine (the bump which can easily be felt over the front part of the hip region). Kicking sports such as American football or soccer with strong contraction of the rectus femoris can cause avulsion of the anterior inferior iliac spine (front part of the hip region just below the anterior superior iliac spine). Running sports may cause avulsion of the ischial tuberosity (the bone we sit on) with strong contraction of the hamstrings.

Identification

Symptoms of avulsion fracture include sudden onset of pain localized to the area of injury. Often the acute pain is associated with an audible snap or pop. Tenderness to the touch occurs over the fracture, and pain is elicited by range of motion of the hip.

Treatment

Treatment of fractures to the front part of the hip is conservative with analgesics, ice, and activity restriction until the fracture heals. Surgery appears to offer no advantage. Some controversy exists concerning appropriate treatment of ischial tuberosity avulsion fractures. Complications such as strength deficits and callus formation with pain have been reported with larger ischial tuberosity avulsions. Some physicians suggest that large fragments that are displaced more than one to two centimeters should undergo early surgical repair.

Return to Action

Athletes may return to their sport once they have recovered strength in the associated muscles and there is callus formation in the fracture. Isokinetic testing can be used to accurately compare strength, and X-rays can assess maturing callus. Return time is generally six weeks to four months.

SNAPPING HIP SYNDROME

Common Causes

A snapping hip can be caused by several pathologic processes that result in a characteristic snapping sensation when tendons in the hip region pop over bony prominences. Snapping hip occurs in runners, triathletes, cheerleaders, dancers, and occasionally recreational athletes. The snapping usually results from the iliotibial band (the muscle along the outer part of the thigh) moving over the greater trochanter (the bump on the outer side of the hip). Other causes include acetabular labrum tears within the hip joint, iliopsoas tendon snapping over the pectineal eminence, and intraarticular loose bodies. With all these conditions, motion creates a "bow string" effect, causing an audible or palpable snap or click.

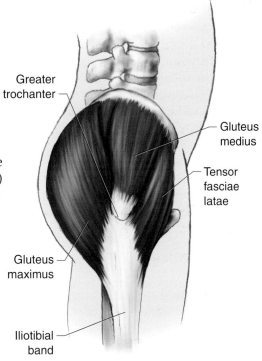

Greater trochanter

Gluteus medius

Tensor fasciae latae

Gluteus maximus

Iliotibial band

Identification

Snapping from intraarticular pathology will likely cause gait abnormalities and pain with weight bearing. If an athlete has significant pain or instability with hip range of motion, diagnostic imaging should be performed to rule out intraarticular bone fragments or a tear of the acetabular labrum. Extraarticular snapping may be felt over the greater trochanter with passive ranging of the hip or while walking. A trainer can walk with the athlete with a hand over the greater trochanter to detect any snapping. Secondary trochanteric bursitis causes tenderness over the greater trochanter and pain when lying on the affected side. Examination involves rotation of the hip while held in an adducted position to feel the iliotibial band snapping over the greater trochanter. Extending the hip from a flexed position might provoke snapping of the iliopsoas tendon over the pectineal eminence.

Treatment

Treatment for snapping hip focuses on stretching and strengthening of the hip abductors and adductors, hip flexors, and iliotibial band. The athlete should rest and avoid activities associated with the snapping. Anti-inflammatory medications might be required for pain or associated bursitis. Persisting problems might require cortisone shots into the bursa or region of snapping. Continued hip problems may require surgical repair.

Return to Action

With an aggressive and consistent stretching and strengthening program, most athletes will be less symptomatic and ready to return to activity in two to three weeks. Failure to improve in that time frame warrants corticosteroid injection and a referral to physical therapy for a formalized stretching program.

Common Causes

Hip pointers (also known as iliac crest pain) are contusions that occur along the pelvis, particularly the iliac crest's anterior and lateral hip area. This injury is generally caused by direct trauma to the iliac crest by another player (such as being struck by a helmet in American football, kicked by a foot in soccer, checked by a lacrosse stick, or hit by a pitch in baseball) or colliding with a hard playing surface (checked into the boards in hockey, tackled onto frozen turf, pushed to the basketball court, or sliding forcefully in baseball).

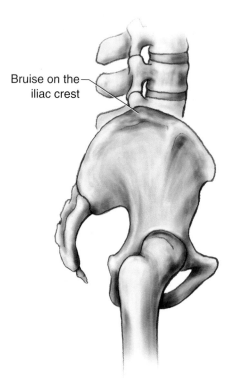

Bruise on the iliac crest

Identification

The hallmark symptom of hip pointer injuries is focal pain along the bony iliac crest, usually on the lateral side of the pelvis where it is covered by very little soft tissue. Hip pointers can also occur at any of the other bony prominences around the pelvis. Typically, the injured athlete reports pain while performing a sit-up or with resisted trunk rotation or resisted hip abduction (moving the leg out laterally away from the midline).

Swelling and bruising over the injury site usually indicates a more significant injury. Irritation to touch and severe bruising suggest an underlying fracture and warrant prompt referral to a physician for diagnostic evaluation. MRI best determines which structures are involved and to what degree, information that affects the design of a rehab program.

Treatment

Initial treatment includes prompt application of ice, alternating 5 minutes on and 5 minutes off, for 30 to 40 minutes four times per day. These applications should continue for 72 hours as needed for pain and to control superficial swelling and hematoma formation, and a compression wrap should be worn between applications. Gentle stretching of the hip muscles follows unless there is extensive bruising, in which case it is deferred for up to one week. Treatment by an athletic trainer or physical therapist might then include electrical stimulation to contract the injured surrounding muscle to reduce edema and retard atrophy. At 7 to 10 days postinjury, ultrasound may be added to promote deep warming of the injured tissues, making them more compliant to stretching and increasing blood flow to the region.

HIP POINTER

Occasionally, hip pointers are so severe that they make walking very painful. In such cases the use of crutches for protected weight bearing on the affected limb for a week or so often proves helpful. If extensive bruising occurs and a large hematoma is suspected, refer the athlete to a rehab physician or orthopedist. Large hematomas might benefit from early aspiration (withdrawing the pooled blood with a needle and syringe) to reduce tissue distension, promote more complete resorption, and speed healing.

Return to Action

Simple, small hip pointers might resolve within one week to allow comfortable weight bearing and full pain-free range of motion of the hip and trunk. In such cases, athletes may immediately return to play. More severe hip pointers, particularly those with associated hematoma formation or small tears of the surrounding muscle, can take two to four weeks to heal to the extent that motion is pain free and strength is returned to surrounding muscle. The affected iliac crest should be protected by viscoelastic or other compression-resistant padding for a month or so following the injury. On a limited basis (game day only), use of a long-acting anesthetic agent injected into the painful region might allow return to play earlier without risking much further injury. This is not recommended for high school athletes.

OSTEITIS PUBIS AND ATHLETIC PUBALGIA

Common Causes

Osteitis pubis is an inflammatory or degenerative condition of the pubic symphysis, the juncture where the right and left pubic bones meet in the front of the pelvis. Athletic pubalgia is another cause of pain in this region and is related to strains or tears of numerous tendons or weakness of musculature that attach and act on the pelvis, causing instability. Osteitis pubis and athletic pubalgia can occur independently, or one condition can influence the development of the other. By definition athletic pubalgia is a painful condition, but the degenerative changes of the pubic bones of osteitis pubis may or may not be painful.

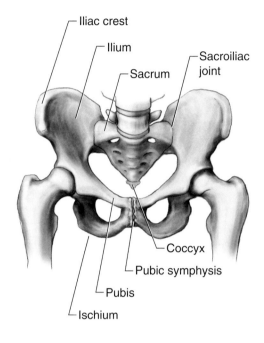

Iliac crest
Ilium
Sacrum
Sacroiliac joint
Coccyx
Pubic symphysis
Pubis
Ischium

Osteitis pubis and athletic pubalgia are frequently seen in athletes who play contact sports such as American football, rugby, and hockey and non-contact sports such as soccer, cross-country running and skiing, and figure skating. Athletic pubalgia is also seen in tennis, squash, and basketball players and, more rarely, swimmers.

The cause of injury in osteitis pubis is likely repetitive stress and shearing at the pubic symphysis when the pelvis is briefly supported on one leg and the other leg is swinging forcefully, such as when kicking a soccer or football, sprinting or cutting while running or during hockey or skating, and jumping in figure skating. Impaction of the pubic symphysis by a helmet or compression of the pubis by a forceful tackle or fall on one side are also possible causes of injury.

Athletic pubalgia is believed to arise more commonly in elite athletes who suffer strains or tears to the tendons that attach the abdominal muscles to the front of the pelvis, primarily the rectus abdominis tendon. This tendon might be injured through repetitive combined trunk rotation on an abducted and extended hip, such as while swinging a bat, or by a single forced extension (backward bending) of the trunk, such as when a running back is tackled full-on while changing direction (cutting) or when a quarterback has his back leg planted and is brought down by a head-on tackle. Similar trauma can occur when a hockey player is skating quickly toward the opposing goal and is forcefully "stood up" when checked by an opposing defenseman.

Identification

Osteitis pubis, when symptomatic, is indicated by a gradual onset of focal pain localized over the pubic symphysis. The pain might be accompanied by slight swelling but rarely any bruising unless the onset is associated with a direct blow to the region. Injured athletes with this condition report pain during attempts to walk briskly, jog, or run, and particularly with resisted hip adduction (the athlete attempts to cross his or her legs, and the physician, trainer, or therapist attempts to push the legs apart) or when lying on their back they lift one leg up against resistance. All these maneuvers place strain on the injured pubic symphysis, causing pain.

Athletes with athletic pubalgia typically have an acute, rather than gradual, onset discomfort in the mid- to lower-abdominal region initially and, if left untreated, might begin to experience pain in either or both medial thighs and inguinal (groin) regions. One theory suggests that tears of the abdominal rectus muscle tendon weaken and redistribute the balance of support the abdominal and hip girdle muscles have on the stability of the pelvic joints, thereby causing the adductor longus, gracilis, and other hip girdle and lower-abdominal muscles to strain to maintain pelvic stability. In rare cases, pain radiates to the perineum, the region between the genitialia and anus. Performing resisted hip adduction, double-leg lifts, or resisted trunk rotation will replicate the pain. Only 25 percent or so of athletes with athletic pubalgia have concurrent tenderness over the pubic symphysis, and 33 percent experience tenderness along the inferior portion of the pubis where the adductor tendons insert. On examination by a physician, the injured athlete might have pain and tenderness along the inguinal canal, but rarely is a true hernia found.

Diagnostic tests might include X-rays, which could reveal degenerative changes of the pubic symphysis indicative of osteitis pubis, or concurrent hip osteoarthritis, another cause of groin and medial thigh pain. MRI of the pelvis might reveal asymmetry or strain of the abdominal rectus muscles, inflammation or tear of the distal rectus abdominis tendon, irregularity or inflammation of the pubic symphysis, and other nonspecific findings, which when correlated could provide helpful information.

Treatment

Initial treatment for both osteitis pubis and athletic pubalgia involves rest from the offending activities (forceful side-to-side kicking, trunk rotation to extremes, sprinting, and jumping), acetaminophen or ibuprofen, and either intermittent ice or warm packs, as comfort dictates. This conservative treatment should last for up to 14 days. If the athlete is still in pain after that time, formal rehabilitative therapies should be started by a certified athletic trainer or registered physical therapist, or as prescribed by a physician.

Physical modalities such as ultrasound with concurrent stretching of the adductor muscles and the hip joint might help restore flexibility and motion to these structures, thereby reducing pull on the pubic symphysis and lower-abdominal muscles. Interestingly, therapeutic massage can be helpful to these conditions, presumably by further stretching of the fasciae and muscle, resetting the stretch reflex, and reducing edema in the affected muscles. Therapeutic massage may be added about four weeks postinjury. Should symptoms persist, a corticosteroid may be injected to the pubic symphysis in the case of osteitis pubis or to the proximal adductor tendon insertion on the lower portion of the pubic bone in the case of athletic pubalgia.

Once symptoms have subsided, reconditioning exercises may begin. Stationary cycling, water walking or jogging, and walking on level ground should be initiated. When the athlete can perform resisted hip adduction exercises on several consecutive

(continued)

days without immediate or residual next-day pain, then strengthening and balancing of the hip girdle and abdominal muscles may begin. The treating health care professional should take care to assess the entire leg from foot to hip and the abdomen and spine for strength, range of motion, and flexibility deficits because any weakness along this course (the kinetic chain) might result in persistent or recurrent injury.

Athletes begin initial strengthening exercises in a neutral position (hips and trunk aligned with no rotation) and both feet supported on the ground or training equipment. These exercises are followed by exercises allowing the limb off the ground. Finally running, cutting, and sport-specific training are added in succession as strength allows.

If athletes do not respond favorably to the treatment regimen described here within six to eight weeks, they should receive a thorough medical examination to rule out other causes of pain, including genitourinary infections, colorectal tumors, and occult hernias in either gender; endometriosis, ovarian cysts, or benign or cancerous uterine or ovarian tumors in women; and prostatitis or prostate or testicular tumors in men.

In rare instances the degenerative changes of osteitis pubis result in such significant instability of the pubic symphysis that surgical fusion is required. In cases of athletic pubalgia resistant to conservative treatment measures, referral to a general surgeon experienced in this condition is warranted for possible surgical repair and reattachment of weakened abdominal and pelvic floor musculature. For persistent medial thigh pain, a release of the adductor fascia (firm connective tissue that surrounds the muscle) is also performed. Rarely do abdominal braces or pelvic straps prove helpful in either osteitis pubis or athletic pubalgia.

Return to Action

Return to play is permitted when the athlete achieves a pain-free state both at rest and throughout each stage of the rehabilitative course. The athlete must be able to perform every aspect of the specific sport in practice at full effort before being allowed to return to competitive play. Rehabilitative efforts should extend beyond the return-to-play date to maximize core and hip girdle strength in hopes of preventing a recurring injury.

COCCYXGEAL FRACTURE

Common Causes

The coccyx, commonly called the tailbone, is comprised of four fused segments and is attached to the lowest portion of the sacrum by the sacrococcyxgeal ligament and to the pelvis by the sacrospinal ligaments. The coccyx maintains motion (albeit minimal motion) through a flexible fibrocartilaginous connection between itself and the sacrum. The coccyx is rarely injured except through direct trauma such as a fall onto a hard surface in the sitting position and landing squarely on one's buttocks or when struck by a swift-moving object such as a lacrosse ball, baseball, hockey puck, or shoe. A coccyxgeal fracture is not uncommon in gymnasts who fall onto the edge of a bar or balance beam, or in cyclists who hit their tailbone on the bar of the bike.

Identification

Fractures of the coccyx are generally associated with injury to the connecting sacro-coccyxgeal ligament. Fractures might be initially missed by X-rays because the fracture segments might not be displaced. MRI or a CT scan can provide a definitive diagnosis of fracture and surrounding soft-tissue injuries but is rarely needed unless pain symptoms persist for over a month. Dislocation of the coccyx also occurs due to trauma and may be seen clearly on X-ray. At the time of injury, athletes with a coccyxgeal fracture or dislocation will have moderate to severe pain along with bruising and swelling. Initially, simple walking can prove difficult because of pain, but this generally subsides within a day or so. The injured athlete is then left with pain in the region while sitting on firm surfaces or when pivoting at the hips. Some also find it painful to pass a large or hard stool for a few days or to wipe the rectum after a bowel movement. Wearing of a male dancer's belt and tight leotard can irritate this injury. Intercourse may also be temporarily uncomfortable.

Treatment

Treatment of this condition aims at reducing pain and swelling with ice compresses and over-the-counter pain relievers. Sitting with weight more forward on the ischial tuberosities or on a pillow, inflatable donut, or foam wedge with a relief cut out beneath the coccyx will be more comfortable than normal sitting. Sitting slumped backward tends to cause pain. If symptoms last longer than four weeks or continue to get worse, the athlete should see a physician. Persistent cases might benefit from an injection of an anesthetic and lidocaine. Manual therapies (via rectal exam) can be done to realign a malaligned coccyxgeal segment. This technique may be extremely helpful in reducing pain. Only in the most stubborn chronic conditions should the athlete refer to a surgeon for possible coccyx excision.

Return to Action

Return time is based solely on the athlete's tolerance to the pain. As long as the athlete does not repeat the same kind of fall, this injury will not be exacerbated by athletic activity.

SPORTS HERNIA

Common Causes

Sports hernia is a condition characterized by chronic groin pain caused by weakness of the posterior inguinal wall. The onset is usually slow and gradual, delaying diagnosis and treatment. Sports hernia is believed to have multiple causes, including shear forces across the pelvis, overuse, and muscle imbalance. Sports hernias are caused by a weakness in specific muscles within the abdomen. Even athletes with strong abdominal muscles are subject to a potential sports hernia because the hernia does not result from weakness in the thick muscle tissue, the rectus abdominis, but rather from abdominal wall tissue that is too thin. Confusion often exists between athletic pubalgia and a sports hernia. Specifically, a sports hernia occurs through a defect in the transversalis fascia or the conjoint tendon. Athletic pubalgia occurs because of a weakness of the rectus abdominis. The constant pulling, jumping, and twisting that occur in sports apply a repetitive stress on these congenitally thin tissues and may lead to a herniation or protrusion of tissue inside the lower abdomen. For instance, a defect in the transversalis fascia (the posterior barrier in the inguinal region) can allow the bladder oe bowel to protrude or push forward into the inguinal area.

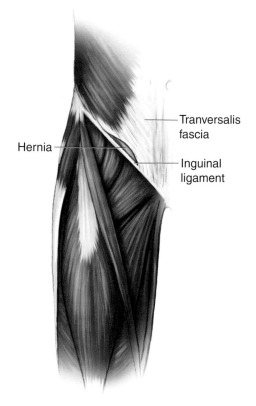

Identification

Symptoms associated with sports hernia include gradually worsening lower-abdominal or groin pain that might be confused with an adductor strain. In males, pain may be present in the testicle, commonly due to injury to the ilioinguinal nerve in the pelvic area. This nerve lies on the transversalis fascia and stretches when this tissue is stretched. Pain is exacerbated by kicking, running, cutting, or jumping and can radiate along the inguinal ligament, rectus muscles, adductors, and testicles. Valsalva, such as with cough, sneeze, or bowel movement, can worsen symptoms. Athletes might have tenderness of the groin and spasm of the adductors.

While many people think of a hernia as having a palpable mass that can be felt when coughing or bearing down, this is not always the case. More often, the mass is not palpable at all. A doctor must evaluate the symptoms and perform tests to rule out other potential causes of the symptoms before arriving at a diagnosis of sports hernia. An ultrasound is commonly used to diagnose a hernia.

SPORTS HERNIA

Treatment

Conservative treatment of sports hernias with PRICE and gradual return to activity is usually unsuccessful. Physical therapy can sometimes be helpful. If these conservative measures fail, surgical intervention can be considered. Surgical repair results in about 90 percent of athletes returning to full activity. Operative repair involves open or laparoscopic exploration with repair of the posterior inguinal wall defect. After surgery, stretching and strengthening regional muscle groups is imperative.

Return to Action

After surgery, athletes may return to sports once cleared by the operative physician. Return time varies widely, depending on the extent of surgery. Athletes might miss as little as six weeks and as much as six months of participation. Most athletes can return to action about six to eight weeks after surgical correction of the hernia. There should be only minimal discomfort, if any, upon return to activities.

SACROILIAC JOINT INJURY

Common Causes

The sacroiliac joint is made up of the lowest segment of the spine (the sacrum) and forms a joint with each of the adjacent iliac bones. The joint is held together by a very strong and diffuse complex of ligaments, which make the joint extremely stable. Injury to the sacroiliac joint might occur with an abrupt single trauma, such as missing a landing while skateboarding, snow skiing, or skating; being struck by a helmet in American football; or through repetitive trauma, such as in long-distance running, cross-country skiing, or rowing.

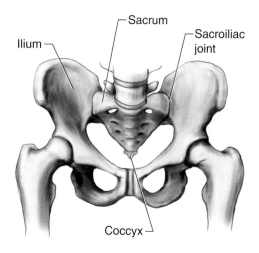

Identification

The sacroiliac joint helps transfer, absorb, and distribute the forces of impact from the ground that travel up through the leg and hip to the pelvis and on to the spine. During the act of running, several times the body's weight is generated in upward force each time the heel strikes the ground. Despite the partial absorption of these forces by the muscles and joints of the foot, leg, and thigh, there are still considerable forces acting across the sacroiliac joint. With repetitive activity, strain and injury to the ligaments and joint itself can occur. Injury can also occur to the sacroiliac joint when it is forced to bear heavy weight, such as while performing squats, or when subject to long-lever torsion stresses, as in lunging or hurdling and the sweeping high kicks of martial arts. Direct trauma to the joint is more likely to damage the joint surface, precipitating early osteoarthritis, and less likely to cause disruption of the ligaments, although minor malalignments can occur. Pregnant women (who have high levels of the hormone relaxin, which increases the elasticity of the pelvic ligaments in preparation for the delivery of a child) and individuals who have a hereditary hyperlaxity syndrome are more susceptible to injury of the sacroiliac joint.

The pain of this injury is usually located on one or both sides of the sacrum, just lateral to the central crease of the buttocks. The pain is usually dull but can be sharp if acutely injured and might radiate through the buttock and back of the thigh, even rarely continuing to the top of the posterior calf. Pain might also radiate around the thigh to the outer (lateral) portions of the groin. Unlike the pain of a pinch or inflamed lumbar nerve root, which has an often similar pattern of radiation, this pain is not associated with any numbness, tingling, or weakness other than pain-limited strength. Symptoms are generally worse with prolonged sitting and motions that cause the spine to extend (backward bending) because these increase load on the joint. The injured athlete might point to a small skin dimple (dimple of Venus) on the painful side of the sacrum or buttocks as the most painful spot in this condition. Unless the joint itself suffers direct trauma, bruising and swelling of the overlying soft tissues are frequently absent. In acute cases, pain can be exacerbated by hopping on the leg of the affected side or by brisk trunk and hip motions.

SACROILIAC JOINT INJURY

Treatment

Treatment of sacroiliac joint injuries begins with assessing the extent of injury to the joint and surrounding tissues. If the athlete cannot stand alone on the leg of the injured side of the joint without excruciating pain, or if extensive swelling or bruising occurs, the athlete should be evaluated immediately by a physician (because an underlying fracture of the sacrum or iliac bones might have occurred). If the athlete has associated numbness or tingling to the genital, rectal, or lower leg, an injury to the adjacent lumbar spine or sacral nerve roots should be suspected; again, the athlete should see a doctor. In the absence of these symptoms, apply ice compresses for up to 20 minutes each hour (five minutes on and five minutes off) for the first 72 hours and use acetaminophen or ibuprofen as needed. If running or other impact activities are the suspected cause of the injury, the athlete should avoid these activities until walking is pain free.

At this juncture, gentle stretching of the hip girdle muscles can begin to address flexibility deficits in the legs and pelvis and strength imbalance of the thigh and hip muscles, both of which adversely affect the function of this joint. Take care not to use the legs as long levers to stretch the hip girdle (sitting with legs stretched and feet resting on a stool or coffee table) because this puts too much strain on the joint. This also applies to the use of ankle weights, which when coupled with the length of the leg generates considerable strain on the sacroiliac joint. Hip girdle strengthening (including exercises such as bridges with the hips and spine aligned in neutral and planks) is excellent for strengthening the surrounding muscles.

If symptoms persist for a few weeks, the athlete should see a physician who is skilled in manipulation (osteopathic, allopathic, or chiropractic) or a physical therapist experienced in manual therapies. Such therapy can help in correcting any underlying malalignment, leg-length discrepancies, or associated muscular pain or spasm. In cases of hyperlaxity of this joint, the use of a sacroiliac joint compression belt might prove helpful in reducing symptoms and maintaining alignment. Should pain persist despite these measures, a sacroiliac joint corticosteroid and anesthetic may be injected with X-ray guidance to reduce pain and inflammation. Rarely, in chronic cases of this condition in which joint laxity persists, the injection of agents to purposely scar and tighten the ligaments (prolotherapy or sclerotherapy) is helpful. In instances of severe disruption of the joint, surgical fusion might be necessary, but such cases are rare.

Return to Action

Return to sports following a sacroiliac joint injury depends on symptoms when at rest and on the gradual gains made through prescribed exercise. Generally, flexibility deficits and strength imbalances should be corrected before the athlete attempts a return. Once he or she can do sport-specific activities without postexercise or delayed-onset pain, a return may be initiated. Runners and rowers should gradually work up to their preinjury distances over a course of weeks rather than days. Weightlifters should gradually increase their weights and should avoid single-leg squats for no less than a month after achieving a pain-free state. A sacroiliac joint belt or taping techniques might prove helpful initially for instability-related pain, but they cannot be counted on to reliably protect the sacroiliac joint from injury during running or other impact activities.

PELVIC NERVE INJURY

Common Causes

A traumatic blow to the abdominal wall sustained in a contact sport such as American football or rugby can cause a pelvic nerve injury, such as an affliction to the ilioinguinal nerve or genitofemoral nerve. Athletes might become symptomatic some time after the traumatic event when scarring or fibrosis develop. Less common nerve entrapments causing hip pain involve the cluneal nerve and lateral femoral cutaneous nerve (LFCN).

Identification

Symptoms of ilioinguinal nerve injury include burning pain over the lower abdomen that might radiate down the thigh and into the genitalia. Tenderness of the nerve as it passes medial to the anterior superior iliac spine might occur. Genitofemoral nerve injury can cause numbness or burning of the medial thigh or genitalia. Symptoms might be exacerbated by extension of the hip or thigh. Maintaining a flexed posture can alleviate these symptoms. Nerve blocks might be required for definitive diagnosis. Lateral femoral cutaneous injury can cause numbness or burning of the anterior lateral thigh.

Treatment

As is true of most nerve injuries, treatment consists of restricting activity and resting to allow time for recovery. Trying to return too soon might cause more significant nerve damage. Topical applications such as a lidocaine patch might be helpful when placed over the region of burning pain. Symptoms of LFCN injury can be alleviated with a cortisone injection to the nerve near the anterior superior iliac spine (ASIS). In rare cases, surgical release of the nerve from surrounding compressive tissues might be required.

Return to Action

Athletes should expect recovery to take four to six weeks. If pain persists and surgical decompression was performed, the athlete may be sidelined for three months. Conservative and postoperative rehabilitation focuses on range-of-motion exercises and core strengthening.

CHAPTER 12

Thigh and Hamstring Injuries

Lisa M. Bartoli, DO, MS, FAAPMR

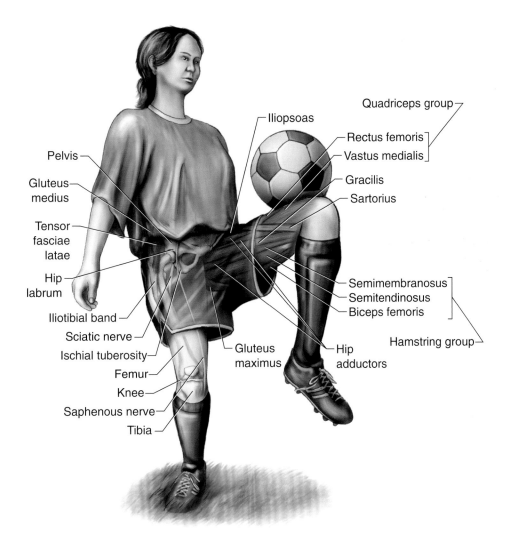

Thigh injuries are extremely common in sports, occurring in the hamstrings and quadriceps muscle groups. Any sports activity requiring explosive bursts of speed or quick changes in direction might cause injury to these muscle groups. Early and complete rehabilitation makes for a faster return to play and reduces recurrence of these injuries.

Thigh and Hamstring Injuries

HAMSTRING AVULSION

Common Causes

An avulsion is a tearing away. Avulsion injuries are less common than strains of the musculotendinous junction and often occur when the hip is forced into flexion while the knee maintains full extension, as happens in water skiing. Commonly the entire tendon is avulsed from the ischium. Adolescents tend to have a higher incidence of bony avulsion injuries in general.

Identification

Athletes with avulsion injuries have significant functional deficits, including a loss of speed, power, and agility as well as a poor return to prior functional level. They will have persistent pain, pain with sitting, weakness in full flexion, and poor leg control, especially when descending stairs or walking downhill. Sciatic nerve injury is also a possibility. X-rays can usually identify a bony avulsion injury. MRI can identify the avulsion as well as the extent of tendon disruption or tearing.

Treatment

Treatment for acute avulsions follows the PRICE protocol (protect, rest, ice, compression, and elevation) common for all acute injuries. If the displacement of the hamstring tendon from the ischium is greater than 2.5 centimeters (1 inch), or if conservative treatment has failed, the athlete will almost certainly require surgery. The current trend is to surgically repair acute avulsion injuries even when displacement is less than 2.5 centimeters. The earlier surgery occurs, the argument goes, the sooner the athlete can return to sport. For many athletes, early surgery is preferable to prolonged conservative treatment that might lead to additional weeks of downtime.

Return to Action

Return to play follows the same criteria as described for hamstring strains (see p. 194). Surgical repair calls for a prolonged rehab under the supervision of a physical therapist. The surgeon must clear the athlete before he or she returns to sport.

HAMSTRING STRAIN

Common Causes

A strain is a degree of tearing of the muscle fiber. The tearing or straining of hamstring muscles, particularly the long head of the biceps femoris, occurs frequently in athletics, particularly in sports that require brisk accelerations of speed and cutting, such as rugby, American football, soccer, and tennis. Although complete tears can occur, most tears are partial and occur at the myotendinous junction as a result of a failed lengthening of the muscle (eccentric contracture).

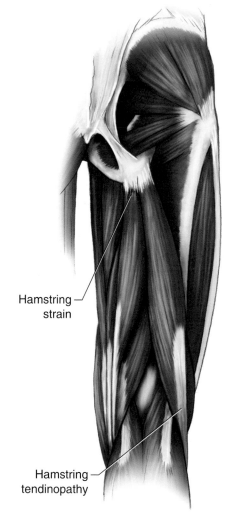

Hamstring strain

Hamstring tendinopathy

The hamstring muscle group includes three distinct muscles: the biceps femoris, the semitendinosus, and the semimembranosus. This group crosses two joints: the hip and the knee. Injuries to the hamstrings generally occur at the musculotendinous junction. Of the three muscles in the hamstring group, the biceps femoris is most likely to be injured. Factors that predispose an athlete to hamstring strains include insufficient warm-up, fatigue (strains tend to occur later in training or competition and later in the competitive season), poor muscular coordination, excessive pelvic tilt, prior hamstring injury, and imbalance in muscle strength between the hamstring and quadriceps (in which the hamstring is weaker).

Poor flexibility of the hip flexors and quadriceps alters the lumbopelvic mechanics by causing the pelvis to tilt anteriorly and increases the degree of lumbar lordosis (the curve in the low part of the back), which places extra tension on the hamstrings. Poor running mechanics in which the athlete has excess forward lean causes the gluteus maximus, the prime hip extensor in sprinting, to function poorly. This results in overstriding, increasing the hamstring length and making strain more likely.

Hamstring tendinopathy, a related injury, is an overuse injury resulting in dense fibrosis (thickening of muscle fibers) and occasionally, hyaline degeneration at the attachment of the hamstring to the ischium. It differs from tendinitis in that tendinopathy represents more of a chronic injury whereby the actual muscle fibers begin to degenerate and undergo structural changes. In tendinitis, the muscle fibers are intact but there is local inflammation due to acute injury. This injury is commonly seen in middle- and long-distance runners.

HAMSTRING STRAIN

Identification

The athlete often becomes aware of the injury by hearing or feeling a pop in the area of the hamstrings followed by immediate pain in the posterior thigh. This generally occurs during sprinting activities.

A palpable defect can often be detected in the area of injury. The athlete might feel tenderness in a focal area, especially soon after the injury. By 24 hours after the injury, the tender area becomes more diffuse and difficult to localize. The easiest way to isolate the area of tenderness is to palpate (explore via touch) the hamstring with the athlete prone and the knee flexed. Resisted knee flexion generally reproduces discomfort in the area of injury. A mass in the proximal posterior thigh might appear, especially in more severe strains. Functionally, if an athlete with a hamstring injury attempts to run, he or she shortens the stride length to reduce pain. Grade III strains, involving complete tearing of the musculotendinous unit and causing severe functional deficits and significant weakness, often occur at the origin of the hamstrings on the ischium and might even be accompanied by a fracture at this site (see hamstring avulsion, p. 193).

Perform a slump test to eliminate the possibility of neural injury as a cause of the posterior thigh pain. To perform the test, ask the athlete, while seated, to extend each leg individually. Then ask him or her to tuck the chin into the chest and repeat the extensions. If pain is exacerbated on the involved side when the leg is extended and the chin is tucked (rather than when the chin is not tucked), the slump test is positve and signifies a nerve problem. Some athletes experience a back-related hamstring injury in which a more gradual onset of pain occurs; in such cases, MRI typically reveals no hamstring injury. Injuries to the L5/S1 level and hypertrophy of the lumbosacral ligament tend to be more common in older athletes. Such injuries result in irritation of the L5/S1 nerve roots, leading to a higher incidence of hamstring and calf strains in athletes over the age of 30.

Diagnosis of a hamstring injury is made primarily by obtaining details of the cause of the injury from the athlete and by performing a physical examination. Initially, the injured athlete will have worsening pain with either a passive stretch or resisted contracture of the hamstring. Often an area of point tenderness and a palpable fascial defect or balling of the torn muscle appear. Bruising below the level of the tear can be quite impressive and widespread. In instances in which a complete tear of the hamstring muscle or proximal tendon is suspected, MRI of the thigh will more clearly define the extent of injury and help determine treatment. Typically, MRI is extremely useful in localizing and detailing the extent of injury as well as in making a prognosis and helping to determine readiness to return to play. Plain X-rays are only helpful in ruling out bony avulsion injury of the ischial tuberosity (see p. 193). Ultrasound might be helpful in identifying the location and extent of a muscle injury.

In the case of hamstring tendinopathy, the sciatic nerve can become entrapped. If this occurs, athletes often complain of pain with sitting, deep buttocks pain, or posterior thigh pain with running at faster speeds. If the sciatic nerve is not compressed, there is usually no pain referral into the thigh, only local discomfort. Direct pressure on the region, such as sitting, can invoke increased symptoms due to compression of nerves and other local structures. MRI is helpful in localizing and outlining the extent of injury.

(continued)

Treatment

Approach treatment of hamstring strains and hamstring tendinopathy in phases. In the first phase, the goal is to decrease the amount of local bleeding, swelling, pain, and inflammation. Nonsteroid anti-inflammatory (NSAID) medications can help limit inflammation and allow earlier rehab, but these should be used for only three to seven days postinjury because they can delay muscle regeneration and interfere with healing.

During the first phase of treatment, acute conservative care of hamstring strains follows the guidelines for most soft-tissue injuries (PRICE; see p. 27). Start icing and light compression with an ace wrap as soon as possible. The injured hamstring should be protected by limiting movement on hills, ramps, stairs, and uneven surfaces. The use of a cane or crutches should help reduce weight bearing, but holding the leg flexed at the knee and off the ground with crutches can aggravate the injury. A flat-foot gait with assistive devices is advocated until the athlete is walking pain free. If formal rehabilitative therapies are available, the use of concurrent electrical stimulation and ice might speed healing.

About seven or eight days after injury, the second phase begins. Most experts agree that electric stimulation, passive range of motion, myofascial release, and isometric exercises can be introduced at this point. The athlete should work on varying the position of the hip and knee during contraction. Stretching the hamstring while maintaining an anterior pelvic tilt, and holding each stretch for 20 seconds, has also been shown to be helpful. Pulsed ultrasound therapeutic massage might further reduce swelling and promote rehabilitation. Once the athlete has regained voluntary control of the muscle, he or she may begin gentle stretching.

Once the athlete has achieved 75 to 80 percent of normal range of motion, he or she begins resisted stretching techniques, such as isometric contract–relax exercises, active isolated stretching, and proprioceptive neuromuscular facilitation (PNF). Initial strengthening through concentric resistive exercises (shortening contractures of the muscle), either isokinetic (constant speed) or isotonic (constant weight), are preferred over eccentric resistive (lengthening contractures of the muscle) exercises because they pose less risk for reinjury. Swimming and cycling on a stationary bicycle may be added at this time if pain allows. All exercises should be performed within pain-free range of motion.

The third phase is the remodeling phase and occurs anywhere from one to six weeks after the initial injury. Pain-free static stretching of the hamstring, psoas, and quadriceps continues to be important to the rehab program. Eccentric strengthening, isokinetic strengthening, and proprioceptive neuromuscular facilitation is also introduced. Some of the stretching and strengthening exercises should include hip rotation. This is important because many sport movements such as pivoting, cutting, or changing direction involve hip rotation, both internal and external, with hip extension, which places stress on the hamstring.

In the final phase of treatment the goal is returning the athlete to sport. This phase includes sport-specific activities, emphasizing increasing hamstring strength and flexibility to preinjury levels or better. The athlete progresses from jogging to sprinting;

he or she performs cutting and pivoting activities as well as drills that incorporate rapid acceleration and deceleration.

Other modes of treatment that are beneficial for hamstring strains include ultrasound (late in the treatment), deep friction massage, and neuromobilization. Acupuncture is also helpful and may be used as soon as the injury occurs and throughout the rehab program.

For athletes with complete proximal hamstring tendon tears who have persistent strength deficits despite conservative treatment, surgical repair and subsequent rehab have been shown to restore near complete strength and promote a return to athletic activities.

Return to Action

For hamstring strain and tendinopathy, the athlete is cleared to return to play when he or she can participate in sport-specific activities pain free. Some professionals advocate return when isokinetic testing reveals strength within 10 percent of the sound leg at slow and fast speeds with equal flexibility and endurance. To prevent recurrence of the injury, the athlete should continue regular stretching and strengthening and should always warm up properly. Faithful compliance with hamstring and other hip girdle musculature stretching and continued balanced strengthening of the quadriceps and hamstrings will help prevent reinjury.

One of the greatest risks for hamstring strain is prior hamstring strain, so complete and continued rehabilitation is necessary. Recovery can occur as quickly as one week or take six weeks or more, depending on the grade of the strain.

FEMORAL STRESS FRACTURE

Common Causes

Fractures of the neck of the femur occur in only 1 to 10 percent of all lower-extremity stress fractures, and femoral shaft stress fractures are even less common. Stress fracture can occur anywhere in the medial femoral shaft but happens most commonly at the junction of the proximal and middle third. The femur is bowed anteriolaterally at this junction; it is also the site of origin of the vastus medialis and the insertion point for the adductor muscle group.

The cause of femoral neck stress fractures might be unclear, but biomechanics, hormonal influences, and alterations in bone mineral content likely play a part. Typically, athletes involved in endurance sports such as running and soccer experience such injury. Risk factors for the development of femoral neck and shaft stress fractures include increases in mileage, intensity, or frequency of running. A new running surface or new shoes might also be implicated, as might low bone mineral density, and in those with a short and thin femoral shaft, poor alignment, leg-length differences, weak lower-extremity muscles, and in those who are overweight, and, in females, amenorrheic (Brunet and Hontas 1994; Provencher, Baldwin, Gorman, Gould, and Shin 2004). Coxa vara (hip deformity) is a likely risk factor for development of femoral neck stress fractures.

Identification

Because of the high rate of complications with femoral neck fractures (avascular necrosis, fracture displacement, malunion, and nonunion), the earlier the diagnosis, the better. Athletes with femoral neck stress fractures generally experience pain in the groin or hip. Athletes with femoral shaft stress fractures might experience thigh or knee pain, which decreases with rest and increases with activity.

Physical exam findings for femoral fractures are often limited. Tenderness might be noted in the area but is usually limited because of overlying muscle. Femoral shaft fractures can be diagnosed using various clinical tests (fulcrum test, fist test, or single-leg hop test) but imaging is the best. Femoral neck fractures might cause pain or limited movement with hopping, hip internal rotation and flexion, and resisted hip extension.

X-rays may not reveal a fracture line early on; the fracture site may not be visible in plain X-ray until the repair process begins (2 to 12 weeks after initial pain) and callus formation occurs. At this time a lucent fracture line might be revealed. Radionucleotide bone scan, which can immediately reveal a fracture, has long been considered the gold standard for early detection of stress fractures.

Treatment

Fractures to the neck of the femur occurring on the compression or medial side are considered more stable and can be managed conservatively. Athletes usually use crutches to avoid weight bearing on the limb. X-rays can then help monitor healing. Tension-side (outer-lateral) femoral neck fractures have a high rate of displacement, and internal fixation is recommended. Surgical fixation often requires placing pins through the fracture site to stabilize the fragments. For some nondisplaced tension-side stress fractures, strict bed rest and weekly X-rays have good results. Athletes with stress fractures that are not well aligned should be referred to an orthopedic surgeon for emergent reduction and fixation.

With a femoral shaft stress fractures on the inner (medial) side, the athlete uses crutches and is allowed only toe-touch weight bearing for one to four weeks based on demonstration of healing (through X-ray) and no pain in walking. For fractures on the outer lateral (tension) side, if surgery was not done, no weight bearing is allowed for a minimum of six to eight weeks.

Return to Action

Return to running generally occurs 8 to 16 weeks after the onset of pain. Monthly X-rays for three months are recommended to ensure healing and nondisplacement. Before the athlete resumes training, the cause of the stress fracture should be determined. Amenorrheic females should undergo bone density testing and treatment for the amenorrhea before returning to sport. Training errors should be corrected and caution taken against a rapid increase in training mileage and intensity. Before athletes resume running they should be pain free during a fairly intense activity, such as cycling, swimming, or pool running.

Athletes should restrict themselves to three to five miles for weeks one to three. If they remain pain free, they can increase distance gradually back to half their normal distance over the next two weeks. If symptoms return, the athlete should stop and return to the previous activity that did not cause pain (e.g., if running caused pain, the athlete returns to biking or swimming).

QUADRICEPS CONTUSIONS

Common Causes

Quadriceps contusions result from blunt trauma (usually from a knee or thigh) to the thigh. Initially, symptoms might seem minor, but significant swelling and pain and decreased range of motion can occur over the next 24 hours. The blunt trauma generally results in damage to the muscular layer adjacent to the bone, thereby injuring deeper muscle than is normally involved in strains. This injury is common in American football, rugby, karate, judo, soccer, hockey, and lacrosse.

Identification

Contusions are generally classified as mild, moderate, or severe; most are mild to moderate. This classification is made 24 to 48 hours postinjury, when swelling and hematoma have stabilized. Classification is based on knee range of motion and physical findings. Mild contusions of the quadriceps have greater than 90 degrees of knee flexion and mild tenderness. Moderate contusions of the quadriceps have 45 to 90 degrees of knee flexion and enlarged, tender thighs. Severe contusions have less than 45 degrees of knee flexion and significant swelling and pain with quadriceps contraction. If there is less than 45 degrees of knee flexion, along with severe pain and swelling, the contusion is considered severe, and compartment pressure testing should be considered to rule out compartment syndrome (see p. 204).

Initial X-rays can rule out a fracture. At two to four weeks postinjury, X-rays can also rule out traumatic myositis ossificans (see p. 203). MRI should reveal the specific injury as well as the size and exact location.

Treatment

Early and aggressive treatment is the key for quick return to play and minimal complications. Athletes can return only when knee flexion is at 120 degrees. Thus, the key is to treat the athlete early, when he or she still has 120 degrees of knee flexion. At that point, the knee is passively flexed and wrapped to maintain 120 degrees of flexion. The athlete is braced or wrapped in this position for 24 hours and uses crutches (Aronen and Chronister 1992). Placing the quadriceps under tension should slow the intramuscular bleeding and maximize the quad stretch.

After 24 hours, the brace or wrap is removed; icing, electric stimulation, and passive pain-free quad stretching follow. The athlete is encouraged to perform this passive stretch frequently throughout the day. Athletes use the crutches until they can perform a pain-free isometric quad contraction and until swelling has diminished and the thigh has returned to normal size (Aronen and Chronister 1992). Strengthening begins with flexion and proceeds to extension. Progress exercises as motion and strength return.

If the athlete is not treated until after swelling and muscle spasm have occurred (thus making it difficult or extremely painful to attain 120 degrees of knee flexion), a modified approach to treatment is attempted. The prone athlete performs pain-free isometric knee-extension exercises until the quad fatigues, causing the spasms to decrease. Once fatigue sets in, begin passive pain-free stretching of the quad. This pain-free extension, relaxation, and stretching exercise is initially performed three times. The knee is then immobilized in a hinged knee brace at the maximum degree of pain-free flexion. Ice and electric stimulation are added at the next treatment, and the procedure is repeated. The athlete wears the brace continuously until he or she has 120 degrees of full-knee flexion (Aronen and Chronister 1992).

Return to Action

Athletes can return to action once they attain full range of motion, and strength is equal to the noninjured leg. Return time is often within one week for mild to moderate contusions. The athlete is fitted with a protective pad, which should be worn for the remainder of the season. Failure to treat a thigh contusion aggressively can delay return time up to four weeks.

QUADRICEPS STRAIN

Common Causes

The quadriceps consists of the four muscles located on the anterior thigh: the vastus medialis, vastus lateralis, vastus intermedius, and rectus femoris. Only the rectus femoris crosses two joints (the hip and knee) and functions as both a hip flexor and knee extensor. The other three muscles are responsible for knee extension only.

Quadriceps strains are common in American football, rugby, soccer, track, basketball, hockey, and other sports that require repetitive sprinting, kicking, and jumping. Strains generally occur with a forceful (near maximal) contraction or forceful stretching of the quadriceps. Quadriceps strains generally occur at the musculotendinous junction and can be partial or complete. Grade I strains involve minor muscle fiber disruption. Grade II strains involve more extensive tearing of the muscle fiber with accompanying hemorrhage, and grade III strains are full tears of the musculotendinous junction. The rectus femoris muscle is most often strained, followed by the vastus intermediate and vastus lateralis.

Identification

If the athlete experiences more pain with knee flexion when the hip is extended than with the hip flexed, the rectus femoris is involved. Feeling the muscle can help localize the injury site. Defects, or a mass that occurs with knee extension, are more commonly seen with grade II and III strains. It is difficult to palpate a defect in the muscle once swelling or hematoma formation has occurred. MRI is considered the standard for imaging muscle strain injuries. In most cases, MRI can identify the exact location and severity of the strain.

Treatment

Treatment for quadriceps strains is similar to treatment for hamstring strains and follows a similar phase-based approach (see p. 194). Once the athlete's treatment has progressed to pain-free motion, he or she begins isometric exercises at full extension and progresses to 90 degrees of knee flexion. Straight-leg raising exercises should be avoided early on because these place the greatest stress on the rectus femoris. Gentle and cautious active stretching is initiated in this phase. Stretching generally starts with the athlete in a prone position, actively flexing the knee against gravity as tolerated. During the final stage of rehabilitation, force absorption and production exercises are added—for example, jumping down from a one-foot box, absorbing the force, and then jumping back up from that position.

Acupuncture (see chapter 16) is also helpful in decreasing pain and swelling, which in turn promotes increased range of motion and gets the athlete through rehab faster. Acupuncture should be used as early as possible and continued through the rehab process.

Return to Action

The athlete returns to sport when range of motion is full and pain free, when isokinetic strength testing is within 10 percent of the uninjured leg, and when the athlete can complete agility testing and sprinting without difficulty. The athlete should continue using compression sleeves with protective padding throughout the season. Return to full activity generally occurs two to three weeks after injury.

MYOSITIS OSSIFICANS

Common Causes

Myositis ossificans—the formation of heterotopic (misplaced) bone in a surrounding muscle—is a complication that often occurs with grade II and III quadriceps contusions, most commonly adjacent to the femur. In a study of military recruits with thigh contusions, myositis ossificans developed in 20 percent of treated contusions (Brunet and Hontas 1994).

Identification

A firm mass developing three to four weeks postcontusion might be myositis ossificans. X-rays should confirm diagnosis. It appears as a whitish collection on X-ray. This mass might or might not be connected to the femur. Generally, it takes three to six months to mature (cease forming). Ultrasound can detect the formation of myositis ossificans before it appears on X-ray.

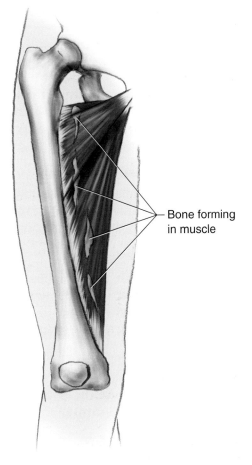

Bone forming in muscle

Treatment

Treatment is essentially the same as for contusions (see p. 200). If left untreated, persistent loss of range of motion, painful bony mass, and significant limitations in athletic function can result. Ultrasound may help to break up the myositic collection.

Additional treatments to consider are single low-dose radiation and the use of NSAIDs (specifically Indocin or Naprosyn) for two to six weeks (Larson, Almekinders, Karas, and Garrett 2002; Wang, Lomasney, Demos, and Hopkinson 1999). Both are advocated to inhibit the formation of further heterotopic bone. Radiation may help in heterotopic bone breakdown.

In rare instances, surgical excision is needed. If so, it is imperative that the bone formation reach full maturity, which takes about six months, before being surgically excised. If the formation is cut out before it reaches maturity, it might return even greater than its original size. If surgery is done, the athlete may be advised to begin a postoperative course of radiation to inhibit the re-accumulation of heterotopic bone.

Return to Action

Myositis ossificans can delay return time beyond what is required for a contusion. A physician or physical therapist should make the call.

COMPARTMENT SYNDROME

Common Causes

In this condition, the "compartment" refers to the fascia or covering of the quadriceps muscle group that encircles the muscle. Compartment syndrome occurs in contact sports when a knee, helmet, or other hard object forcefully contacts the quadriceps or anterior muscle group. Rarely, excessive bleeding and edema following a quadriceps contusion can result in compartment syndrome. When the swelling in the anterior compartment increases, compartmental pressure rises. This fascia does not have the ability to expand a great deal. Thus, a large amount of swelling causes an increase in pressure, which ultimately deprives the muscle of an adequate blood supply, effectively starving the muscle of oxygen and nutrients. If this process is allowed to continue, it can result in muscle death.

Identification

Clinically, pain out of proportion to the injury, pain at rest, pain with passive knee flexion, and a diffusely tender and tense thigh suggest the possibility of compartment syndrome. Sensory deficits might occur along the saphenous nerve (medial knee and tibia). Motor deficits and absent pulses are late findings that imply more severe and permanent muscle damage.

Diagnosis is made by obtaining compartment pressures from the anterior thigh compartment. The critical pressure duration that can lead to permanent damage ranges from four to eight hours.

Treatment

The treatment for acute thigh compression is fasciotomy, or surgically cutting the fascia to allow the muscle to receive an adequate blood supply. The fascia is surgically closed again once the swelling resolves. Following surgical decompression, early rehab is begun to limit swelling, pain, and atrophy as well as to improve range of motion.

Return to Action

Following a complete rehab program, most athletes can return to their sports within 8 to 16 weeks, once they are cleared by their physician.

CHAPTER 13

Knee Injuries

Michael Kelly, MD; Yvonne Johnson, PT

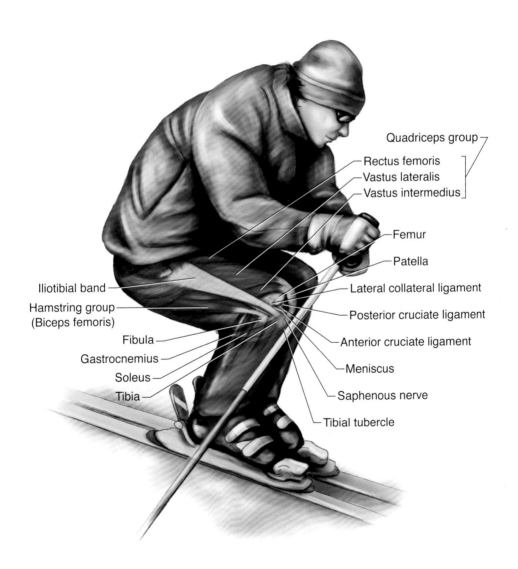

Quadriceps group

Rectus femoris
Vastus lateralis
Vastus intermedius

Iliotibial band

Hamstring group
(Biceps femoris)

Femur

Patella

Lateral collateral ligament

Posterior cruciate ligament

Fibula

Anterior cruciate ligament

Gastrocnemius

Soleus

Tibia

Meniscus

Saphenous nerve

Tibial tubercle

Knee injuries will soon match and likely surpass in incidence the most common injury in the weekend warrior, which is back pain. Injuries to the knee can be debilitating, but thanks to terrific advances in diagnosis and both nonoperative and operative treatments, the athlete can often return to play in a relatively timely manner.

Knee Injuries

PATELLOFEMORAL PAIN

Common Causes

Patellofemoral pain, also known as anterior knee pain, is the most common complaint of pain in the knee and is most associated with athletic overuse. Patellofemoral pain spans all age groups and all sports and is aggravated by flexed-knee activities such as sitting, climbing stairs, and driving.

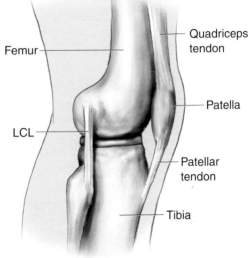

Femur

Quadriceps tendon

Patella

LCL

Patellar tendon

Tibia

Identification

The athlete typically has pain in the anterior knee, but this pain might radiate posteriorly in the case of associated patellofemoral degenerative changes (more common in the older athlete). Significant swelling is unusual, though knee buckling might occur.

Localized tenderness might spread over any aspect of the patella. Tenderness at the anterior medial joint line is common. Patellofemoral tracking should be evaluated. The angle formed by the pull of the rectus femoris and patellar tendon is called the quadriceps angle and might be increased in athletes with poor tracking. Ligament tests can help rule out ACL injury. A physical exam should include an overall evaluation of the lower extremity alignment as well as the ipsilateral hip. An X-ray might show patellofemoral malalignment and bony dysphasia as well as degenerative changes.

Treatment

The vast majority of patellofemoral disorders improve with nonoperative treatment. Typically, either a home exercise program or formal physical therapy is recommended. These programs focus on increasing flexibility and strengthening both the quadriceps and hamstring muscle groups. Ultrasound and electrical stimulation might assist in rehabilitation. If swelling or severe pain occurs, nonsteroidal anti-inflammatory medication might be useful. Some athletes might also find an adjustable brace helpful. During rehab, the athlete should avoid locking the knees. Any extreme positions of bending (cross-legged sitting, kneeling, or squatting) or straightening (supporting the leg on a coffee table) should also be avoided. If the patient is not doing well after six months of treatment, MRI can help evaluate the other possible causes of symptoms. Surgical results for patellofemoral pain problems are variable.

Return to Action

Typically athletes refrain from the involved activity for a few weeks up to six months. Athletes who have surgery might take three to six months to recover before returning to sports. Athletes must be able to perform motions mimicking their sport without significant pain before returning. If pain or weakness remains, more therapy is recommended. Patellofemoral braces are available, but these are adjuncts, not remedies.

ILIOTIBIAL BAND SYNDROME

Common Causes

Irritation of the iliotibial band (ITB) as it crosses the lateral aspect of the knee to its insertion on the tibia is often related to overuse activity of the knee and is frequently diagnosed in cyclists, runners, and triathletes. ITB is most commonly associated with increases in training volume.

Identification

The pain is localized to the ITB in the lateral side of the knee; the remainder of the knee might be asymptomatic. The athlete usually experiences the pain at some distance into a training session, making the session difficult or impossible to complete. Typically, little pain occurs at the onset of activity and there is no complaint of swelling.

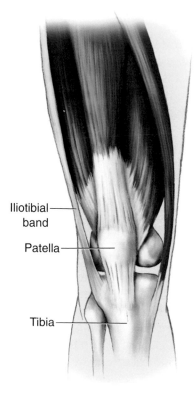

Iliotibial band

Patella

Tibia

Diagnosis for this injury is the physical exam. Well-localized tenderness spreads over the iliotibial band as it crosses the lateral aspect of the knee. There is typically no localized soft tissue swelling. The ITB might be tight and irritated by front-to-back movement of the band during the flexion–extension movement of the knee. Occasionally, proximal tenderness of the band in the hip area might also occur. The area of lateral knee tenderness should be differentiated from the lateral patella and lateral joint line. Range of motion is normal, and the remainder of the knee exam is normal. Some localized soft tissue irritation might be present in the area of the ITB. Knee X-rays, usually normal, should be run to rule out other injuries.

Treatment

Treatment of ITB syndrome is almost always nonoperative and begins with rest. Supervised physical therapy is very useful in treating this disorder. ITB stretching is difficult for the athlete to perform adequately on his or her own, so it is best to have a physical therapist assist. In addition to stretching the ITB, local modalities such as ultrasound and electrical stimulation to the area of tenderness adjacent to the lateral femoral epicondyle (on the outer side of the knee) are helpful. The athlete might try a 10-day course of anti-inflammatory medications with the proper precautions. A cortisone injection might also be of benefit. Stretching the lower-limb muscles helps to eliminate tension and irritation of the ITB. Ice massage several times a day, using an ice cube directly over the outer border of the knee, should help eliminate symptoms. The athlete should work on maintaining and improving strength in the lower limbs, emphasizing the hip muscle.

Return to Action

This is one disorder in which exercise technique (especially in cyclists) might contribute significantly to the problem. Serious cyclists might want to work with cycling specialists who can examine their biking position and suggest changes to decrease the irritation of the ITB during the cycling motion. For runners, examining the feet and possibly altering the running shoe or adding an orthotic might prove beneficial. Once symptoms have subsided and the athlete has returned to exercise, a continued program of ITB stretching should be incorporated into training. Mending time for an ITB injury is at least 6 weeks and might take up to 12 weeks. When pain is absent or minimal during daily activities, such as stair climbing or pedaling a stationary bicycle, athletes may consider returning to athletic participation. Return must be gradual and may progress as long as there is no pain.

MENISCAL TEAR

Common Causes

Medial meniscal tears occur in every age group. Athletes under 30 who tear their medial meniscus tend to do so in the course of a traumatic injury to the knee; in extreme situations they might be unable to fully extend the knee (known as a *locked knee*.) In 30- to 60-year-olds, the athlete may not recall any specific injury but report only that pain developed after a particular activity. Although medial meniscal tears largely outnumber lateral meniscal tears, they are both caused by twisting. Basketball, American football, and soccer have high rates of meniscal injuries.

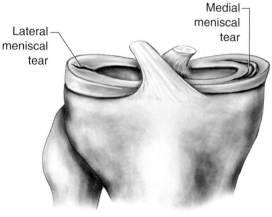

Lateral meniscal tear

Medial meniscal tear

Identification

Localized pain with a small amount of swelling after activity is the most frequent complaint. Pain is often aggravated by any rotational leg activity or extremes of motion. Athletes might experience positional pain in the knee while sleeping. They often have difficulty returning to their sport of choice but are not disabled by their symptoms (though if a loss of knee extension occurs, this should be immediately addressed). Almost all injuries that result in painful knees make for discomfort or pain in descending stairs.

Check for localized tenderness at the involved joint line. The medial meniscus is located in the medial joint line of the knee, and the lateral meniscus is located in the lateral joint line of the knee. (As a reminder, the medial side of the knee is the side closest to the other knee, whereas the lateral side of the knee is the outside of the knee.) Rotary maneuvers such as flexing and extending the knee while externally and internally rotating the limb can help diagnose a meniscus tear if these actions reproduce pain or symptoms. Hearing a click when rotating the knee might indicate a mobile flap of meniscus.

Lateral meniscus tears are sometimes associated with a meniscal cyst, which can be felt as a firm, tender soft tissue swelling at the mid-lateral joint line of the knee. Older athletes with coexisting osteoarthritis might have a mild angular deformity at the knee. Standard X-rays are typically normal, though they might show degenerative changes in older athletes. MRI testing is quite accurate in confirming the diagnosis of a meniscal tear.

Treatment

Blood circulation to the menisci is quite limited, so little biologic healing occurs with these injuries. Occasionally athletes do reasonably well with nonoperative treatment, but in most cases surgery is required. During arthroscopic surgery, doctors remove the least amount of meniscal tissue required to solve the problem. The success of arthroscopic partial meniscectomy is quite good in the absence of associated degenerative joint disease. Long-term issues of degenerative joint disease following partial meniscectomy might be related to the amount of meniscus removed, and these effects are minimized with current arthroscopic techniques.

Surgery is typically an outpatient procedure with a swift recovery. Athletes often return to full function within six weeks. A home exercise program or supervised physical therapy speeds recovery. Exercise should focus on lower-limb strengthening, with emphasis on hip exercises to reduce stress on the knee joint.

Return to Action

With conservative care (no surgery), about 30 percent of athletes do well. They can return to sports in about 8 to 12 weeks and are limited by occasional pain and instability. Following surgery, athletes often return sooner, sometimes within four weeks. Although some professional athletes have returned sooner (in as little as two weeks), keep in mind that these athletes are rehabilitating five to six days per week for several hours each day. As with many knee injuries, the use of a knee sleeve or soft brace usually depends on the athlete's desire to wear one. These devices usually offer more proprioceptive support than actual mechanical support.

Athletes returning to sport should progress slowly and monitor swelling and pain. If either occurs, decrease the activity level while continuing with a lower-limb strengthening program with emphasis on hip exercises. Hip strength is critical in supporting the entire lower limb. Ice after exercise to reduce swelling and pain.

MEDIAL COLLATERAL LIGAMENT TEAR

Common Causes

The typical cause of a mild to moderate isolated medial collateral ligament (MCL) tear (or sprain) involves either a contact or noncontact injury with a valgus force directed at the knee (placing the knee in a "knock-knee" position). These injuries occur in athletes of all ages (particularly those 16 to 50) but are relatively uncommon in older athletes. Injury to the MCL is common in skiers as well as in American football and soccer players. Athletes are at risk when they are positioned with their knees together with a force pushing from the outer side toward the inner side of the knee.

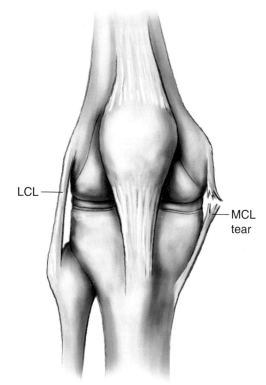

LCL

MCL tear

Identification

The athlete often reports hearing a pop or feeling a tearing sensation in the knee. The pain is typically localized to the inner (medial) side of the knee, particularly at the MCL origin on the upper aspect of the knee. Physical examination of the knee with an isolated MCL injury reveals little, if any, swelling. The athlete might have occasional limited range of motion, especially the final 10 degrees of extension, because of pain in the area of the MCL. Localized tenderness occurs along the course of the MCL that might include the medial joint line. It is common that the most significant tenderness is at the MCL insertion on the upper knee.

MCL stress testing and a ligamentous exam can verify an MCL diagnosis and help determine if there is an associated anterior cruciate ligament (ACL) tear or other ligament injury. MRI can also verify if the injury is isolated to the MCL or if the ACL is involved. Rotary stress testing at the knee might be painful. These tests are typically positive in athletes with meniscal tears but will also cause pain in those with an MCL sprain.

Treatment

Virtually all isolated MCL injuries can be managed nonoperatively (though combined multiple-ligamentous injuries might require surgery). For a low-grade MCL injury, begin active–passive range of motion immediately, with local ice massage, exercise bicycle as tolerated, and exercises to strengthen the quadriceps. Supervised physical therapy should accelerate recovery. No bracing is required, but a medial–lateral sleeve might provide additional comfort. Athletes must make sure to move the knee to regain full range of motion (even when painful) so the knee does not become stiff.

MEDIAL COLLATERAL LIGAMENT TEAR

They must not sleep with a pillow under the knee because this might hinder the ability to straighten the knee while walking.

For more severe isolated MCL injuries, a period of bracing might be necessary to assist in ligament healing. The brace starts at 30 degrees in a hinged locked brace that is gradually unlocked to allow increased motion and physical therapy as healing progresses. Discontinue bracing after four to six weeks. It is uncommon with this injury to have an associated meniscal tear, but if progress remains limited at three months, check for additional tears with MRI.

How stiff the knee is at the onset of therapy will depend on the extent of the tear and how long the knee has been braced. Initially, the goal is to regain full range of motion, which may be painful and stiff at the outset. As progress is made, the athlete should complete an exercise program for lower-limb strengthening with emphasis on the hip muscles. When doing inner and outer thigh strength exercises, the athlete should take care not to stress the medial collateral ligament. Ice should be applied after exercise to reduce swelling and pain.

Return to Action

Recovery might take three months. Return to sport depends on restoration of range of motion, strength, and absence of pain. Athletes will typically use a knee sleeve with supports on the medial and lateral sides as they return to activity. They should progress slowly and gradually increase the amount of time spent in their sport. Athletes should master running and cutting drills before beginning full participation.

ANTERIOR CRUCIATE LIGAMENT TEAR

Common Causes

Rupture of the anterior cruciate ligament (ACL) occurs more often in females than in males, from adolescents to older adults. Noncontact injuries to the knee are responsible for most ACL tears. Pivoting and cutting sports (soccer and basketball) are the most common scenarios for noncontact ACL injuries, whereas most direct contact ACL injuries occur in American football. ACL tears can be associated with meniscal tears or collateral ligament injuries.

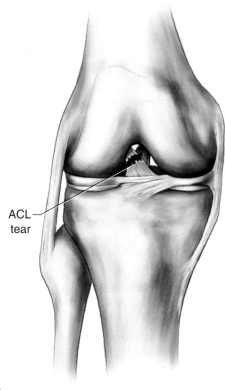

ACL tear

Identification

Most athletes who have torn their ACL will hear or feel a pop accompanied by pain and, soon after, swelling, though in rare cases little swelling occurs. Rapid swelling in the knee is typically caused by bleeding associated with the injury. The pain might subside quickly after an ACL injury, but this does not mean the tear or strain is healing. An athlete will experience instability with an insecure sensation while pivoting or loading the knee; an occasional sense of hyperextension of the knee is also common. Tenderness often occurs at the lateral joint line.

Critical to diagnosis of the ACL tear is the Lachman test, which evaluates the ACL laxity at 30 degrees of knee flexion and includes the uninjured knee for comparison. If the ligament is intact, there will be an endpoint feeling like tensing a string. Absence of this firm sensation typically signals an ACL tear. The medial, lateral, and posterior ligaments are tested as well. Evaluating range of motion is especially important. Standard X-rays are required but seldom reveal much. Occasionally, a small piece of bone that has pulled off of the lateral aspect of the tibia might show up on X-ray. This indicates an avulsion fracture and is typically associated with an ACL tear. MRI is quite accurate in diagnosing ACL tears. Typically, MRI findings with a torn ACL include bone bruises at the end of the thigh bone, femur, and posterior tibia; swelling; and an abnormal ACL at the femoral attachment. It is not uncommon to have an associated meniscal injury (see p. 210) with an ACL tear, and this is also diagnosed with MRI.

Treatment

Age, occupation, desired activity, sports involvement, and associated injuries to the knee are all taken into consideration when deciding on treatment for an ACL tear. Nonoperative treatment includes supervised physical therapy to restore range of motion, decrease swelling, and restore strength. With return to activities, athletes in more vigorous sports might use a derotational ACL brace.

Thanks to recent advances in arthroscopic ACL reconstructive procedures and more rapid postop recovery and return to sports, surgery for ACL tears is a much more attractive option than it once was. In the very young patient with open growth plates, surgery might be delayed until bone maturation, but there is some controversy about this. In the patient older than 60 years, nonoperative treatment is generally recommended but certainly the octagenerian who skis on a regular basis may opt for surgical reconstruction of the ACL. Whereas nonoperative treatment might be considered in any age group for isolated ACL injuries, it is typically less successful in active and athletic patients.

Postsurgery, athletes typically return to school or sedentary work within a week. Athletes will use crutches for one to two weeks and begin physical therapy almost immediately. Physical therapy and a strengthening program continue until the injured knee has 90 percent of the strength of the other knee. Training focuses on strengthening the hamstring and quadriceps muscle groups as well as the other lower extremities. The hamstring muscles are particularly important because they add stability to the injured knee. Hamstring contractions pull the tibia backward, which helps counter the inherent ACL instability, which is a forward glide of the tibia. Also, full-knee extension is critical for long-term knee function and should always be a priority in treatment. Clinical results of ACL reconstruction are quite good, with very low reinjury rates. The most common complication is some residual anterior knee pain. Strengthening the hip muscles during therapy is also extremely important in helping to restore stability in the lower limbs and decrease strain on the reconstructed ligament.

Return to Action

With surgery and rehab, athletes can usually return to sport in about six months. Bracing might be initially beneficial upon return. The decision to brace usually depends on athlete preference and whether any instability remains in the rehabilitated knee. Some medical professionals evaluate the post-ACL athlete via a series of functional tests to assess the knee's strength and stability. Devices such as isokinetic strength-testing machines and a series of hopping tests are used. Athletes must progress slowly in resuming sport activity and perform exercises such as running, cutting, twisting, and jumping to mimic the movements of the sport before beginning full participation.

POSTERIOR CRUCIATE LIGAMENT TEAR

Common Causes

Injuries to the posterior cruciate ligament occur when a front-to-back force is directed straight onto the upper tibia. This injury typically occurs during a fall onto a flexed knee, after trauma to the front part of the extended knee, or when the knee is hyperextended. PCL injuries are most common in contact sports such as American football and in cutting and pivoting sports such as basketball, in which knee hyperextension could occur. These injuries are often overlooked and undiagnosed because pain might be the only symptom.

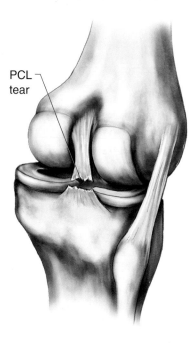

PCL tear

Identification

Posterior cruciate ligament injuries are much less common than ACL injuries. The athlete with an injured PCL complains of local knee pain, might have swelling, and offers little complaint of instability. The injury is debilitating in that it adversely affects an athlete's ability to run all out, either because of pain or a sense of not being able to trust the knee. Athletes might say, "the knee just doesn't feel right." Diagnosis is confirmed via MRI.

Treatment

Most PCL injuries are treated conservatively. Unless associated injuries cause either instability or increased biomechanical stress, surgery is not usually required. However, extensive rehabilitation is necessary. The focus of rehabilitation is strengthening the quadriceps muscles because these muscles add stability to the PCL-deficient knee.

Return to Action

Expect three to six months of rehab with conservative (nonsurgical) treatment of a PCL injury. At least six months are required to rehabilitate the surgically repaired PCL-injured knee. As with the ACL-injured knee, return to athletics is permitted once the knee is relatively pain free, range of motion is good, and the athlete can complete a series of functional knee tests. Bracing is recommended if the athlete wants it or if any knee instability remains. Athletes must progress slowly when returning to sport and perform exercises such as running, cutting, twisting, and jumping to mimic the movements of the sport before beginning full participation.

LATERAL COLLATERAL LIGAMENT TEAR

Common Causes

Injury to the lateral collateral ligament (LCL) usually occurs because of a force directed from the medial (inner side) knee toward the lateral (outer side) knee. This injury can result from a direct blow in contact sports or by a misstep or sharp pivot during pivoting sports.

Identification

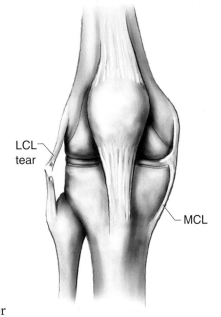

Athletes with an injury to the LCL will have local discomfort along the lateral knee. If the athlete sits and flexes the injured knee and then places the foot of the injured knee over the other knee, pain will flare up at the top of the fibula bone. Feel for a tight band of tissue that travels toward the upper knee—this is the LCL.

LCL stress testing and a ligamentous exam can verify an LCL diagnosis and help check for an associated anterior cruciate ligament (ACL) tear or other ligament injury. MRI may also be used to determine whether or not the injury is isolated to the LCL. Rotary maneuvers involving stress testing at the knee might be painful. These tests are typically positive in athletes with meniscal tears but also cause pain in those with LCL sprains.

Treatment

Virtually all isolated LCL injuries can be managed nonoperatively (though multiple ligament injuries might require surgery). For a low-grade LCL injury, the athlete should begin active-passive range-of-motion exercises immediately, local ice massage, exercise bicycle as tolerated, and quadriceps-strengthening exercises. Supervised physical therapy should accelerate recovery. No bracing is required, but a medial–lateral sleeve can provide some additional comfort. For more severe isolated LCL injuries, bracing might be necessary to assist in ligament healing. The brace starts at 30 degrees in a hinged locked brace that is gradually unlocked to allow increased motion and physical therapy as healing progresses. Discontinue bracing after four to six weeks. If progress remains limited after three months, MRI might be necessary to check for additional injuries.

Physical therapy should emphasize lower-limb strengthening and balance exercises that focus on the hip muscles to reduce stress and strain on the knee. Use caution with hip exercises to avoid stressing the outer leg or lateral collateral ligament.

Return to Action

Overall recovery might take three months. Return to sport depends on restoration of range of motion and strength and resolution of pain. Athletes typically use a knee sleeve with supports on the medial and lateral sides as they return to activity. They should progress slowly and perform exercises that mimic their sport before attempting full participation.

PATELLAR TENDINITIS

Common Causes

Painful knee symptoms associated with patellar tendinitis are commonly related to jumping and repetitive running. This condition is often called "jumper's knee" and is seen most often in basketball players. The injury might also be related to overuse of the knee.

Identification

The hallmark of patellar tendinitis is localized pain in the proximal portion of the patellar tendon near the lower part of the patella. The pain is aggravated by jumping and running and not typically related to any single traumatic event. When pain is severe, athletes might complain of discomfort while stair climbing and sitting. Swelling is uncommon, and the remainder of the knee exam is normal. MRI might reveal changes in the proximal portion of the patellar tendon that are consistent with a partial tear or thickening of the tendon in chronic cases.

Patella

Patellar tendon

Inflammation

Treatment

Most athletes with patellar tendinitis respond to nonoperative treatment. In acute cases, a 10-day course of approved nonsteroidal inflammatory medications (if tolerated) is recommended. The athlete should begin an exercise program emphasizing quadriceps stretching and strengthening. Ice massage might have some benefit. The athlete should avoid all jumping activities. Most athletes will respond to this conservative treatment. Surgical treatment for patellar tendinitis is quite uncommon. On rare occasions, the athlete who has not responded to more than six months of nonoperative treatment and has an abnormal patellar tendon on MRI might consider surgery. Surgical treatment is usually followed by a three- to six-month recovery period. Cortisone shots are not recommended for this injury. Cortisone may hasten degeneration of the patella tendon.

Return to Action

Return time following nonoperative treatment of patellar tendinitis is highly variable. The condition rarely improves before six weeks. Chronic symptoms are not uncommon and often require repetitive treatment. Some athletes report improvement of symptoms and ability to play using a strap at the level of the mid-patellar tendon, similar to the strap used for tennis elbow. The rare athlete who requires surgical treatment might not return to action for six months. Because there is no guarantee for success of this procedure, return time could be much longer.

PATELLA FRACTURE

Common Causes
Fracture of the patella is almost always caused by a direct blow to the knee. This injury can occur in any sport and causes significant disability.

Identification
Fracture of the patella causes immediate pain, swelling, and reduced motion. Weight bearing is difficult. If a patella fracture is suspected, the athlete should be immediately transported to an emergency room; consultation with an orthopedist is encouraged. X-rays should aid diagnosis and provide information on which to base treatment options.

Treatment
If the fracture does not cause significant misalignment of the patella, four to six weeks of immobilization (via bracing or casting) might be recommended. Following this, a progressive course of physical therapy can restore motion, strength, and overall knee function. If surgery is required, the knee is immobilized postoperatively for a shorter time, which allows earlier range-of-motion exercises. Weight bearing should be avoided for about four to six weeks, which could cause atrophy and weakness in the knee. It is thus important to maintain lower-limb strength via straight-leg raises in all positions at least four times a week, adding resistance as tolerated. Begin with resistance above the knee and progress to the ankle as long as no stress is felt on the knee.

Return to Action
Return to sport takes at least eight weeks. The athlete must have good range of motion and strength in the involved knee before attempting a return. Depending on the sport, recovery time might take three to six months, particularly for contact sports.

PATELLOFEMORAL INSTABILITY

Common Causes

Instability of the patellofemoral joint can be caused by either an acute episode or recurrent subluxations or dislocations. The injury might result from trauma such as a direct hit in American football or from a twisting movement in a noncontact sport. Younger athletes often fall victim to patellofemoral instability. An athlete who has been injured this way once must take precautions because this injury tends to recur.

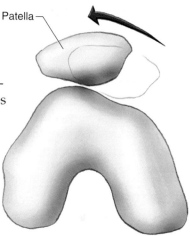

Patella

Identification

Dislocation of the patella is a distinct event that incapacitates the athlete. In many cases, the athlete might recall only that something gave out in the knee because most dislocations occur spontaneously with extension of the knee. Following a patellar dislocation, check for localized tenderness in the medial aspect of the knee relating to an injury to the medial patella or medial patella retinaculum. Tenderness is noted on the inner aspect of the knee and is associated with tearing of the medial patellofemoral ligament, an important medial stabilizer of the patella. Significant dislocation of the patella, in which the patella moves out of its groove, may cause a fracture of the patella or of the underlying femur bone; this is known as an osteochondral fracture.

Treatment

Treatment of an acute patellar dislocation is somewhat controversial. Uncommonly, the athlete must be taken to an emergency room for a closed reduction of the patella. Most athletes can be managed nonoperatively with a two-week period of immobilization followed by an aggressive rehabilitation program emphasizing quadriceps and hip muscle strengthening. X-rays might show a small fleck of bone representing an osteochondral fracture with a loose body. MRI may show effusion, tearing of the medial retinaculum or medial patellofemoral ligament, bone contusions, or possible osteochondral fractures of either the medial patellar or lateral femoral condyle. Athletes who have suffered an osteochondral fracture with a loose body or those with significant tearing of the medial restraints of the patella might require surgical intervention. It is very difficult to repair these fractures because very little residual bone remains. Some athletes require repair of the torn medial structure.

Return to Action

Return time varies depending on the degree of soft-tissue damage. A return to sport might require almost three months, and the athlete wears a patellar-aligning brace during initial activity. A postoperative recovery requires a period of bracing and crutches for six weeks followed by extensive rehabilitation, delaying return time at least six months. Surgery tends to have excellent results in preventing further patellar dislocation, but some athletes might have mild residual pain.

OSGOOD-SCHLATTER'S SYNDROME

Common Causes

Osgood-Schlatter's syndrome is a painful condition affecting growing children. Symptoms tend to be caused by running and jumping activities involving virtually any sport. Pain is related to the growth plate of the tibial tubercle (the bump on the leg just below the knee cap) where the very strong patellar tendon inserts. Once this growth plate closes, symptoms subside. The growth plate closes at a younger age in females than in males.

Identification

Osgood-Schlatter's is characterized by well-localized tenderness of the tibial tubercle. Look for mild soft tissue swelling, warmth, and prominence of the tubercle. Again, the condition is commonly seen in the growing athlete. Rarely, adults with a history of Osgood-Schlatter's might continue to have episodic pain at the tibial tubercle when an infused bone ossicle (a small piece of bone attached to the patellar tendon) persists at the tibial tubercle. This can be seen on a lateral X-ray.

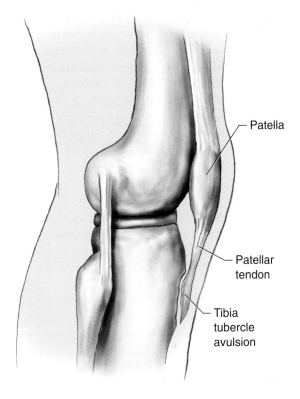

Patella

Patellar tendon

Tibia tubercle avulsion

Treatment

Virtually all cases of Osgood-Schlatter's syndrome can be treated nonoperatively. In the past, immobilization was recommended, but it is not required. Treatment is directed toward the degree of painful symptoms. Options include initial cessation of the related activity, local treatment with ice massage and stretching, and strengthening exercises. If symptoms are severe, a seven-day course of an anti-inflammatory medication can be considered. For an adult patient with a symptomatic tibial tubercle with evidence of an unfused ossicle, surgery might be considered to remove the ossicle. The majority of unfused ossicles are asymptomatic. There should be no surgery for cosmetic reasons on an unusually large tibial tubercle.

Return to Action

Return time is dictated by the degree of symptoms and the young athlete's ability to perform his or her sport. Often they return to sport with mild recurrent symptoms. Again, this condition resolves itself once the growth plate in the maturing athlete closes.

OSTEOCHONDRITIS DISSECANS

Common Causes

Osteochondritis dissecans (OCD) is usually caused by repetitive trauma. A fragment of subchondral bone in the knee joint becomes loose and leads to vague pain and disability. This condition is most common in athletes undergoing repetitive stresses across the knee. Athletes participating in gymnastics and baseball seem most prone to OCD.

Identification

OCD usually occurs below the age of 18 and is twice as common in males as females. The injury is most often seen behind and to the outer side (posterolaterally) of the medial femoral condyle (about 80 percent of cases), and less often seen in the posterior aspect of the lateral femoral condyle. Tenderness occurs along the joint lines, and loading of the joint causes pain. Athletes might sometimes rotate the lower leg when walking to relieve pressure. Pain is most notable during weight bearing and when the involved knee is extended straight. X-rays usually reveal a lesion on the femoral condyle.

Treatment

Because healing of this injury requires as much stress removal as possible, weight-bearing restrictions last longer than usual. Conservative treatments might require several months of bearing no weight on the involved knee, requiring extensive use of crutches. If surgical treatment is selected, a period of a few months of reduced weight bearing is still necessary. With the lack of weight bearing and the use of crutches, the leg atrophies and weakens, so athletes must focus on maintaining lower-limb strength via straight-leg raises in all positions at least four times a week, adding resistance as tolerated. Begin with resistance above the knee and progress to the ankle as long as no stress is felt on the knee.

Return to Action

Whether treatment is conservative or operative, recovery time is at least six months. Return to play is advised only after careful reassessment via X-ray and a clinical exam. Range of motion should be pain free in the involved knee.

CHAPTER 14

Lower-Leg and Ankle Injuries

William G. Hamilton, MD; Andrew A. Brief, MD

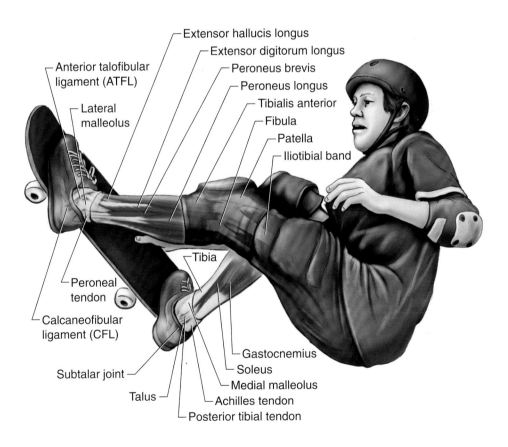

- Extensor hallucis longus
- Extensor digitorum longus
- Peroneus brevis
- Peroneus longus
- Tibialis anterior
- Fibula
- Patella
- Iliotibial band
- Anterior talofibular ligament (ATFL)
- Lateral malleolus
- Peroneal tendon
- Calcaneofibular ligament (CFL)
- Tibia
- Subtalar joint
- Talus
- Gastocnemius
- Soleus
- Medial malleolus
- Achilles tendon
- Posterior tibial tendon

Ankle injuries are extraordinarily common in sports, particularly in pivoting and contact sports such as basketball, soccer, and American football. The unique anatomy and relatively meager support of soft tissue make the ankle joint especially prone to sports injury.

The ankle consists of an ankle bone (talus) held firmly in an upside-down box-like structure called the mortise, as in mortise and tenon joints, formed by the two bones of the lower leg: the shinbone (tibia) and the small bone that runs down the outside of the leg (fibula). The talus moves only up and down, so a second joint under the ankle, the subtalar joint, moves in and out and provides the motion the ankle itself lacks. This motion is powered by the Achilles tendon in back of the ankle; by the posterior tibial tendon on the inside of the ankle; by the peroneal tendons on the outside of the ankle; and by the extensor tendons in the front, which move the ankle in various directions.

The ankle is turned outward by about 10 to 15 degrees in relation to the knee and is built to allow up-and-down motion but very little inward-outward rotation. If inward-outward rotation is forced on the ankle, an injury often results because the joint is not made to move that way. The subtalar joint allows us to walk on uneven ground, such as cobblestones or the side of a hill. This motion of the subtalar joint is surprisingly important and when lost, through arthritis or injury, extremely disabling.

The primary purpose of the ankle (along with the foot) is to absorb energy when landing and then to propel us forward again off the toe. This occurs by means of the subtalar joint beneath the ankle, which transmits the power of the Achilles tendon efficiently through the foot into the ground. Anything that limits or interferes with this motion in the subtalar joint significantly alters the function of the entire lower extremity.

Sports that involve jumping require ankles that absorb energy well, whereas in repetitive sports such as running (there are 1,000 foot strikes in every mile, and each one is almost exactly the same), small differences such as a slight inequality in the length of the legs or stiffness in the subtalar joint can lead to repetitive stress injuries. In this chapter we look at the most common lower-leg and ankle injuries and discuss how to treat them.

Lower-Leg and Ankle Injuries

SHIN SPLINTS

Common Causes

Shin splints and medial tibial stress syndrome (a more severe form of shin splints) are caused by an inflammation of the periosteal sleeve of tissue surrounding the tibia. This type of injury frequently occurs in running or other repetitive cardiovascular activities in which the athlete suddenly increases the distance, duration, or frequency of a training regimen. The muscular insertion of the tibialis anterior, tibialis posterior, and soleus are frequently affected.

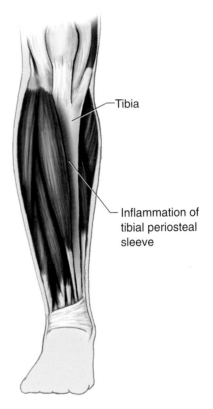

Tibia

Inflammation of tibial periosteal sleeve

Identification

Symptoms typically include a burning or aching pain on the medial (nearer the middle of the body) aspect of the leg or shin after completion of the activity. This pain is a common complaint among runners who are training for a marathon or young athletes who are conditioning at the outset of a new sporting season. The area of pain and tenderness usually spreads out over an area of three-fingers width along the front or back edge of the shinbone. X-rays are usually normal but bone scan reveals localized uptake along the edge of the bone.

Treatment

Treatment for shin splints involves a change in the athlete's training regimen (e.g., decreased mileage, frequency, or intensity of exercise). Icing of the involved area after activity helps in the short term. If pain persists, or gets worse, despite curtailing the level of activity, the athlete should seek professional attention to rule out a more serious injury such as a stress fracture (see p. 227) or exertional compartment syndrome (see p. 226). Examine the athlete's footwear and feet for additional problems. Look for excessive and uneven wear on the soles of running shoes, which may represent biomechanical flaws. Also, if the athlete's feet pronate excessively (the arch flattens as the foot strikes the ground under load), an orthotic may be indicated.

Return to Action

Typically, a one- to two-week layoff from impact exercise allows for a rapid return. A return is recommended when the athlete can practice comfortably and is pain free after vigorous exercise. Taping is seldom useful in achieving a quicker recovery from shin splints.

LOWER-LEG COMPARTMENT SYNDROME

Common Causes

All muscles in the body are grouped into anatomical compartments, each of which is encased with a soft tissue covering called fascia. In these tight compartments, the muscles may swell and expand with vigorous exercise, choking off their own blood supply and endangering the viability of the muscle tissue. This injury usually occurs in distance runners or athletes who engage in continuous running activity.

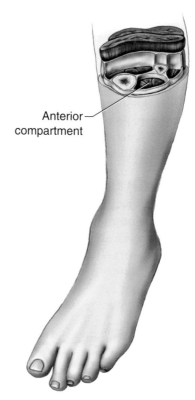

Anterior compartment

Identification

The symptoms of compartment syndrome are more generalized than in other lower-leg conditions. Typically, there is pain, swelling, and sensitivity of the involved muscular compartment that occurs during the peak of exercise. Symptoms typically get worse during the course of a workout and subside afterward. The condition is most accurately diagnosed by measuring the compartment pressures during exercise under local anesthesia.

Treatment

When rest and modifying activity to avoid stressing the lower extremity fail to alleviate symptoms, a minor surgery is required to release the tight fascia surrounding the affected compartment (fasciotomy).

Return to Action

Following surgery, athletes typically return to sport gradually, reaching maximum recovery by four to six months postoperation. Athletes can typically begin lower-extremity workouts two weeks postoperatively. Following conservative treatment, athletes should refrain from running or full sport participation until pain is minimal upon repetitive striding, such as on a treadmill.

LOWER-LEG STRESS FRACTURE

Common Causes

A stress fracture is a process that occurs in response to abnormal stress placed on a normal bone. Such a fracture can occur when a bone is repetitively overloaded for a prolonged period of time. This is particularly apt to occur when a bone is weak to begin with. Patients vulnerable to stress fractures include those with osteoporosis, improper diet, sudden increases in a training regimen, or eating disorders.

Identification

Pain associated with a stress fracture is typically activity related. There is a period of time prior to the actual presence of a fracture in which the bone structure is damaged, but it has not actually cracked yet; this is called a stress reaction. A good analogy is bending a paper clip repeatedly to weaken it (stress reaction) until it breaks (stress fracture). Once the fracture occurs, the pain increases considerably and can be localized (one finger width) on examination to a very specific area. If the bone has been symptomatic for a long time, a small and tender bump might develop on the bone (callus) where it is trying to heal. The most accurate way to diagnose a stress reaction or stress fracture in the early stages is with a bone scan; an X-ray might reveal nothing until the fracture has been there a month or more. There have been several cases of a bone breaking all the way through during running or jumping on a chronic stress fracture.

Treatment

The treatment for both a stress fracture and a stress reaction is usually a marked reduction in activities to allow the fracture to heal. If symptoms are severe, partial weight bearing on crutches and use of a bone stimulator (which may assist in the laying down of new bone and expedite the healing process) might be necessary.

Female athletes with chronic stress fractures should always be checked for symptoms of the female athlete triad: disordered eating, amenorrhea, and osteopenia or osteoporosis. If these related problems are present, the athlete should be treated for them while recovering from the injury.

Return to Action

Once treatment has started, stress fractures tend to take as long to heal as the athlete has been exercising with pain. For some athletes that means three to six months before a return to regular training and competing. However, athletes can often engage in nonimpact types of cross-training (such as deep-water running and some forms of weightlifting) to maintain fitness while the fracture heals.

CALF STRAIN OR TEAR

Common Causes

A calf strain or tear, often called a calf pull, is usually caused by improper stretching before engaging in exercise or sports or by the inability of the calf muscles to accommodate the concentric (muscle-shortening) and eccentric (muscle-lengthening) forces generated by sudden changes in direction of the lower limbs that can occur in many sports. Calf strains are noted in tennis (the strains are sometimes called tennis leg), racquetball, paddle ball, and in most cutting and pivoting sports. Calf strains seem to be more prevalent in weekend warriors and others who do not regularly engage in sport.

Identification

The athlete experiences a popping sensation in the calf, followed by well-localized tenderness over the inside calf muscle in the middle portion of the leg. Because of the immediate pain, athletes often have difficulty putting weight on the affected leg. The severity of this injury ranges from mild (grade I), to moderate (grade II), to severe (grade III) depending on the extent of damage to the muscle belly.

Treatment

The immediate treatment is PRICE (protection, rest, ice, compression, and elevation) followed by an evaluation by a physician. Severe pulls might need cast immobilization or a removable boot. Often, a simple leg sleeve will suffice. After healing is complete, physical therapy is important to restore strength and flexibility and to prevent recurrence. Given time to heal and proper rehab, calf strain is usually a benign injury with a good prognosis. Many people with this condition are more comfortable wearing clogs or shoes with an elevated heel, which takes tension off the Achilles tendon during the healing phase.

Return to Action

The athlete should avoid all cardiovascular exercise for at least a month from the time of injury. Activity should be increased as tolerated thereafter. Taping or strapping of the calf can be applied as needed. The key is not to return too soon. Often athletes are tempted to get back out there after only three weeks, but if the return to sports occurs prematurely, a retear could turn a four- to six-week recovery into a three-month recovery.

ACHILLES TENDON RUPTURE

Common Causes

Achilles rupture is a serious injury that often occurs because of preexisting Achilles tendinitis or inadequate stretching before sports. This injury typically occurs during pivoting or twisting in sports such as soccer, American football, and basketball.

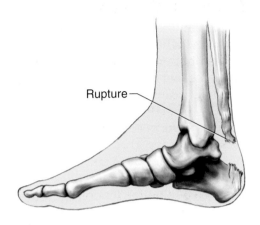

Rupture

Identification

The athlete experiences a pop in the back of the ankle. A gap develops in the tendon that can be felt to the touch, and the tendon no longer functions. When asked to flex the ankle in a downward position ("step on the brake pedal"), injured athletes usually cannot do so. Because of the severity of the pain, athletes often have difficulty putting weight on the affected leg.

Treatment

Again, the immediate treatment is PRICE (protection, rest, ice, compression, and elevation) followed by an evaluation by a physician who will match treatment to the problem. Many Achilles ruptures are missed at the time of the injury if there is only a partial tear or if the examination is performed by an inexperienced clinician.

Two basic treatment approaches are available for a ruptured Achilles tendon: nonsurgical and surgical. Each has its advantages and disadvantages and, interestingly, the two approaches have the same complication rate (19 percent). The nonsurgical approach is cast immobilization in the foot-down position until the tendon heals, which takes six to eight weeks. The advantage here is the avoidance of surgery and all the associated complications, but the disadvantage is loss of strength and a higher likelihood of rupturing the tendon again during the healing period. The surgical approach can restore the normal length and strength of the tendon, but complications can arise in the form of phlebitis and wound infections. The decision as to which approach is best should be made by the athlete and a physician. Either way, rehabilitation plays a major role in the recovery process.

Return to Action

The recovery process following Achilles tendon rupture emphasizes rebuilding of muscle strength and restoration of range of motion. Return to the gym following either treatment approach begins between two and three months from the time of injury. Running can begin at about four months, and pivoting sports at six months. Advise the athlete that full recovery might take up to a year.

ACHILLES TENDINITIS

Common Causes

Achilles injuries are especially common in athletes who allow their Achilles tendons to become tight by not regularly stretching and conditioning the tendon.

Identification

Athletes experience chronic pain in the back and lower part of the calf and ankle that will not subside. A strained Achilles tendon usually occurs in either of two locations: within the tendon itself (usually in the isthmus or narrowest part just behind the ankle), or in the insertion of the tendon in the heel (called Haglund's disease). In the acute phase when the tendon is hot, swollen, tender, and painful, this injury is called tendinitis. In the chronic phase when the inflammatory process has quieted but not gone away, the injury is called tendonosis. The tendon usually develops a painful lump.

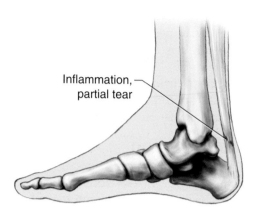

Inflammation, partial tear

Treatment

The healing process for Achilles tendinitis tends to be long and slow. During the healing phase, athletes might prefer to wear clogs or shoes with an elevated heel to prevent further straining of the Achilles. Athletes should avoid stretching until most of the pain is gone. This injury can take months to heal and usually occurs in people who are already very active. You can usually measure the healing by the diminution of the symptoms and the decreased tenderness in the lump. When the condition finally heals, a small, firm lump remains, but it is typically asymptomatic.

Return to Action

Athletes should delay a return to sport until they are completely pain free. At this time, physical therapy and stretching exercises should be emphasized.

ANKLE SPRAIN

Common Causes

In the United States, ankle sprains account for 1 of every 10 visits to the emergency room. Most of these sprains are sustained during contact and pivoting sports.

Identification

Ankle sprains cause a painful, swollen, bruised area on the outside (lateral) aspect of the athlete's ankle. The athlete might not be able to bear weight on the ankle. Ankle sprains are usually classified as mild (grade I), moderate (grade II), or severe (grade III) depending on the extent of the damage. There are two main ligaments on the outside of the ankle that hold it together: the anterior talofibular ligament (ATFL) and the calcaneofibular ligament (CFL) (see p. 223). In most sprains, the ATFL tears first, and then the CFL tears. A grade I sprain is a partial tear of the ATFL, a grade II sprain is a complete tear of the ATFL with the CFL still intact, and a grade III sprain is a complete tear of both the ATFL and CFL. Fortunately, grade III sprains are very rare. An X-ray can help diagnose whether an ankle is fractured or sprained.

Treatment

The treatment of acute ankle sprains is similar to the treatment of most acute injuries: PRICE (protection, rest, ice, compression, and elevation). Many sprains are minor injuries that improve after a few days, and these will usually take care of themselves. However, if pain is considerable and it is difficult to bear weight on the ankle, a physician should have a look at it. These injuries often require the use of crutches and some sort of a brace or support to protect the ankle while it is healing. Recovery usually starts with the healing phase, which involves elevation at night on one pillow to reduce swelling, protected motion, and weight bearing as tolerated. During this phase, ultrasound, massage, acupuncture, and nonsteroidal anti-inflammatory drugs can be useful. As healing progresses, the rehab phase begins with physical therapy to restore motion, strength, proprioception, and function to the ankle.

Sprained ankles often heal with residual weakness. If this weakness is not corrected, a cycle might develop: the weakness of the ankle makes it liable to roll over, and after it rolls over, the ankle is weaker. A common cause of recurrent problems with ankle sprains is incomplete rehabilitation and residual, unrecognized weakness. A sprained ankle that won't heal usually involves one of the following:

- Weak peroneal tendons. These two tendons span the outside (lateral) aspect of the ankle, preventing the ankle from rolling.
- Sinus tarsi syndrome. There is a hollow area on the side of the ankle that can be painful because of scar tissue from a healed sprain.
- Injured peroneal tendons. Chronic unstable ankles can develop partial tears in the peroneal tendons that cause pain and improper function. Tears often don't show up well on MRI. A sonogram might reveal the damage better.

Return to Action

Return to sport for grade I sprains typically takes one to two weeks; grade II sprains take two to four weeks; and grade III injuries take four to six weeks. Taping or ankle braces can provide stability in the acute phases of healing.

ANKLE FRACTURE

Common Causes

Ankle fractures are often the result of high-energy injuries, such as falls from height, motor vehicle accidents, or contact sports.

Identification

Much like ankle sprains only more severe, ankle fractures usually involve a painful, swollen, and bruised ankle. Most athletes cannot bear weight on a fractured ankle.

Treatment

If an ankle is broken, but the bone is not displaced, the injury may be treated without surgery. If the bones are displaced, the fracture will almost always require surgical management to restore stability to the ankle and ensure adequate healing of the fracture.

Return to Action

Much like the recovery following Achilles tendon rupture, recovery from an ankle fracture requires many months of rehabilitation. Typically, an athlete whose broken ankle requires surgery will wear a cast and be unable to bear weight on the ankle for two months. Afterward, physical therapy begins, and return to the gym occurs between two and three months from the time of injury. Running can begin at about three to four months, and pivoting sports at four to six months. The patient should be advised that maximum recovery might not be achieved until one year from the injury.

POSTERIOR TIBIAL TENDINITIS

Common Causes

The posterior tibial tendon (PTT) is the large, strong tendon on the inside of the ankle that holds up the arch of the foot. The tibial strain is commonly seen in pronated (flat-footed) runners or those whose lower legs are rotated outward (duck-footed).

Identification

The athlete often experiences increasing or chronic pain on the inside (medial) aspect of the ankle. He or she might report a progressive worsening flat-footed deformity or collapse of the arch of the foot over time. Another problem related to PTT strain is a painful accessory navicular bone (see p. 241).

Treatment

Treatment usually involves immobilization in a boot, if the pain is bad, and supportive measures such as orthotics and strapping to support the arch of the foot. Cortisone shots are risky because they can damage the posterior tibial tendon within which the accessory navicular bone often lies. In athletes under 40, the injury tends to heal with time and therapy, whereas in athletes over 50, especially in overweight females, it tends not to heal. For these individuals, the tendon inflammation can get progressively worse and lead to slow rupture of the tendon and collapse of the foot (like an old rope that stretches out and eventually comes apart). Surgery may be performed to reconstruct the deficient tendon.

Return to Action

Athletes may return to sport as soon as symptoms subside. They might consider using an orthotic during future sporting activities.

BONE SPURS ON THE ANKLE

Common Causes

Athletes engaged in jumping activities tend to develop bone spurs in the front of the ankle where the bones bang into each other. These form slowly over time.

Identification

Athletes experience persistent pain and swelling at the front of the ankle. The hallmark symptom of this condition is limitation in the upward motion (dorsiflexion) of the ankle caused by impaction of the bone spurs into each other.

Treatment

If symptoms are severe enough, the spurs can be removed with an arthroscope or a small open incision. Less severe cases are treated symptomatically with local icing and medications for pain.

Return to Action

These "cleanout" surgical procedures are usually quite effective, but the ankle is a touchy joint that tends to recover slowly after surgery. It may be several months before athletes are able to return to their usual levels of activity.

CHAPTER 15

Foot and Toe Injuries

William G. Hamilton, MD; Andrew A. Brief, MD

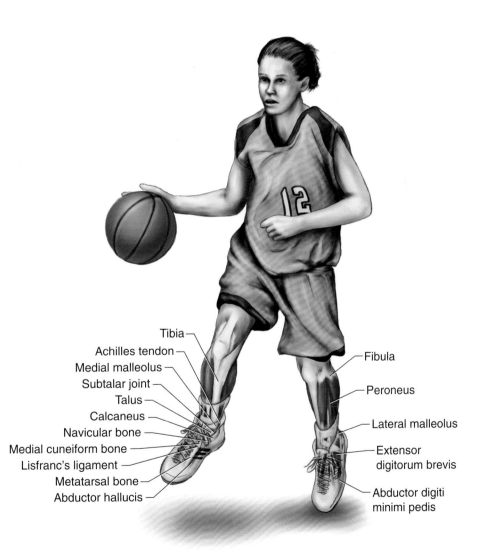

Tibia
Achilles tendon
Medial malleolus
Subtalar joint
Talus
Calcaneus
Navicular bone
Medial cuneiform bone
Lisfranc's ligament
Metatarsal bone
Abductor hallucis

Fibula
Peroneus
Lateral malleolus
Extensor digitorum brevis
Abductor digiti minimi pedis

The foot is made up of 26 bones plus the soft tissues. The soft tissues are the skin, blood vessels, nerves, and connective tissues that include *tendons,* which connect muscles to bones, and *ligaments,* which hold bones together and allow joints to move in only certain directions. The hindfoot is the heel bone (also called the calcaneus). The midfoot or midtarsal bones are solidly packed together like the stones of a roman arch, and the forefoot contains the long bones—the metatarsals—that lead to the toes.

The feet each of us ends up with are the ones we were genetically programmed to have. In terms of the *arch* of the foot, there are three types (see figure 15.1):

- The normal-arched foot—with the arch moderately high off the ground—is the ideal foot to absorb energy; it is neither too rigid nor too flexible.
- The flat foot—low arch—is hypermobile and does not transmit energy well. It is a weak foot that is easily overstrained and tends to tire.
- The cavus foot—high arch—is rigid and does not absorb energy well. It is prone to stress fractures and ankle sprains.

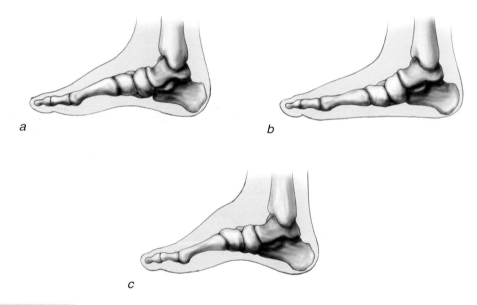

a

b

c

Figure 15.1   The three arch types include *(a)* the normal-arched foot, *(b)* the flat foot, and *(c)* the cavus foot.

In terms of the *shape* of the foot, there are several types (see figure 15.2):

- The Grecian foot is sometimes called the Morton's foot, on which the second toe is the longest.
- The Egyptian foot is one on which the great toe is the longest.

- The Simian foot is a wide foot that forms a bunion.
- The peasant's foot is broad and square with metatarsals of almost equal length; it is very stable and absorbs energy quite well. It is an ideal foot for sports.
- The model's foot is narrow and tapered. Because of the unequal length of the metatarsals, it absorbs energy poorly and is not a good foot for impact sports.

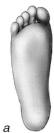 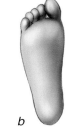 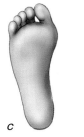 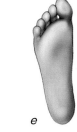

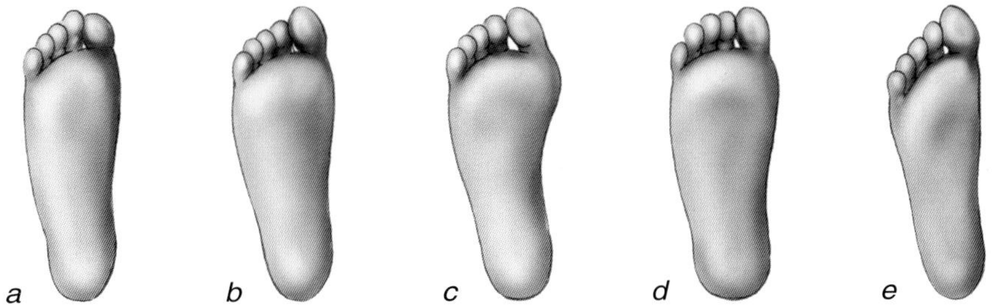

a   b   c   d   e

Figure 15.2   The foot shapes include *(a)* the Grecian foot, *(b)* the Egyptian foot, *(c)* the Simian foot, *(d)* the peasant's foot, and *(e)* the model's foot.

Foot and Toe Injuries

Injury	Page
Bunions	248
Corns	253
Fifth Metatarsal Fractures	245
Forefoot Neuromas	252
Freiberg's Disease	251
Fungal Infections	254
Hallux Rigidus	246
Lisfranc's Sprain	243
March or Dancer's Stress Fracture	244
Painful Accessory Navicular Bone	241
Plantar Fasciitis	238
Purple Toe	257
Navicular Bone Stress Fracture	242
Sesamoid Injury	249
Shoelace Pressure Syndrome	256
Stone Bruise	240
Talon Noir	258
Tarsal Tunnel Syndrome	255
Tennis Toe	250
Turf Toe	247

PLANTAR FASCIITIS

Common Causes

The plantar fascia is a strong, tough band of tissue on the sole of the foot that begins at the ball of the foot and attaches to the bottom of the heel. It can be strained either acutely or chronically, but chronic conditions appear to be more common. Plantar fasciitis is often the result of overuse, either from running too long without rest or jumping on the heel too much. Strains sometimes occur in the midportion of the arch, but are more often seen at the attachment to the heel. Occasionally, the plantar fascia is torn, either partly or completely, during physical activity.

It was once thought that a heel bone spur, often seen on X-ray, was the cause of plantar fasciitis—however, the spur is actually located above the insertion of the fascia rather than in the fascia itself. The spur is likely not the cause of the pain.

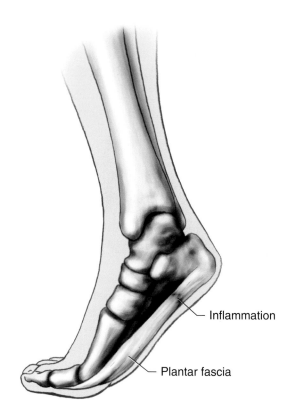

Inflammation

Plantar fascia

Plantar fasciitis must be differentiated from plantar fibromatosis. Although plantar fibromatosis also involves the plantar fascia and causes pain, the problem arises from fibrous lumps that form in the plantar fascia rather than from inflammation. Plantar fibromatosis tends to run in families and is sometimes associated with a similar condition in the palmer fascia of the hand. The condition can be identified by soft, mobile lumps on the sole of the foot that can be painful to the touch and symptomatic during standing or playing sports. These lesions can increase in size over time but typically are not fast-growing tumors. Plantar fibromatosis tumors are benign tumors and are best left alone because they have a very high recurrence rate following surgical removal. The athlete with plantar fibromatosis may participate in sports as tolerated. Following excision, sports should be avoided for at least a month.

Identification

Plantar fasciitis is characterized by localized tenderness on the bottom of the heel and a specific type of pain that occurs in the morning getting out of bed. Athletes often describe this pain as feeling "something like a carpet tack stuck in my heel. For the first few steps I can't get my heel to the floor; then I can slowly get it down." The discomfort during the first few steps may occur because during sleep the foot is held in a plantar-flexed position (toes pointing down). Thus, during the first steps, the toes and foot extend upward (dorsiflexion). This action causes tension on the plantar fascia and irritates the inflamed tissue.

Treatment

Treatment of plantar fasciitis is somewhat controversial because there are dozens of different items available on the market for this common problem. A very good study done by the American Orthopedic Foot and Ankle Society showed that there is a 90 percent healing rate in nine months regardless of treatment. Athletes might try using heel cups, physical therapy, and a night splint worn to hold the foot up at night. This splint usually decreases the morning pain, and once this begins to get better, the condition usually resolves itself. Healing can be slow and frustrating, but the best treatment for planter fasciitis is rest. There are a few cases that fail to get better, and these might need to be treated with steroid injections, shock wave therapy, or surgical release.

Return to Action

The athlete should return to sports only when completely pain free. The timetable for return to sports is variable; it can be as brief as a few weeks or may be an entire year. Postoperatively, athletes can expect several months of downtime before returning to competition.

STONE BRUISE

Common Causes

There are many causes of heel pain; the heel has many nerve endings and is quite sensitive to injury. A stone bruise is caused from a stone or other object that bruises the bottom of the heel. This injury might sound minor, but it can produce severe pain depending on the number of cells that get bruised. Stone bruises are seen most often in athletes and other active people. Many times these bruises are accompanied by a hairline fracture that will not show on an early X-ray but might show up later when the injury begins to heal. In running and other repetitive-type sports, this pain can also be caused by a stress fracture (see p. 227).

Identification

When the bottom of the heel is bruised it is often extremely painful and tends to heal slowly. Pain might be accompanied by swelling and tenderness. The athlete might have difficulty putting weight on the foot.

Treatment

The best treatment for a stone bruise is to curtail walking as much as possible until the injury heals. The foot should be immobilized and placed in a boot until symptoms subside, which might take anywhere from two to eight weeks.

Return to Action

A stone bruise heals slowly. The athlete should return to sports only when completely pain free. This might take as long as eight weeks, and longer if not treated with care.

PAINFUL ACCESSORY NAVICULAR BONE

Common Causes

Roughly 5 to 10 percent of people are born with an extra bone on the inside of the arch of the foot adjacent to the navicular bone. Athletes who have an accessory navicular in one foot have a 50 percent chance of having it in the other foot as well. It is present from birth and frequently causes no trouble other than an abnormal prominence in the arch of the foot. Its presence can render the appearance that the arch is flat, when in actuality it is not.

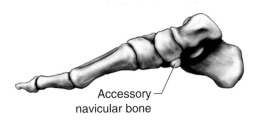

Accessory navicular bone

Identification

Many people with an accessory bone go through their whole lives without difficulty, whereas others have symptoms from an early age. Some experience pain following a sprain or direct blow to the area. Once the area begins to hurt it may eventually stop but often progresses to cause pain or a flat-foot deformity.

Treatment

Initial treatment is immobilization in a boot or cast, with the use of crutches. Some advocate a local cortisone injection to control inflammatory symptoms. If these measures fail, the bone can be removed surgically, but recovery time is often long and frustrating, taking from three to nine months. The younger the athlete is when surgery is done, though, the faster the recovery.

Return to Action

The athlete with a symptomatic accessory navicular should immobilize it until symptoms subside. He or she should return to sports only when completely pain free and might need to wear a medial arch support or orthotic inside the tennis shoe or cleat.

NAVICULAR BONE STRESS FRACTURE

Common Causes

The navicular is a boat-shaped bone directly in front of the ankle that runs across the midfoot. In athletes with a high-arched foot that absorbs energy poorly, this bone is prone to stress fractures.

Identification

The athlete with a navicular stress fracture will typically experience severe midfoot pain without an injury. Like all stress fractures, a navicular stress fracture might not show up on an X-ray, but it is a dangerous fracture because if it is not recognized and treated, the fracture line can propagate and bone fragments will separate. If a navicular stress fracture is suspected, a bone scan will usually pick it up.

Treatment

This injury is potentially serious and needs to be treated aggressively, usually with surgery including screw fixation to promote healing and prevent recurrence.

Return to Action

Following surgery, the athlete will be unable to bear weight on the foot for two months. Expected return to sports is anywhere from six months to one year after surgery.

LISFRANC'S SPRAIN

Common Causes

The middle of the foot is normally quite rigid because it is bound together by a series of strong ligaments. In the forefoot (just beyond the midfoot), there are five rays, each of which has a metatarsal and toe bone (phalange). The ray running to the great toe is the first ray, and the rest follow suit, two through five. At the base of the first ray is a strong ligament (Lisfranc's ligament) that binds the first ray to the other rays. When this ligament is torn, the connection is disrupted, leaving the foot weak and unstable. This sprain is particularly common in American football, soccer, and any sport in which the foot may twist severely.

Identification

This injury comes in several different types and degrees of severity. It is important not to miss it because it can lead to chronic pain and posttraumatic osteoarthritis. The sprain will sometimes show up on a weight-bearing X-ray of both feet, but both MRI and a CT scan might be required to make the diagnosis.

Treatment

Surgery is often needed to stabilize the midfoot and prevent chronic pain. The alternative to surgery is a two-month period of bearing no weight on the foot, which still might not be effective in preventing the onset of osteoarthritis in the future.

Return to Action

The recovery from this injury is prolonged. Following surgery, the athlete is unable to bear weight on the foot for two months. Expect a full return to take anywhere from six months to one year after surgery.

MARCH OR DANCER'S STRESS FRACTURE

Common Causes

The "march fracture" got its name because it was common in Army recruits after a long march. This injury usually occurs in the middle of the second or third metatarsal bone in the forefoot. It is very common in runners who begin training for a marathon. Female ballet dancers, probably because they dance on their toes, get the same fracture, but they sustain it not in the shaft of the bone but at the base of the second metatarsal.

Identification

The pain and tenderness is typically localized over the shaft of the bone, in the middle of the midfoot. As with all stress fractures, it rarely shows up on the initial X-ray but can be seen several weeks later as it begins to heal and lays down new bone. The most reliable way to diagnose a stress fracture early is with a bone scan.

Treatment

Athletes should avoid activity until the bone heals. Dancers who develop this fracture should be screened for the female athlete triad, which includes amenorrhea, disordered eating, and osteopenia or osteoporosis.

Return to Action

Return to weight-bearing exercises typically begins about six weeks from the time of diagnosis. Running can be initiated at three months.

FIFTH METATARSAL FRACTURES

Common Causes

The fifth metatarsal is the small bone on the outside of the forefoot just below the ankle. Injuries to this bone are very common and are usually caused by abrupt twists of the foot during a fall.

Identification

The athlete might feel a pop and have immediate pain, discoloration, and swelling of the area. Fractures occur in four different locations of the bone.

The *tubercle fracture* occurs at the base of the bone nearest the ankle, at which there is normally a bump where a tendon attaches to the bone. This fracture is the most common of the fifth metatarsal fractures and the least serious. The *Jones' fracture* is very near the tubercle but occurs in an area with a poor blood supply and heals poorly. It is the most serious of these injuries. The *spiral oblique fracture* (also called the dancer's acute fracture) occurs further down the shaft of the bone in the distal third. This fracture occurs frequently when dancers who dance up on the ball of the foot roll the foot over. A *boxer's fracture* involves a break at the distal end of the bone, just near the knuckle of the fifth toe joint.

Treatment

Tubercle fractures are usually treated in a firm shoe with crutches until healed. They rarely require surgery. Jones' fractures tend to fail to heal, proceed to a nonunion, and result in chronic pain and disability—especially if the athlete is allowed to walk on the foot. For this reason, many orthopedists favor putting a screw in the bone to secure healing and prevent recurrence. The alternative is to avoid weight bearing and use crutches for six to eight weeks until the fracture has healed. The spiral oblique fracture will usually heal without surgery, although some displacement might occur. Boxer's fractures rarely require treatment aside from PRICE (protection, rest, ice, compression, and elevation) and activity restrictions.

Return to Action

Nonsurgical fifth metatarsal fractures are stable injuries. Athletes typically return to full activity within two months from the time of injury. Athletes with a surgically repaired Jones' fracture return to sport after a few months, when cleared by the surgeon.

HALLUX RIGIDUS

Common Causes

Hallux rigidus is a condition in which the big toe joint begins to wear out and becomes painful, stiff, and arthritic. This can occur in one foot or both and is hardly ever caused by a specific injury. Women often have more trouble with hallux rigidus because the use of high-heeled shoes is painful with this condition.

Identification

Athletes who are bothered by hallux rigidus experience pain and stiffness in the big toe. A bump usually forms on the top of the joint and is frequently mistaken for a bunion (see p. 248). Hallux rigidus is easy to differentiate from a bunion by the painful loss of motion that occurs. Bunions do not usually become stiff, whereas loss of motion is the hallmark of hallux rigidus.

Treatment

Once the condition begins, it usually progresses slowly in spite of treatment. The nonsurgical approach involves footwear that prevents the big toe joint from being forced to move beyond its limited range of motion. This usually means wearing a modified shoe with a stiff sole and a rocker mechanism that allows you to walk or run without forcing the big toe upward.

If conservative measures fail, surgery for hallux rigidus depends on how worn out the joint is. In the early stages, osteoarthritis begins in the uppermost part of the joint and over time destroys the whole surface. Procedures that clean out the arthritis work best in the early stages of the condition, but when all or most of the joint has deteriorated, these measures no longer serve their purpose. Surgical treatment of advanced hallux rigidus presents a difficult problem. An implant of metal or plastic will not hold up over time and has been proven not to work. The traditional treatment is to fuse the two bones on either side of the toe so the joint no longer exists, but this requires up to three months to fuse and might cause some limitations later. For example, cross-country skiing is very difficult, if not impossible, after fusion surgery because the toe joint will not move upward. Additionally, high heels cannot be worn after fusion surgery.

Return to Action

Athletes with this condition can be as active as their discomfort allows. They will often be limited in sports requiring jumping (basketball) or explosive bursts of sprinting (tennis). Following surgery athletes can return to play when cleared by the surgeon.

TURF TOE

Common Causes

Turf toe is a violent injury that happens most often in contact sports such as American football, basketball, and soccer when a player falls on another player's foot and the first metatarsal phalangeal joint is driven upward to an extreme degree, tearing the attachment of the sesamoids under the base of the big toe.

Site of tearing

Identification

Like so many injuries in orthopedics, turf toe is graded I, II, or III, depending on the extent of the damage. Symptoms include, pain, swelling, bruising, and difficulty bearing weight on the ball of the foot.

Treatment

Turf toe is a serious injury with potential for long-term disability. Frequently, surgery is required to restore the normal anatomy. Conservative treatments include taping the toe and wearing solid-sole shoes to reduce motion and encourage healing.

Return to Action

Turf toe injuries require a minimum of one month out of sports. Depending on the severity, return to action can take as long as a year from the time of injury.

BUNIONS

Common Causes

Bunions arise from an inherited disorder that causes a bump to form on the inside of the foot at the base of the big toe. This causes the big toe to drift laterally, sometimes crossing under the second toe. Bunions are much more common in women than men. Tight-fitting cleats or training sneakers might exacerbate this condition, but they do not cause it.

Identification

Many people have bunions and are symptom free all their lives. Others experience pain with footwear and forefoot pain with exercise. Pain is typically present on the bump itself or on the sole of the foot of the second metatarsal, where a callus might have formed. There is a misconception that the deformity is often caused by osteoarthritis, but this is usually not the case.

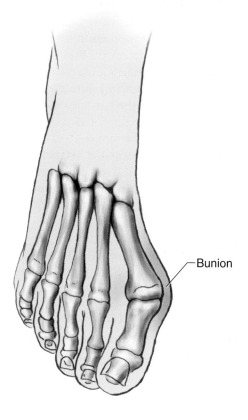
Bunion

Treatment

An athlete with a bunion should wear shoes that accommodate the shape of the feet because most of the pain that occurs is caused by shoe pressure against the bump. Women with bunions often find relief by buying wider sneakers or even men's shoes, which are wider than those made for women. Commercially available toe spacers can be placed between the first and second toes to alleviate pain when wearing shoes. Many people with bunions choose to have them surgically corrected. The results are usually quite good and the complication rate is low.

Return to Action

There is no required downtime in most cases. The athlete can be as active as discomfort or pain allows. Return time to sports after surgery is at least three months.

SESAMOID INJURY

Common Causes

Two small bones beneath the big toe joint are shaped like sesame seeds; these are the sesamoid bones. They lie inside of the tendons of the toe flexors much as the kneecap lies within the quadriceps muscles. When these bones are injured and painful, the condition is called sesamoiditis. Many factors can make the sesamoids hurt, including a fracture or stress fracture, a separation of the bone, avascular necrosis, and osteoarthritis.

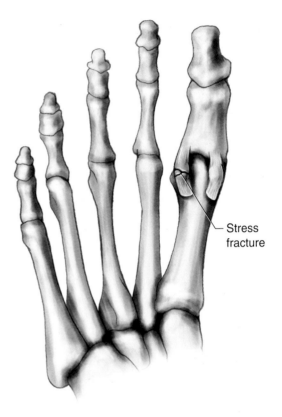

Stress fracture

Identification

With sesamoiditis, the athlete experiences progressively increasing pain beneath the great (big) toe. The onset is typically spontaneous and not caused by an injury. The condition is relatively easy to diagnose because of the characteristic symptoms and the specific location of the tenderness on physical exam. However, determining whether the problem was caused by fracture, separation or sprain of a two-piece sesamoid (many people are born with the sesamoid in two pieces instead of one), or avascular necrosis of the sesamoid can be difficult. In avascular necrosis, for reasons that are poorly understood, the sesamoid dies and can be painful for months before the problem shows on X-ray. Avascular necrosis often follows a stress fracture when the bone, rather than healing, disintegrates. Osteoarthritis of the sesamoids can be painful in older athletes. Exact diagnosis frequently requires a bone scan or MRI.

Treatment

Treatment depends on the diagnosis and can involve anything from an orthosis, which limits the motion in the joint and takes weight off the painful area so it can heal, to a walking boot, crutches, or a bone stimulator. Surgery should be a last resort, but removal of one of the two sesamoids can be safely performed when nonsurgical options have failed.

Return to Action

There is no required downtime in most cases. The athlete with a sesamoid injury can be as active as discomfort or pain allows. Return time to sports after surgery is at least a month.

TENNIS TOE

Common Causes

Tennis toe is a black toenail that forms as the result of a contusion or bruise under the toenail, usually of the second toe, or whichever toe is longest. The condition is really a blood clot caused by wearing shoes that are too small or by not lacing the shoe up tightly enough to hold the foot back in the shoe. As a result, the toe slips forward and hits the tip of the toe box.

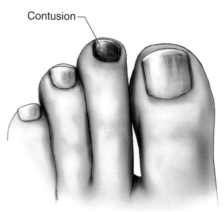

Contusion

Identification

Diagnosis is made on inspection of the foot once the toenail turns black. The athlete experiences pain, but the injury is not serious.

Treatment

The best treatment is to leave the toe alone. The nail will come off once a new nail has grown in beneath it.

Return to Action

There is no required downtime with tennis toe. The athlete can be as active as discomfort allows.

FREIBERG'S DISEASE

Common Causes

In Freiberg's disease, the head of the second metatarsal dies. This condition is most commonly seen in female athletes in their 20s. The precise cause is unknown, but the disease is an example of avascular necrosis—death of bone caused by lack of blood supply. You sometimes see this occur in other bones in the body, including the foot, ankle, knee, or wrist.

Identification

Freiberg's disease is characterized by chronic pain and stiffness in the middle of the forefoot. Weight bearing and sports activity can be painful. Initial X-rays might be normal, but repeat X-rays taken several months later because of persistence of symptoms might show the disease. When Freiberg occurs in the foot, it is *not* associated with problems elsewhere.

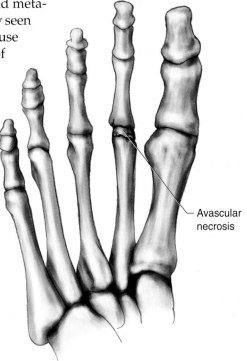

Avascular necrosis

Treatment

If orthotic management is unsuccessful, surgery might be required to correct the problem.

Return to Action

There is no required downtime in most cases. Athletes may be as active as their pain or discomfort allows. Return to sport after surgery takes at least two months.

FOREFOOT NEUROMAS

Common Causes

A neuroma is caused by a pinched or irritated nerve. Several different types of neuromas can occur throughout the body. Morton's neuroma is common in women. It usually occurs in the third web space of the foot between the third and fourth toes (80 percent), and less frequently (20 percent), in the second web space between the second and third toes. Morton's neuroma is usually caused by wearing shoes that are too tight. Joplin's neuroma occurs adjacent to the medial sesamoid below the inside of the big toe; it is commonly seen in runners who pronate or roll in with their stride.

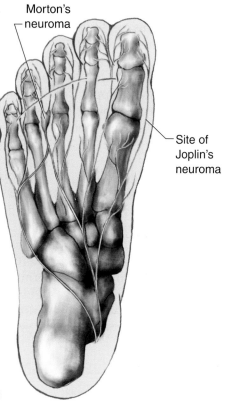

Morton's neuroma

Site of Joplin's neuroma

Identification

Neuromas cause a distinctive and localized pain, often described as numbness, tingling, stinging, or pain radiating either up or down the foot. In the case of Morton's neuroma, the pain radiates into the toes and is characteristically relieved by removing shoes and massaging the foot. Joplin's neuroma is often confused with sesamoid pain (see p. 249); the pain in this case tends to radiate up and down the medial side of the foot.

Treatment

Initial treatment consists of wearing wide shoes or orthoses. If this fails, cortisone injections are recommended. If these measures fail, surgical removal is recommended. Results from surgery are not always good. A study at the Mayo Clinic with large numbers showed an 80 percent success rate. Treatment for Joplin's neuroma includes wearing wider shoes to prevent rubbing of the shoe against the irritated nerve.

Return to Action

There is no required down time with this condition. Athletes may be as active as pain or discomfort allows. Recovery time after surgery is at least a month.

CORNS

Common Causes

Among the several types of corns are hard corns, soft corns, and seed corns. Hard corns form on the surface of the toes where friction occurs between the skin and the shoe. They tend to build up with time. Soft corns occur in the web spaces between the toes, usually between the fourth and fifth toes. They are caused by wearing shoes that squeeze the toes together. Seed corns, which are related to cholesterol plaques, are a particular kind of corn typically found on the sole of the foot.

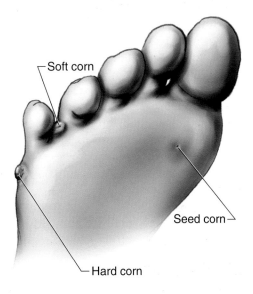

Identification

All corns tend to cause significant pain and discomfort. Hard and soft corns usually build up in layers like onion skin. A seed corn, however, dives inward and forms a little white nidus that acts much like a splinter. Seed corns are easily identified by the presence of a little white dot in the center of the corn.

Treatment

Hard corns can be controlled by wearing corn pads and rubbing the corns down occasionally with a pumice stone. They usually will need to be trimmed and can often be controlled by wearing lamb's wool or cotton between the toes. In chronic conditions, surgery might be required. Immediate relief is obtained for seed corns when the little white nidus is removed by a professional in the office setting.

Return to Action

There is no required downtime with this condition. Athletes may be as active as pain or discomfort allows.

FUNGAL INFECTIONS

Common Causes

Athlete's foot and onychomycosis are both caused by fungal infections. Athlete's foot is usually spread in moist areas such as locker rooms and showers. Onychomycosis is a specific type of athlete's foot that grows under the toenails and is *very* resistant to treatment. It is typically not a serious problem, but it is an unsightly one.

Athlete's foot

Identification

Athlete's foot causes dry, itchy, and flaking skin between the toes. More severe cases may include scaling and blistering or pain and swelling. If untreated, the symptoms may spread to the sole and top of the feet and the toenails. Scratching the feet and then touching other parts of the body can spread the infection to these areas (e.g., groin, knees, elbows, or underarms). Athletes with onychomycosis typically have a deformed, discolored, and rigid toenails that resist normal grooming.

Treatment

Good foot hygiene should be maintained. Keep the feet clean and dry, change socks on a daily basis, allow shoes to air out before wearing again, and wear sandals or flip-flops when walking in potentially contagious areas such as the locker room. Topical antifungal medications are often required. Depending on how chronic and severe the symptoms are, an oral antifungal medication may be prescribed.

Many varieties of local medications have been tried for the problem of onychomycosis, but all have failed. The only effective way to get rid of this infection is to take an oral antifungal medication regularly for at least three to six months. However, these drugs are potentially damaging to the liver, so people taking this medicine need to have their liver function tested every six weeks to ensure they are not harming the liver. Because of this potential side effect, many people feel the cure is worse than the problem.

Return to Action

During treatment, athletes with athlete's foot or onychomycosis should avoid walking barefoot in locker rooms to prevent spreading the infections. Otherwise, they may be as active as pain or discomfort allow.

TARSAL TUNNEL SYNDROME

Common Causes

There are two bumps (malleoli) on the ankle, one on the inner side and one on the outer side. Behind the inner bump, there is a tunnel through which several structures pass, including the posterior tibial nerve. Tarsal tunnel syndrome occurs when this tunnel is compressed and the posterior tibial nerve becomes irritated. Common causes of tarsal tunnel syndrome are altered biomechanics and trauma. Contributing factors include excessive pronation, posttibial deficiency, and congenital flat feet.

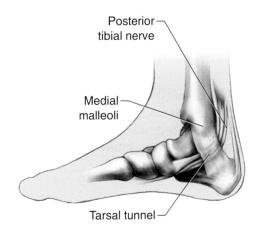

Identification

Athletes with tarsal tunnel syndrome typically experience vague pain on the inner side of the ankle. Numbness, tingling, burning, and a "funny" sensation on the inner side of the ankle may also be present. These symptoms may radiate into the arch of the foot. Symptoms usually improve with rest and worsen with running or other activities.

Treatment

Orthotics can be helpful to correct symptoms stemming from a biomechanical problem such as hyperpronation or flat feet. Sometimes an injection of steroid into the tunnel helps calm the inflammation. If conservative treatment is not effective, surgical decompression of the tunnel may be necessary.

Return to Action

Return to sport following tarsal tunnel syndrome depends on the underlying cause. Return to sport may occur once the athlete has full, pain-free range of motion and activity does not bring back the symptoms. Conservative treatment allows the athlete to return to sports in as little as two to three weeks, as symptoms abate. Depending on the type of procedure, surgical treatment may require that the athlete be out for two to three months.

Robert S. Gotlin, DO, contributed this injury text.

SHOELACE PRESSURE SYNDROME

Common Causes

Shoelace pressure syndrome occurs when the athlete ties his or her shoelaces too tight or when the tongue and top of the footwear is too snug.

Identification

Shoelace syndrome causes pain, numbness, or tingling at the top of the foot where the shoelaces are tied. The symptoms may radiate toward the toes.

Treatment

Once other causes of the symptoms are ruled out by appropriate diagnostic studies, simply tying the shoelaces less tightly may relieve the symptoms. Remember, the feet swell during the course of the day. Athletes should purchase running or athletic shoes late in the day and wear socks that are similar to those that will be worn during running or participation in their sport.

Return to Action

If no other problems exist, the athlete may return to sport with shoes that fit properly.

Robert S. Gotlin, DO, contributed the injury text on this page.

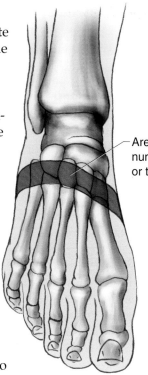

Area of pain, numbness, or tingling

PURPLE TOE

Common Causes

Purple toe, similar to tennis toe (p. 250) but affecting the entire toe rather than just the nail, results from repetitive banging of the nail into the front of the shoe. This repetitive trauma results in minimal bleeding beneath the nail bed. It is seen in long-distance runners and in those who wear shoes with rigid toe boxes.

Identification

Purple toe causes a purple discoloration of the toe and throbbing pain in the toe. The toe may also be somewhat swollen. The first and second toes are most often affected.

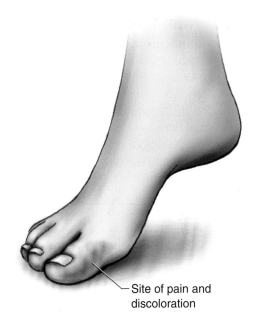

Site of pain and discoloration

Treatment

PRICE is helpful. Appropriate modification of footwear is often necessary to provide more support and take pressure off the toe. The toe box should not be too rigid. An orthotic may also be required. Often, this condition is solely related to overuse (i.e., too many strides).

Return to Action

Once the athlete has full, pain-free range of motion and the underlying cause has been addressed (e.g., footwear, biomechanics), he or she can return to sport.

Robert S. Gotlin, DO contributed the injury text on this page.

TALON NOIR

Common Causes

Repetitive jumping, cutting, twisting, or turning can lead to shear stresses on the small blood vessels within the skin of the heel. When these blood vessels bleed, they cause a darkening in the heel, which is known as talon noir, or black heel. It is most commonly seen in young athletes and in runners, weightlifters, tennis players, and mountain climbers.

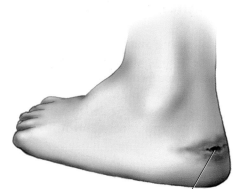

Site of bleeding blood vessels

Identification

Talon noir typically causes painless blue-black dots or discolorations on the back or bottom of the heel. Although they may not feel them, athletes may notice them and be worried about them.

Treatment

No treatment is generally required for these asymptomatic discolorations, but a heel pad may help the lesion disappear more quickly. Athletes should consult a physician if the lesion persists for more than a week to make sure that it is not something more serious such as a malignant skin cancer.

Return to Action

The athlete may continue to participate in sports with this asymptomatic lesion.

Robert S. Gotlin, DO, contributed the injury text on this page.

CHAPTER 16

Integrative Medicine Treatments

Roberta Lee, MD

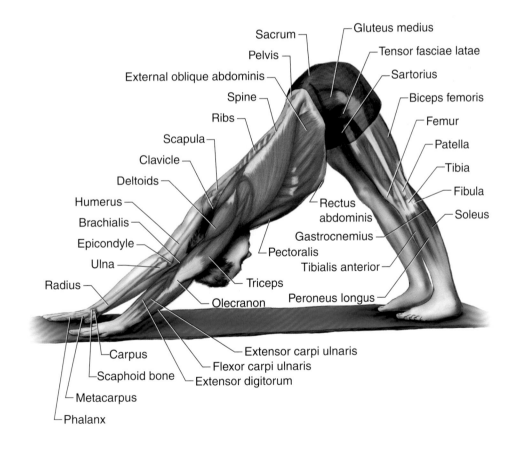

Integrative medicine (IM) is a relatively new direction in the approach to disease management and health maintenance that fuses alternative and conventional medical practices. Integrative medicine, founded by Andrew Weil, MD, in the 1990s, is "a healing oriented medicine that takes account of the whole person (body, mind, and spirit), including all aspects of lifestyle. It emphasizes the therapeutic relationship and makes use of all appropriate therapies, both conventional and alternative" (Weil 2001). Given this definition, IM adds value to sports medicine by addressing not only the medical ailments or injuries of a person but also lifestyle factors such as nutritional needs, exercise patterns, and stress effects on health.

Sports medicine is a discipline that focuses on enhancing athletic performance and reducing injury from sports-related trauma (Roy and Irvin 1983), and its preemptive prevention-oriented objectives are in alignment with many of the approaches found in complementary and alternative modalities (CAM). CAM therapies are defined in most studies as "those modalities and practices neither taught widely in medical schools nor generally available at U.S. hospitals" (Eisenberg et al. 1993; Barnes et al. 2004). The integrative medicine approach of combining CAM interventions with conventional sports medicine can benefit the treatment of acute and chronic management of injuries—by reducing pain and inflammation.

The most common of CAM modalities, classified as CAM therapies, include the following:

- **Botanical medicine.** The field of botanical medicine encompasses a wide variety of botanical preparations used for medicinal purposes. Some forms of botanical use are derived from complex indigenous medical practices such as Chinese medicine. In other situations, the use of plant-based medicines are derived from herbalists' experience and knowledge, as is the case of Western herbalism practiced in Europe. Athletes using these preparations should be aware that the ingredients can interact with other medications, as is true of conventional medications, and ensure that all of their health care providers are aware of their use of botanical medicine.

- **East Asian medicine and other indigenous systems.** Chinese medicine, East Asian medicine, and other indigenous medical treatments often define health in terms of function. These medical systems have existed for thousands of years, and many experts suggest that their treatment plans tend to be effective. Thus, in some situations, including incidents of acute injuries, treatments by practitioners of these systems might be useful.

- **Musculoskeletal manipulation.** Whether performed by a chiropractor or osteopathic physician, musculoskeletal manipulation can enhance the flexibility or improve the mobility of an athlete and thus aid in treatment or rehabilitation in a variety of musculoskeletal injuries.

- **Yoga and tai chi.** Flexibility can be enhanced through the introduction of a daily regimen including yoga or tai chi, movement practices derived from the ancient medical systems of Ayurveda and traditional Chinese medicine.

- **Mind–body practices.** Mind–body or mental imaging modalities such as hypnosis, meditation, and guided imagery are other alternative therapies that can be useful in enhancing sport performance. These practices can encourage the subconscious to focus on desired goals in sports and can also assist in reducing anxiety.

The nutritive contribution of diet is one area in which the shared preventive goals of conventional medicine and alternative medicine, heretofore labeled as integrative medicine, can reduce the vulnerability of the athlete to a variety of health ailments. It is well recognized that the increased nutritional needs of physical exertion in athletes creates a demand for increased caloric consumption. Yet, this increased demand should be addressed by thoughtful food choices that meet the requirements of muscular restructuring and tissue repair.

For athletes of all ages, food sources providing empty calorie content should be replaced with foods of equal caloric value that are rich sources of antioxidants and minerals. At a minimum, coaches should advise all athletes to take a general multi-vitamin and an omega-3 fatty acid supplement to provide increased antioxidant and essential fatty acid support. In this way, sports nutrition can play a central role in an integrated sports medicine approach. Although this chapter doesn't cover the details of sports nutrition, some excellent resources for athletes on nutrition can be found in *Nancy Clark's Sports Nutrition Guidebook*, *Nutrition in Sport* by the IOC Commission, and in other sports nutrition texts.

It is useful to think of integrative therapies as interventions that can be administered in a layered fashion. For example, if an athlete has a mild ankle sprain, in addition to implementing medications such as a nonsteroidal anti-inflammatory (NSAID) and proper mechanical support (e.g., splints and braces), acupuncture can also be initiated. Acupuncture may provide shorter recovery time, reduced pain, and more rapid symptom resolution. Taking this example one step further, if the athlete with this injury has poor gastrointestinal tolerance to NSAIDs, botanical preparations such as turmeric (*Curcuma longa*) or ginger (*Zingiber officinale*) can be used as alternative options for healing and reducing inflammation. Furthermore, if the injury is related to repetitive motion, work with an osteopathic physician for gait assessment and subtle limb-length discrepancies could be added.

There are many treatments and indigenous medical systems that are not discussed in this chapter. Rather than being a comprehensive review of alternative treatments and modalities, this chapter is designed to give a general sense of an integrative approach of traditional and alternative medicine's applications in sports medicine. Ultimately, the preferences of the athlete, existing available expertise, and medical conditions will dictate the best course of action. However, the inclusion of alternative treatments in an integrative medicine approach, with its increased emphasis on nutrition, flexibility, and musculoskeletal support, can greatly enhance physical well-being and reduce vulnerability to injury. The judicious inclusion of many alternative treatments and anti-inflammatory alternatives might also enhance pain management in acute and chronic sport-related injuries.

Botanical and Dietary Supplements

About $11.9 billion is spent annually on sport-related supplements in the United States, and these supplements are widely used by the public. In the United States, supplements and botanicals are regulated as foods rather than drugs, so the quality of these products should be evaluated and monitored by consulting with knowledgeable professionals or verifying the product quality through other means (such as text references and independent testing labs). The regulation of products through Dietary Supplement Health and Education Act (DSHEA) has created a situation in which product quality is variable—mainly because quality control over the product is primarily at the discretion of the manufacturer. Nevertheless, reputable botanical and supplement companies are available, and a growing body of research is emerging suggesting that selected supplements might have medicinal value, particularly for treating sports injuries. Those choosing to implement botanical alternatives should be aware that it might take one to two months to achieve maximal therapeutic benefit. Compared with conventional mediciations, botanical alternatives contain lower doses of pharmacologically active ingredients found in natural substances. These lower doses require more time to reach a therapeutic range. Additionally, as with all oral preparations, idiosyncratic allergic reactions and interactions with conventional medications must be considered. All too often people erroneously assume that because many supplements are "natural" they pose no risk. But there have been reports of dramatic interactions and misuse of supplements that have caused great harm through misinformation and poor judgment in dosing.

Anti-Inflammatory Botanicals

Many anti-inflammatory botanical alternatives might be useful for sports injuries. Because botanicals can take two months to achieve maximal therapeutic benefit, one strategy might be to implement a botanical supplement in the subacute phase of injury, introducing its use after beginning anti-inflammatory control with a conventional NSAID. For more information on many of the botanicals discussed in the following sections, see www.naturaldatabase.com.

Turmeric

One of the five spices found in curry is turmeric (*Curcuma longa*), a root whose active ingredients have significant anti-inflammatory properties. The active constituents in this spice, known as curcumoids and turmerones, influence prostaglandins, leukotrienes, and cyclooxygenase enzymes in the same way that conventional non-steroidal anti-inflammatory medicines do. The customary oral dose of turmeric is 500 milligrams four times daily. Adding this spice to the diet will have some positive anti-inflammatory influence, but to maximize the medicinal effects of this natural aspirin-like spice, a concentrated turmeric supplement should be taken. No equivalent dose in cooking is recommended, although the average Asian consumption of turmeric is approximately 2 grams a day, a dose thought to have some degree of anti-inflammatory influence.

Ginger

Another rhizome with anti-inflammatory abilities is ginger (*Zingiber officinale*). Several small clinical trials have suggested that ginger is effective in reducing pain in those with osteoarthritis (Srivastava and Mustafa 1992). In another trial, it was effective in reducing pain in those with rheumatoid arthritis (Srivastava and Mustafa 1989). Given the results of these studies, we can extrapolate that ginger taken as a dietary supplement would be useful for any sports injury in which inflammation plays a part or in which one would normally suggest the use of nonsteroidal anti-inflammatory medicines. Ginger's active ingredients are gingerdione and shogoals, which are concentrated in the root. Ginger is generally well tolerated, but if consumed in doses over 5 grams per day, heartburn is likely. The recommended dose as an anti-inflammatory botanical is 250 milligrams twice a day as a dietary supplement. Another dietary source of ginger that may have an anti-inflammatory influence is candied ginger, which is full of the shogoals that reduce inflammation.

Devil's Claw

A native plant of Africa, devil's claw (*Harpagophytum procumbens*) is another promising botanical for the treatment of anti-inflammatory conditions. It has been investigated for use either alone or in conjunction with NSAIDs, and preliminary results suggest modest reduction in pain symptoms from osteoarthritis. In addition, a study combining devil's claw with NSAIDs lowered the need for a high-dosing schedule of the NSAID (Chantre et al. 2000). Recently, the 2006 Cochrane review of lower-back pain found strong evidence that daily doses standardized to 50 to 100 milligrams of harpagosides were better than placebo for short-term improvements for pain and rescue medication.

Devil's claw is also known to mildly reduce glucose, increase stomach acid, lower blood pressure, and increase bile production. Thus, the adverse effects of hypoglycemia, gastroesophageal hyperacidity, and hypertension might be improved by the use of this supplement. Like other NSAIDs, devil's claw has the potential to exacerbate gastroesophageal reflux disease (GERD). However, because it has weaker NSAID activity, it is less likely to induce or exacerbate this problem. For those with borderline hypertension, or acid reflux, using devil's claw might be doubly beneficial. Usual dosing for the treatment of osteoarthritis is 2.6 grams daily, providing 57 milligrams of the harpagoside equivalent and 87 milligrams of the iridoid glycosides daily as a dietary supplement.

Stinging Nettle

Another herbal medicine that has some clinical evidence suggesting efficacy as an anti-inflammatory alternative is stinging nettle (*Urtica dioca*). This herb has a long history of use by the Greek physicians, Dioscorides and Galen, as a diuretic and laxative. As with other botanicals discussed in this section, stinging nettle's aboveground parts have been proven through in vitro studies to reduce inflammation and minimally lower glucose and blood pressure (Randall et al. 2000). The dose for anti-inflammatory use is 9 grams per day as a dietary supplement. Because stinging nettle has a large amount of vitamin K, athletes who are taking Coumadin should be watched closely by their physicians.

Willow Bark

A natural anti-inflammatory historically used by European herbalists, willow bark (*Salix alba*) has been investigated for use in reducing back pain and found to be effective at concentrations of 240 milligrams daily. This herb has also been shown to have a modest effect on patients with osteoarthritis, though it is not as efficacious as other NSAIDs, such as diclofenac. As with those who take conventional NSAIDs, athletes who use willow bark should be monitored for excessive bleeding. The dose for willow bark should provide 120 to 240 milligrams daily of salicin. Those taking anticoagulants and antiplatelet medications should be monitored closely for increased bleeding.

S-Adenosyl-L Methionine

A naturally occurring molecule in the body, S-adenosyl-L methionine (SAME) is involved in biochemical reactions ranging from modification of the brain chemicals related to depression (serotonin) to the activation or metabolism of proteins, hormones, and nucleic acids. SAME has been shown to reduce pain and inflammation at levels of 400 milligrams daily. Its anti-inflammatory effect is related to a number of reactions. It appears to be important in the restoration of glutathione in the liver, indirectly decreasing inflammation. Additionally, preliminary evidence in vitro suggests that SAME might stimulate cartilage growth and the repair of damaged tissue from inflammation. SAME also has antidepressant properties, increasing serotonin turnover, dopamine, and norepinephrine. Caution should be used in concomitantly prescribing SAME in people using depression medications and other pharmaceuticals known to increase serotonin (e.g., Prozac). The recommended dose for SAME as an anti-inflammatory alternative is 400 to 600 milligrams daily from a dietary supplement.

Capsicum

Derived from chili pepper, capsicum (*Capsicum annuum*) has been found with topical use to reduce pain or discomfort from shingles, postherpetic infections, sprains, bruises, tissue damage from blunt trauma, generalized muscle aches, fibromyalgia, and more. The fruit contains capsaicin, a chemical that creates the sensation of hotness when eaten. When applied to the skin, capsaicin depletes a substance known to transmit the sensation of pain to the brain, known as substance P. Creams with capsaicin are widely available in drug stores over the counter as well as in health food stores and are useful in relieving aches and pains from sprains or muscle aches from overuse during sporting activities (Takahashi et al. 2001). Usually capsaicin is prescribed for sports-related injuries as a topical preparation. Athletes should be aware of the potential for skin irritation with topical use.

Performance-Enhancing Dietary Supplements

Several supplements are used by athletes to enhance physical endurance or to build muscle mass and strength. Athletic performance drugs range from steroids to vitamins. Anything suggesting the desired outcome of enhanced performance is enticing, especially to teenagers. An example of the power of the promises made about these substances is reflected in a survey performed by the National Institute of Drug Abuse, which found that an estimated 3.5 million teenagers used steroids for performance enhancement (Evans 2004). Unfortunately, most claims are not substantiated by clinical trials. As many researchers realized long ago, the use of steroids often comes with great risk to the body.

Creatine

A chemical naturally found primarily in skeletal muscle, creatine is also present in the heart, brain, testes, and other tissues. The body synthesizes 1 to 2 grams per day in the liver, kidneys, and pancreas from food sources of creatine, primarily meat and fish. The intestinal absorption of creatine is extremely bioavailable, as nearly 100 percent is absorbed in the intestine as food. To date, studies in animals and humans are inconsistent in their findings. There seems to be no consistent benefit of creatine supplements for endurance exercises. Possible adverse reactions include gastrointestinal pain, nausea, diarrhea, and weight gain. Renal dysfunction has been reported but is rare in those with healthy kidney function. Creatine is typically acutely loaded at 20 grams per day (.3 gram per kg) for five days followed by a 2-gram maintenance dose. During supplementation water intake should be 64 ounces a day to reduce kidney damage from the dehydration that occurs with the use of creatine. Creatine is allowed by the International Olympic Committee (IOC) and the National Collegiate Athletic Association (NCAA), but the NCAA no longer allows colleges and universities to supply it to their students with school funds.

Whey Protein

A by-product of cheese manufacturing, whey protein contains carbohydrates, minerals, and proteins. As noted by Kelly and Bongiorno, "Whey contains 24 branch chain amino acids that are readily used by the body for energy." Whey protein is also rich in glutathione, a powerful antioxidant that diminishes with exercise (Kelly and Bongiorno 2006). In terms of adverse reactions, whey protein is usually tolerated with minimal difficulty. High doses of 2 to 6 grams per day can cause bloating, nausea, thirst, cramps, fatigue, and headache. Those with a bovine milk allergy should avoid using whey protein.

Phosphatidylserine

A fat-soluble phospholipid, phosphatidylserine occurs naturally and is most abundant in the human brain. A supplement form is being used by resistance-training athletes because it is presumed to prevent muscle tissue degradation and exercise-induced stress (Fahey and Pearl 1998). With the use of phosphatidylserine, significant rises in plasma epinephrine, cortisol, and growth hormone have been noted during exercise. In one study, subjects given phosphatidylserine at 800 milligrams per day for 10 days blunted cortisol but not growth hormone in response to physical exercise (Monteleone et al. 1992). Although the results of preliminary work are promising, more research is needed to substantiate these claims. Because of concerns about bovine sources, most manufacturers now use only soy or cabbage as their sources for phosphatidylserine. Adverse reactions are rare. Gastrointestinal upset is more likely with doses over 300 milligrams per day, and insomnia has been reported with doses of 600 milligrams per day. Typical doses for prevention of muscle fatigue are in the range of 300 to 600 milligrams per day (Kelly and Bongiorno 2006).

Other supplements such as glutamine, ornithine alpha ketoglutarate, boron, chromium, selenium, zinc, ginseng (*Panax ginseng*), Siberian ginseng (*Eleutherococcus senticosus*), carnitine, choline, coenzyme Q10 (ubiquinone), pyridoxal-alpha ketoglutarate, and pyruvate have been used by athletes based on the belief that they can enhance endurance or strength. The research for many of these supplements, although somewhat promising, is too limited to warrant recommendation for use in sports medicine at this time.

East Asian Medicine and Acupuncture

East Asian medicine, which includes the traditional medical practices of China, Japan, and Korea, represents an ancient form of medicine that is nearly 2,000 years old. Even today these systems serve as primary healthcare practices in many developing countries. The practices are founded on principles that focus more on maintaining health than reacting to or modifying a disease. The fundamental approaches to health maintenance include the implementation of changes in diet and attitude. Acupuncture (insertion of needles), a form of massage called tui-na, energy work called qi-gong, and other East Asian treatments are used to treat injury or disease. Although this section highlights acupuncture, East Asian medicine is actually a mixture of practices encompassing a variety of treatments that include botanical medicines and therapeutic lifestyle interventions. Refer to the additional resources section (p. 271) for more information.

Acupuncture has been increasingly incorporated into Western medicine since the 1970s and is being more and more accepted as an effective treatment for many conditions and ailments. In 1997, a scientific panel sponsored by the National Institutes of Health (NIH) convened to provide consensus on the merits of acupuncture. Their conclusion notes that in addition to other uses, "needle acupuncture is efficacious for adult postoperative nausea and vomiting" and that "there are reasonable studies (although sometimes only single studies) showing relief of pain with acupuncture on diverse pain conditions" (National Center for Complementary and Alternative Medicine 2002). In an integrated sports medicine regimen, acupuncture might be helpful for the following conditions:

- Nausea
- Pain from fractures, bruises, blunt trauma, or contusions
- Myalgia from muscle strain
- Acute inflammation of the joints from overuse
- Joint inflammation caused by degenerative or inflammatory joint disease

The practice of acupuncture involves the insertion of fine solid 32 to 36 gauge needles in a variety of precise spots located on channels of energy flow known as meridians. There are 365 points described in classic acupuncture texts. The primary principles governing treatment include the idea that wellness and illness result from the balance and imbalance of *yin* and *yang*. *Yin* represents the feminine aspect of life: nourishing, cool, deficient, inside, receptive, protective, soft, and yielding. *Yang* represents the masculine aspects: hard, dominant, energetic, upper, hot, excessive, outside, and creative. The movement between each seemingly opposite force is identified as *Qi*, which is the essential element in the healing process. The needles "unblock" Qi's vital force, which in a healthy state flows ceaselessly through the meridians.

The mechanisms of action of acupuncture remain incompletely understood. Skeptics have asserted that acupuncture's effectiveness is derived from the placebo effect, citing that needle insertion sites do not correlate with any anatomical or physiological phenomenon that provides a clear explanation for the asserted effects. However, it has been observed that the acupoints are located at sites that have a high density of neurovascular structures that are on the edges of muscle groups (Helms 1996). Based on a review of studies published on acupuncture analgesia, Pomeranz and Stux (1989) have proposed that three mechanisms contribute to its effects:

1. Acupuncture needles stimulate nerve fibers in muscles that block the signaling of pain to the spine and brain.

2. Acupuncture signals areas within the brain that release neurohormones into the spine to inhibit the pain signals where pain might have been perceived.

3. Acupuncture stimulates pituitary release of endorphins, neurohormones that create feelings of well-being.

Although many people assume that pain reduction through acupuncture is subjective in nature, recent functional magnetic resonance angiography (MRA) during acupuncture has shown that specific brain structures are activated during needling. These findings have given many scientists a greater appreciation of acupuncture's direct physiological effects in pain reduction (Cho et al. 2002).

Other organizations such as the American Academy of Medical Acupuncture (AAMA) report similar indications on their Web site (www.medicalacupuncture.org). In regard to sports medicine, the benefit of acupuncture on acute and chronic musculoskeletal injuries has become fairly well accepted. However, many conditions show little to no improvement with acupuncture, including spinal cord injuries, neurodegenerative diseases, thalamically mediated pain, severe chronic fatigue, chronic inflammatory pain, and immune mediated disorders with progression involving the use of corticosteroids (Helms 1998).

Acupuncture during pregnancy should be avoided because it might stimulate uterine contraction. Additionally, acupuncture should not be initiated during menses and should be avoided in those with needle phobia, those who cannot sit still, and those whose behavior is not well controlled, such as patients who are in delirium. People who have known metal allergies, who are taking anticoagulants, and who have bleeding disorders should be considered for acupuncture on a case-by-case basis.

Reported adverse effects include pneumothorax, cardiac tamponade, damage to neurovascular structures, infection, hematoma formation, and broken needles with remnant migration (Kaptchuk 2002). These reports are extremely rare and generally occur with inexperienced practitioners. The overall combined data from prospective and retrospective publications indicates that acupuncture is safe when administered by competent practitioners (Vincent 2001).

In clinical practice, some health professionals readily use acupuncture for pain reduction and musculoskeletal injuries, whereas others are likely to use it only as a last resort. Sierpina and Frenkel have suggested that "a more rational approach would be to recognize the potential role of acupuncture earlier in the treatment of potentially disabling illnesses" (2005). A series of 4 to 10 sessions should be adequate for a trial; those who do not respond can be considered for other therapeutic interventions.

Musculoskeletal Manipulation

Musculoskeletal manipulation involves passive manual maneuvers by skilled practitioners that "extend the patient's range of motion beyond the elastic barrier but do[es] not exceed the anatomic barrier" (Greenman 1996). Two of the most well-known practices of this nature are osteopathic medicine and chiropractic, both founded in the 1890s. Each has distinct medical models as the basis of its manipulative treatments.

Osteopathic Medicine

Osteopathic medicine views the dysfunction of the musculoskeletal system as the basis for the evolution of most diseases. "There exists a similarity between osteopathic thought and traditional Chinese medicine in the awareness that cause is a susceptibility of the host to outside influences" (Grimshaw 2002). Changing the pattern of disease includes dietary modification and lifestyle choices as well as skeletal manipulation. A variety of techniques are used in osteopathic medicine and are described on the Web site maintained by the American Academy of Osteopathy. What follows is in an overview of manipulation techniques (for more information, visit http://osteohome.com):

- **Hands-on contact.** All healers acknowledge that touch has therapeutic value. When manipulation by a DO, a doctor of osteopathy, is initiated, no matter what the diagnosis is, it is felt that healing through physical contact has begun.

- **Soft-tissue technique.** This therapy applies rhythmic pressure, traction, and stretching along the spine. The aim is to redistribute excess tissue fluid from the swollen area and reduce tension in the muscles and fibrous tissue at sites where injury or physical stress is sustained.

- **Myofascial release.** This therapy refers to the manual massage technique for stretching the fascia (connective tissue) and releasing bonds between fascia and muscles and bones with the aim of balancing the body, eliminating pain, and increasing range of motion. Myofascial release treatment (MRT) mobilizes myofascial structures engaging the restrictive barrier. This position is held with constant force until a "release" occurs. After the release is achieved, the dysfunctional tissue is guided or "reeducated" through passive movement to achieve flexibility.

- **Cranial osteopathy.** The dura (tissue covering the brain) and tissues of the central nervous system that produce and hold cerebrospinal fluid generate a cranial rhythmic impulse (CRI), which is also referred to as the third wave impulse. The philosophy of cranial sacral osteopathy suggests that when injuries occur in the body, this inherent rhythm or third wave impulse is disturbed and injured. Gentle manual maneuvers in craniosacral therapy restore the natural rhythm to the head and spine and thereby restore wellness throughout the body.

- **Lymphatic technique.** This technique is a manual procedure of stimulating lymphatic fluid movement. It involves the use of pressure by the physician using his or her hands over the lymphatic system. Hand movement is directed toward the upper chest while the athlete is lying prone. When the athlete inhales, hand pressure is increased; when he or she exhales, pressure from the hands is removed. This activity generates a negative pressure and reinforces the natural movement of the lymphatic fluid to drain back into the right atrium via the thoracic duct.

- **Thrust technique.** The thrust technique is a high-velocity maneuver in which the objective is the restoration of natural joint movement. Neural reflexes are "reset" by this manipulation. This therapy restores joint movement and reduces pain, stiffness, and tenderness.

- **Muscle energy technique.** Muscle energy technique is a manual intervention in which the athlete assumes a precise muscle position. The physician then applies a counterforce that changes or resets the neuromuscular asymmetry of the injured area to restore joint mobility and range of motion.

- **Counterstrain.** This manual procedure is used with acute injuries in which more aggressive manipulation cannot be undertaken because of pain or severe restriction of movement. The pracitioner moves the athlete from the restricted position generated by the injury to a position of comfort. The athlete is without pain, and in this painless state the practitioner generates "strain." This maneuver resets restricted range of motion and increases flexibility (McPartland 2004).

Review of the medical literature suggests that in relation to sports injuries, osteopathic manipulation would be appropriate for acute nonsurgical back strain and neck strain and other areas with acutely derived sports-related muscle tension or plantar fasciitis (Grimshaw 2002). The risk of either osteopathic or chiropractic manipulation is vertebral artery syndrome, an injury to the intimal lining of the vertebral artery caused by sudden thrusts that combine rotation and extension of the cervical spine. The injury results in formation of a thrombus that extends upward, moving into the posterior inferior cerebellar artery. There are no tests available to help predict who is at risk from this injury. The frequency of the injury is estimated to be one in one million manipulations that use high-velocity, low-amplitude maneuvers (Assendelft, Bouter, and Knipschild 1996).

Osteopathic manipulation should not be used to treat people with certain conditions such as unusual hypermobility or ligamentous laxity. For example, people with severe rheumatoid arthritis in the cervical area should not undergo osteopathic manipulation because of the risk of ligament rupture with potential for paralysis. Similarly, athletes with joints that show obvious signs of sepsis (an illness caused by overwhelming bacterial infection) or active bleeding should not receive osteopathic treatment until they have been conventionally evaluated and stabilized. The same is true for those with joints at risk of increased intracranial pressure.

Chiropractic

Chiropractic is a healthcare profession founded by Daniel Palmer, a self-taught naturalist healer who observed that spinal manipulation seemed to help a variety of ailments. Therapeutic chiropractic interventions involve spinal manipulation but also include lifestyle counseling, nutritional management, and the use of many physiotherapeutic treatments, such as ultrasound, electrical muscle stimulation, traction, heat, and manual therapy. Conditions reported in the literature indicate improvement through chiropractic manipulation of acute or subacute lower-back and neck strain and other areas of muscle tension and soreness caused by overuse during sports participation.

Complications reported from chiropractic manipulations are rare, but they include vertebrobasilar (involving decreased blood flow to the brain) and cerebral reactions, disc herniation, and cauda equine syndrome (involving compressed, paralyzed nerves). Half the cases of cauda equine syndrome resulted from manipulation under anesthesia—an uncommon practice rarely performed by chiropractors. A RAND report estimated the rates of cervical complications as 5 to 10 in 10 million manipulations for vertebrobasal events and 3 to 6 in 10 million for major impairment with fewer than 3 fatalities per 10 million manipulations (Coulter et al. 1996). Cases in which chiropractic manipulation is contraindicated (should be avoided) are the same as those for osteopathy.

Yoga and Tai Chi

Yoga, a discipline that began evolving over 4,000 years ago in the Indus River Valley, is an essential practice of Ayurveda, a complete medical system that uses diet, herbal medicine, contemplative mind–body practices (breathing exercises and meditation), and yoga. Yoga is more than the practice of physical postures for fitness. In its highest form of practice, yoga embodies the conscious discipline of spiritual reflection in conjunction with physical well-being.

There are many types of yoga. Some are more physically demanding (ashtanga, bikram, Iyengar), and others are more contemplative (integral and kripalu). Hatha yoga, the most popular form in the United States, focuses primarily on a gentle mixture of postures, breath work, and meditation. Yoga applies to sports medicine first and foremost in its promotion of flexibility. Yoga that is slower and more contemplative speaks to the mental aspect of athletics by promoting calmness and serenity during physical activity. Carefully chosen postures with supportive props such as chairs and pillows can be incorporated to enable athletes with mobility limitations to perform appropriate postures and engage in a form of conditioning without causing injury or discomfort. The more vigorous and physically demanding types of yoga can be used in sports to build up physical endurance. The benefits reported from yoga include improvement in chronic pain, headaches, lower-back and musculoskeletal problems, asthma, fibromyalgia, and dysmenorrhea (Greenfield 2002).

Tai Chi, developed by the Chan family in 1820, has many styles. Although its movements are derived from martial arts, its purpose is to enhance longevity and health. The postures of a Tai Chi practitioner encourage softness, which is far different from the objective of postures in martial arts practiced primarily for self-defense; defensive martial arts postures emphasize a substantial amount of muscle tension in each pose.

Like yoga, Tai Chi reinforces calmness, agility, and balance. Tai Chi requires the ability to hold postures as in yoga, but Tai Chi postures are executed only in a standing position. For athletes who have difficulty sitting still but need to develop calmness, balance, and concentration during sports activities, Tai Chi might prove rewarding.

Mind-Body Practices

There are many potential uses for mind–body practices—hypnosis, for example—in sports medicine. Hypnosis is a state of awareness that is naturally accessible by all individuals. The trance state can be accessed with or without the conscious awareness of the individual but cannot be easily induced without permission of the individual. Hypnosis experts have suggested that individuals who are able to achieve a trance state have either explicitly or implicitly given permission to the hypnotist to bring out this state of mind, even if permission was not consciously perceived by the individual hypnotized. Individuals who have been certified to practice hypnotism have a professional code of ethics outlining the rules for inducing this state in others, and trying to put an unwilling individual into a trance is considered unprofessional conduct.

Hypnosis can be used to promote successful outcomes in athletic performance, reduce performance anxiety, reduce pain perception in states of chronic pain, and enhance healing in states of acute and chronic injury. Individuals who experience physical or psychological trauma should be carefully screened before hypnosis is used as a therapeutic intervention because hypnotic states can reintroduce to conscious memory experiences that have been repressed.

Additional Resources

The follwing resources offer credible, in-depth information on topics such as botanical medicine, nutrition, osteopathy, stress reduction, and mind–body medicine.

Integrative Medicine and Natural Medicine Texts

Kligler, B., and R. Lee. 2004. *Integrative medicine: Principles for practice.* New York: McGraw-Hill.

Pizzorno, J. and M. Murray. 2006. *Textbook of natural medicine* (3rd ed.; vol. 1 and 2). London: Churchill Livingstone / El Sevier.

Rakel D. 2003. *Integrative medicine.* Philadelphia: Saunders.

Botanical Resources

Blumenthal, M.A. Goldberg, and T. Kunz. 2003. *The ABC clinical guide to herbs.* Austin, TX: The American Botanical Council.

Fugh-Berman, A. *The Five-Minute Herb & Dietary Supplement Consult.* 1998. Eclectic Medical Publications.

HerbalGram: www.herbalgram.org

The University of Maryland herbal database: www.umm.edu/altmed/ConsLookups/ Herbs.html

Medline Plus: Herbs and Supplements www.nlm.nih.gov/medlineplus/druginfo/ herb_All.html

Supplement Watch: www.supplementwatch.com

Acupuncture Resources

Acupuncture and Oriental Medicine Alliance (AOMA): www.acuall.org
American Academy of Medical Acupuncture (AAMA): www.medicalacupuncture.org
Acubriefs: www.acubriefs.com

Yoga and Tai Chi Resources

Yoga Internet Resources: www.holisticmed.com/www/yoga.html
American Yoga Association: www.americanyogaassociation.org
Yoga Research and Education Foundation: www.yref.org
QiGong Institute: www.qigonginstitute.org

Osteopathic and Chiropractic Resources

American Academy of Osteopathy: www.academyofosteopathy.org
American Chiropractic Association: www.amerchiro.org
American Medical Massage Association: www.americanmedicalmassage.com
The Touch Research Institute: http://www6.miami.edu/touch-research/
The Upledger Institute: www.upledger.com
Medical Center: www.umassmed.edu/cfm/index.aspx

Mind-Body Resources

American Society of Clinical Hypnosis: www.asch.net

Acknowledgment: Special thanks to Ms. Marsha Handel for her assistance with the text of this chapter.

WORKS CONSULTED

CHAPTER 1 Body Conditioning and Maintenance

Blahnik, J. 2004. *Full-body flexibility.* Champaign, IL: Human Kinetics.

Bompa, T.O. 1999. *Periodization training for sports.* Champaign, IL: Human Kinetics.

Boyle, M. 2004. *Functional training for sports.* Champaign, IL: Human Kinetics.

Chek, P. 2000. *Movement that matters.* Encinitas, CA: C.H.E.K. Institute.

Chek, P. 2002a. Lost in space. In *Chek marks for success.* Vol. 2. Edited by Cara Burke, Penthea Crozier, Holli Spicer, and Bryan Walsh. Encinitas, CA: C.H.E.K. Institute.

Chek, P. 2002b. Should athletes train like body builders? In *Chek marks for success.* Vol. 1. Edited by Cara Burke, Penthea Crozier, Holli Spicer, Bryan Walsh, and Christina Walsh. Encinitas, CA: C.H.E.K. Institute.

Chu, D.A. 1998. *Jumping into plyometrics.* Champaign, IL: Human Kinetics.

Cook, G. 2003. *Athletic body in balance.* Champaign, IL: Human Kinetics.

Dudley, G. and R.T. Harris. 2000. Neuromuscular adaptations to conditioning. In *Essentials of strength training and conditioning* (2nd ed.). Edited by Thomas R. Baechle and Roger W. Earle. Champaign, IL: Human Kinetics.

Fleck, S.J. and W. J. Kraemer. 1997. *Designing resistance training programs.* Champaign, IL: Human Kinetics.

Frederick, A. and C. Frederick. 2006. *Stretch to win.* Champaign, IL: Human Kinetics.

Gambetta, V. 2007. *Athletic development.* Champaign, IL: Human Kinetics.

Gotlin, R. 1997. The lower extremity. In *Sports medicine: principles of primary care.* Edited by G. Scuderi, P. McCann, P. Bruno. Philadelphia: Mosby.

Gray. G. 2002. Functional Video Digest Series *Wynn Marketing News Articles.* www.functionaldesign. com.

Gray, G.W. 2000. Functional biomechanics. *Wynn Marketing News Articles.* www.functionaldesign. com/wynn_marketing/newsarticles_5.htm.

Gray, G.W. with Team Reaction. 2001. *Total body functional profile.* Adrian, MI: Wynn Marketing.

National Academy of Sports Medicine. 2003. *Advanced sports fitness course* (2nd ed.). Calabasas, CA: National Academy of Sports Medicine.

Potach, D.H. and D.A. Chu. 2000. Plyometric training. In *Essentials of strength training and conditioning* (2nd ed.). Edited by Thomas R. Baechle and Roger W. Earle. Champaign, IL: Human Kinetics.

Radcliffe, J.C. and R.C. Farentinos. 1999. *High-powered plyometrics.* Champaign, IL: Human Kinetics.

Romanov, N. 2004. *Pose method of running.* Miami, FL: Pose Tech Press.

Verstegen, M. and P. Williams. 2004. *Core performance: The revolutionary workout program to transform your body and your life.* New York: Rodale.

Wharton, J. and P. Wharton. 1996. *The Wharton's stretch book.* New York: TimesBooks (Random House).

CHAPTER 2 Prevention and Treatment Toolbox

American Academy of Orthopaedic Surgeons. 2003. *The use of knee braces.* Position Statement of the American Academy of Orthopaedic Surgeons. http:// www.aaos.org/about/papers/position/1124.asp

Arnold, B.L. and C.L. Docherty. 2004. Bracing and rehabilitation—what's new. *Clin. Sports Med.* January. 23(1):83-95.

Bruckner, P. and K. Khan. 1993. *Clin. Sports Med.* Sydney: McGraw-Hill.

Fleck, S.J. and W.J. Kraemer. 1997. *Designing resistance training programs* (2nd ed.). Champaign, IL: Human Kinetics.

Fox E.L., R.W. Bowers, and M.L. Foss. 1988. *The physiological basis of physical education and athletics* (4th ed.). Dubuque, IA: Brown.

Frontera, W.R. 2003. *Rehabilitation of sports injuries: Scientific basis.* Malden, MA: Blackwell Science.

Gaesser G.A. and L.A. Wilson. 1988. Effects of continuous and interval training on the parameters of the power-endurance time relationship for high-intensity exercise. *Int J. Sports Med.* Dec. 9(6):417-21

Kibler, W.B. and T.J. Chandler. 1994. Sport-specific conditioning. *Am. J. Sports Med.* 22 (3):424-432

Kraemer, W.J. 2003. Strength training basics: designing workouts to meet patients' goals. *Phys. Sportsmed.* 31(8):39-45.

Krivickas, L.S. 1999. Training flexibility. In *Exercise in rehabilitation medicine*. Edited by W. Frontera, D. Dawson, D. Slovik. Champaign, IL: Human Kinetics.

Martin, T.J. and Committee. 2001. Technical report: Knee brace use in the young athlete. *Pediatrics* 2001; 108:503-507.

McIntosh, A.S. 2005. Preventing head and neck injury. *Brit. J. Sports Med.* 39(6):314-18.

Meredith, R.M. and J.D. Butcher. 1997. Field splinting of suspected fractures: Preparation, assessment, and application. *Phys. Sportsmed.* October. 25(10):29.

Mujika I. and S. Padilla. 2001. Muscular characteristics of detraining in humans. *Med. Sci. Sports Exerc.* 33 (8):1297-1303.

Okuyama, H., Y. Ichikawa, Y. Fujii, and M. Ito. 2005. Changes in dietary fatty acids and life style as major factors for rapidly increasing inflammatory diseases. *World Review Nutr. Diet* 95:52-61

Orchard J., H. Seward, J. McGivern, and S. Hood. 2001. Intrinsic and extrinsic factors for anterior cruciate ligament injury in Australian footballers. *Am. J. Sports Med.* 29(3):196-200.

Protective Eyewear Certification Council http://www.protecteyes.org/

Renstrom, P. 1993. *Sports injuries: Basic principles of prevention and care*. Boston: Blackwell Science.

Renstrom, P. 1994. *Clinical practice of sports injury prevention and care*. Boston: Blackwell Science.

Schwellnus, M. 2003. Flexibility and joint range of motion. In *Rehabilitation of sports injuries: Scientific basis*. Edited by W.W. Frontera. Malden, MA: Blackwell Science.

Sharpe, S.R., J. Knapik, and B. Jones. 1997. Ankle braces effectively reduce recurrence of ankle sprains in female soccer players. *J. Athl. Train.* January. 32(1):21-24.

Verhagen E.A.L.M., W. van Mechelen, and W. de Vente. 2000. The effect of preventative measures on the incidence of ankle sprains. *Clin. J. Sports Med.* October. 10(4):291-296.

Wilkerson, G.B. 2002. Biomechanical and neuromuscular effects of ankle taping and bracing. *J. Athl. Train.* December. 37(4):436-445.

Wilkinson, J.G. 1997. Carbohydrate metabolism. In *Nutrition in Exercise and Sport*. Edited by I. Wolinsky. Ann Arbor Michigan: CRC Press.

Wilmore J.H. and D.L. Costill. 2005. *Physiology of sport and exercise* (3rd ed.). Champaign, IL: Human Kinetics.

Witvrouw, E., N. Mahieu, L. Danneels, and P. McNair. 2004. Stretching and injury prevention: an obscure relationship. *Sports Med.* 34(7):443-449.

CHAPTER 3   Injury Types and Assessments

Gotlin, R. 2005. The lower extremity. In *Sports medicine: A comprehensive approach*. (2nd ed.). Edited by G. Scuderi and P. McCann. Philadelphia: Mosby.

Hirata, I. 1968. *The doctor and the athlete*. Philadelphia: Lippincott.

Klafs, K.E. and D.D. Arnheim. 1969. *Modern principles of athletic training*. Philadelphia: Mosby.

O'Donoghue, D.H. 1984. *Treatment of injuries to athletes*. (4th ed.). Philadelphia: W.B. Saunders.

Rawlinson, K. 1961. *Modern athletic training*. Englewood Cliffs, NJ: Prentice Hall.

Williams, J.G.P. and P.N. Sperryn. 1976. *Sports medicine*. Baltimore: Williams and Wilkins.

CHAPTER 4   Concussions and Head Injuries

Aubry M., R. Cantu, J. Dvorak, T. Graf-Bauman, K.M. Johnston, J. Kelly, M. Lovell, P. McCrory, W. Meeuwisse, and P. Schamasch. 2002. Summary of the first international conference on concussion in sport. *Clin. J. Sports Med.* 12:6-11.

Cantu, R.C. 1993. Functional cervical spinal stenosis: A contraindication to participation in contact sports. *Med Sci Sports Exer.* 25:316-317.

Cantu, R.C. 1997. Stingers, transient quadriplegia and cervical spinal stenosis: Return to play criteria. *Med. Sci. Sports Exer.* 29:S233-235.

Cantu, R.C. 1998. Return to play guidelines after a head injury. *Clin. Sports Med.* 17(1):45-60.

Cantu, R.C., J.E. Bailes, and J.E. Wilberger Jr. 1998. Guidelines for return to contact or collision sport after a cervical spine injury. *Clin. Sports Med.* 17(1):137-146.

Cantu, R.C. and R. Voy. 1995. Second impact syndrome: A risk in any contact sport. *Physician and Sportsmed.* 23:27-34.

Collins, M.W., M. Field, M.R. Lovell, G.L. Iverson, K.M. Johnston, J.C. Maroon, and F.H. Fu. 2003. Relationship between post-concussion headache and neuropsychological test performance in high school athletes. *Am. J. Sports Med.* 31:168-73.

Collins M.W., G.L. Iverson, M.R. Lovell, D.B. McKeag, J. Norwig, and J.C. Maroon. 2003. On-field predictors of neuropsychological and symptom deficit following sports-related concussion. *Clin. J. Sports Med.* 13:222-229.

Collins, M.W., M.R. Lovell, G.L. Iverson, R.C. Cantu, J.C. Maroon, and M. Field. 2002. Cumulative effects of sports concussion in high school athletes. *Neurosurg.* 51:1175-1181.

Grant H.D., R.H. Murray Jr., and J.D. Bergeron. 1986. *Emergency care.* (4th ed.). Englewood Cliffs, NJ: Prentice Hall.

Guskiewicz, K.M., N.L. Weaver, D.A. Padua, and W.E. Garrett Jr. 2000. Epidemiology of concussion in collegiate and high school football players. *Am. J. Sports Med.* 28(5):643-650.

Kelly, J.P., J.S. Nichols, C.M. Filley, K.O. Lillehei, D. Rubinstein, and B.K. Kleinschmidt-DeMasters. 1991. Concussion in sports. Guidelines for the prevention of catastrophic outcomes. *JAMA* 266(20):2867-2869.

Pavlov, H., J.S. Torg, B. Robie, and C. Jahre. 1987. Cervical spinal stenosis: Determination with vertebral body ratio method. *Radiology* 164:771-775.

Pickles, W. 1950. Acute general edema of the brain in children with head injuries. *NEJM.* 242:607-611.

Takeda T., K. Ishugami, S. Hoshina, T. Ogawa, J. Handa, K. Nakajima, A. Shimada, T. Nakajima, and C.W. Regner. 2005. Can mouthguards prevent mandibular bone fractures and concussions? *Dental Traumatol.* 21(3):134-140.

Torg, J.S., T.A. Corcoran, L.E. Thibault, H. Pavlov, B. Sennett, R.J. Naranja, and S. Priano. 1997. Cervical cord neuropraxia: Classification, pathomechanics, morbidity, and management guidelines. *J. Neurosurg.* 89:687-690.

Torg, J.S., R.J. Naranja, H. Pavlov, B. Galinat, R. Warren, and R. Stine. 1996. The relationship of developmental narrowing of the cervical spinal canal to reversible and irreversible injury of the cervical spinal canal in football players: An epidemiological study. *J. Bone Joint Surg. Am.* 78:1308-1314.

Torg J.S. and J.A. Ramsey-Emrhein. 1997a. Management guidelines for participation in collision activities with congenital developmental or post-injury lesions involving the cervical spine. *Clin. Sport Med.* 16:501-530.

Torg J.S. and J.A. Ramsey-Emrhein. 1997b. Suggested management guidelines for participation in collision activities with congenital, developmental, or post-injury lesions involving the cervical spine. *Med, Sci. Sports Exer.* 29(suppl):S256-S272.

Torg J.S., B. Sennett, H. Pavlov, M.R. Leventhal, and S.G. Glasgow. 1993. Spear tackler's spine: An entity precluding participation in tackle football and collision activities that expose the cervical spine to axial energy inputs. *Am. J. Sports Med.* 21:640-649.

Quality Standards Subcommittee. 1997. Practice parameter: The management of concussion in sports. *Neurology* 48:581-585.

Vaccaro A.R., B. Watkins, T.J. Albert, W.L. Pfaff, G.R. Klein, and J.S. Silber 2001. Cervical spine injuries in athletes: Current return to play criteria. *Orthopedics* 24:699-703.

White, A.A., R.M. Johnson, M.M. Panjabi, and W.O. Southwick. 1975. Biomechanical analysis of clinical stability in the cervical spine. *Clin Orthop.* 109:85-96.

Wojtys, E.M., D. Hovda, G. Landry, A. Boland, M. Lovell, M. McCrea, and J. Minkoff. 1999. Concussion in sports: *Am. J. Sports Med.* 27: 676-686.

CHAPTER 5   **Neck and Cervical Spine Injuries**

Cantu, R.C. 1993. Functional cervical spinal stenosis: A contraindication to participation in contact sports. *Med Sci Sports Exer.* 25:316-317.

Cantu, R.C. 1997. Stingers, transient quadriplegia and cervical spinal stenosis: Return to play criteria. *Med. Sci. Sports Exer.* 29:S233-235.

Cantu, R.C., J.E. Bailes, and J.E. Wilberger Jr. 1998. Guidelines for return to contact or collision sport after a cervical spine injury. *Clin. Sports Med.* 17(1):137-146.

Pavlov, H., J.S. Torg, B. Robie, and C. Jahre. 1987. Cervical spinal stenosis: Determination with vertebral body ratio method. *Radiology* 164:771-775.

Torg, J.S., T.A. Corcoran, L.E. Thibault, H. Pavlov, B. Sennett, R.J. Naranja, and S. Priano. 1997. Cervical cord neuropraxia: Classification, pathomechanics, morbidity, and management guidelines. *J. Neurosurg.* 89:687-690.

Torg, J.S. and T.A. Gennarrelli. 1994. Head and cervical spine injuries. In *Orthopaedic sports medicine: Principles and practice.* Edited by J.C. DeLee and D. Drez. Philadelphia: Saunders.

Torg, J.S., R. J. Naranja, H. Pavlov, B. Galinat, R. Warren, and R. Stine. 1996. The relationship of developmental narrowing of the cervical spinal canal to reversible and irreversible injury of the cervical spinal canal in football players: An epidemiological study. *J. Bone Joint Surg. Am.* 78:1308-1314.

Torg J.S., and J.A. Ramsey-Emrhein. 1997a. Management guidelines for participation in collision activities with congenital developmental or post-injury lesions involving the cervical spine. *Clin. Sport Med.* 16:501-530.

Torg J.S., and J.A. Ramsey-Emrhein. 1997b. Suggested management guidelines for participation in collision activities with congenital, developmental, or post-injury lesions involving the cervical spine. *Med, Sci. Sports Exer.* 29(suppl):S256-S272.

Torg J.S., B. Sennett, H. Pavlov, M.R. Leventhal, and S.G. Glasgow. 1993. Spear tackler's spine: An entity precluding participation in tackle football and collision activities that expose the cervical spine to axial energy inputs. *Am. J. Sports Med.* 21:640-649.

Vaccaro A.R., B. Watkins, T.J. Albert, W.L. Pfaff, G.R. Klein, and J.S. Silber. 2001. Cervical spine injuries in athletes: Current return to play criteria. *Orthopedics* 24:699-703.

White, A.A., R. M. Johnson, M.M. Panjabi, and W.O. Southwick. 1975. Biomechanical analysis of clinical stability in the cervical spine. *Clin Orthop.* 109:85-96.

CHAPTER 6 Shoulder Injuries

Bracker, M. 2001. *The 5-minute sports medicine consult.* Philadelphia: Lippincott Williams & Wilkins.

Brukner, P. and K. Khan. 1993. *Clinical sports medicine.* Roseville, Australia: McGraw-Hill.

Itoi, E., R. Sashi, H. Minagawa, T. Shimizu, I. Wakabayashi, and K. Sato. 2001. Position of immobilization after dislocation of the glenohumeral joint. A study with use of magnetic resonance imaging. *J Bone Joint Surg Am.* 83-A (5):661-7.

Joffe, H.V. and S.Z. Goldhaber. 2002. Upper-extremity deep vein thrombosis. *Circulation* 106:1874-1880.

Johnson, T. 1997. Shoulder. In *Essentials of musculoskeletal care.* Edited by Robert Snider. Rosemont, IL: American Academy of Orthopaedic Surgeons.

Moorman III, C., R. Warren, and D. Altchek. 1996. Shoulder Instability. In *Sports medicine, The school-age athlete.* (2nd ed.). Edited by Bruce Reider. Philadelphia: Saunders.

Norris, T. 1997. *Orthopaedic knowledge update, shoulder and elbow.* Rosemont, IL: American Academy of Orthopaedic Surgeons.

Safran, M., S. Salyers, and F. Fu. 1996. Injuries Involving the Clavicle. In *Sports medicine, The school-age athlete.* (2nd ed.). Edited by Bruce Reider. Philadelphia: Saunders.

Warren, R., C. Edward, and D. Altchek. 1999. *The unstable shoulder.* Philadelphia: Lippincott-Raven.

CHAPTER 7 Arm and Elbow Injuries

Benjamin H.J., I. Boyarsky, C. Rank, and E.R. Washington. 2005. Little League elbow syndrome. *Emedicine Sports Medicine online textbook.* Available at www. emedicine.com.

Bradshaw D.Y. and J.M. Shefner. 1999. Ulnar neuropathy at the elbow. *Neurol Clin.* 17(3):447-61.

Cain, E.L. Jr. and J.R. Dugas. 2004. History and examination of the thrower's elbow. *Clin. Sports Med.* 23(4):553-566.

Chumbley, E.M., F.G. O'Connor, and R.P. Nirschl. 2000. Evaluation of overuse elbow injuries. *Am. Fam. Physician* 61(3):691-700.

Creighton R.A., B.R. Bach Jr., and C.A. Bush-Joseph. 2006. Evaluation of the medial elbow in the throwing athlete. *Am J. Orthop.* 35(6):266-269.

Disabella, V.N. 2005. Elbow and forearm overuse injuries. *Emedicine Sports Medicine online textbook.* Available at www.emedicine.com.

Kibler, W. and A. Sciascia. 2004. Kinetic chain contributions to elbow function and dysfunction in sports. *Clin. Sports Med.* 23(4):545-552.

Kibler, W.B. and M. Safran. 2005. Tennis injuries. *Med Sport Sci.* 48:120-37

Parziale, J.R. and W.J. Mallon. 2006. Golf injuries and rehabilitation. *Phys Med Rehabil Clin N Am.* 17(3):589-607

Perkins, R.H. and D. Davis. 2006. Musculoskeletal injuries in tennis. *Phys Med Rehabil Clin N Am.* 17(3):609-31.

Sciascia, A. and W.B. Kibler. 2006. The pediatric overhead athlete: What is the real problem? *Clin J Sport Med.* 16(6):471-7.

Washington, R.L. and D.T. Bernhardt. 2001. American Academy of Pediatrics: Risk of injury from baseball and softball in children. *Pediatrics.* 107(4):782-784.

CHAPTER 8 Hand and Wrist Injuries

Cabrera J.M. and F.C. McCue III. 1986. Nonosseous athletic injuries of the elbow, forearm, and hand. *Clin Sports Med.* Oct 5(4):681-700.

Kahler D.M., and F.C. McCue III. 1992. Metacarpophalangeal and proximal interphalangeal joint injuries of the hand, including the thumb. *Clin Sports Med.* Jan 11(1):57-76.

McCue, F.C. III, W.H. Baugher, D.N. Kulund, and J.H. Gieck. 1979. Hand and wrist injuries in the athlete. *Am J Sports Med.* Sep-Oct 7(5):275-286.

McCue, F.C. III, M.W. Hakala, J.R. Andrews, and J.H. Gieck. 1974. Ulnar collateral ligament injuries of the thumb in athletes. *J Sports Med.* Mar-Apr 2(2):70-80.

McCue, F.C. III, R. Honner, M.C. Johnson, and J.H. Gieck. 1970. Athletic injuries of the proximal interphalangeal joint requiring surgical treatment. *J Bone Joint Surg Am.* Jul 52(5):937-956.

McCue, F.C. III and V. Mayer. 1989. Rehabilitation of common athletic injuries of the hand and wrist. *Clin Sports Med.* Oct 8 (4):731-776.

McCue, F.C. III and K. Meister. 1993. Common sports hand injuries. An overview of aetiology, management and prevention. *Sports Med.* Apr 15(4):281-289.

McCue, F.C. III, T.M. Webster, and J. Gieck. 1972. Clinical effects of proteolytic enzymes after reconstructive hand surgery. A double-blind evaluation of oral trypsin-chymotrypsin. *Int Surg.* Jun 57(6):479-482.

McCue, F.C. III and S.L. Wooten. 1986. Closed tendon injuries of the hand in athletics. *Clin Sports Med.* Oct 5(4):741-755.

Redler, M.R. and F.C. McCue III. 1988. Injuries of the hand in athletes. *Va Med.* Jul 115(7):331-336.

Saliba, S. and F.C. McCue III. 2005. Wrist, hand, and finger pathologies. In *Athletic training and sports medicine* (4th ed.). Starkey and Johnson editors. Sudbury, MA: Jones and Bartlett.

CHAPTER 9 Chest and Abdominal Injuries

Abrogast, K.B., J. Cohen, L. Otoya, and K. Winston. 2001. Protecting the child's abdomen: A retractable bicycle handlebar. *Accident Analysis & Prev.* 3(6):753-757.

Ashrafian, H. 2003. Sudden death in young athletes. *NEJM.* 349(11):1064-1075.

Bundy, W., and D.M. Chilton. 2003. Delayed hemothorax after blunt trauma without rib fractures. *Military Med.* 68(6):501-502.

Drake, D.F., S.F. Nadler, L.H. Chou, S.D. Toledo, and V. Akuthothau. 2004. Sports and performing arts medicine, traumatic injuries in sports. *Arch Phys Med Rehabil.* 85(3suppl1):S67-71.

Geddes, L.A. and R.A. Roeder 2005. Evolution of our knowledge of sudden death due to commotio cordis. *Am. J. of Emergency Med.* 23(1):67-75.

Gregory, P.L., A.C. Biswas, and M.E. Batt. 2002. Musculoskeletal problems with chest wall in athletes. *Sports Med.* 32(4):235-250.

Nicholls, R.L., B.C. Elliott, and K. 2004. Miller. Impact injuries in baseball: Prevalence, etiology and the role of equipment performance. *Sports Med.* 35(1):17-25.

Pilato, M.L. 2005. Seemingly innocuous blunt chest trauma as a cause of death in athletics (commotio cordis), *J. Emergency Med.* 28(2):228-9.

Rifat, S.F. and R.P. Gilvydis. 2003. Blunt abdominal trauma in sports. *Current Sports Med. Reports* (2):93-97.

Ryan, J.M. 1999. Abdominal injuries in sports. *Br. J. Sports Med.* 33(3):155-160.

Wan, J., T.F. Corvino, S.P. Greenfield, and C. Discala. 2003. Kidney and testicle injuries in team and individual sports: Data from National Pediatric Trauma Registry. *J. Urol.* 170(4PT2):1528-1533.

CHAPTER 10 Lower-Back Injuries

Andersson, G.B. and R.A. Deyo 1996. History and physical examination in patients with herniated lumbar discs. *Spine* 15:21(24 Suppl):10S-18S

Bellah, R.D., D.A. Summerville, S.T. Treves, and L.J. Micheli. 1991. Low back pain in adolescent athletes: Detection of stress injury to the pars interarticularis with SPECT. *Radiology* 180:509-512.

Braddom, R.L. 2000. *Physical medicine and rehabilitation* (2nd ed.). Philadelphia: Saunders.

Cacayorin E.D., L. Hochhauser, and G.R. Petro. 1987. Lumbar and thoracic spine pain in the athlete: Radiographic evaluation. *Clin. Sports Med.* 6:767-783.

Day A., W. Friedman, and P. Indelicato. 1987. Observations on the treatment of lumbar disc disease in college football players. *Am. J. Sports Med.* 15:72.

DeLee, J.C. and D. Drez. 2003. *DeLee and Drez's orthopaedic sports medicine* (2nd ed.). Philadelphia: Saunders.

DeLisa, J. A., B.M. Gans, N.E. Walsh, W.L. Bockenek, W.R. Frontera, L.H. Gerber, S.R. Geiringer, W.S. Pease, L.R. Robinson, J. Smith, T.P. Stitik, R.D. Zafonte. 2005. *Physical medicine and rehabilitation: Principles and practice* (4th ed.). Philadelphia: Lippincott Williams & Wilkins.

Denis, F. 1984. Spinal instability so defined by the three-column spine concept in acute spinal trauma. *Clin. Orthop.* 189:65.

Fortin, J.D., P.A. Dwyer, W. West, and J. Pier. 1994. Sacroiliac joint: Pain referral maps upon applying a new injection/arthrography technique, part I: Asymptomatic volunteers. *Spine* 19(13): 1475-1482.

Frontera, W.R. 2002. *Essentials of physical medicine and rehabilitation* (1st ed.). Philadelphia: Hanley & Belfus.

Jackson, D. 1979. Low back pain in young athletes. *Am. J. Sports Med.* 7:364.

Jackson, D., L. Wiltse, R. Dingeman, and M. Hayes. 1981. Stress reactions involving the pars interarticularis in young athletes. *Am. J. Sports Med.* 9:305.

Jacobs, R.R., M.A. Asher, and R.K. Snider. 1986. Thoracolumbar spine injuries. *Spine* 5:463.

Kortelainen, P., J. Puranen, E. Koivisto, and S. Lahde. 1985. Symptoms and signs of sciatica and their relation to the localization of the lumbar disc herniation. *Spine* 10: 88-92.

Kujala, U.M., J.J. Salminen, S. Taimela, A. Oksanen, and L. Jaakkola. 1992. Subject characteristics and low back pain in young athletes and nonathletes. *Med. Sci. Sports Exerc.* 24(6):627-632.

Micheli, L. 1979. Low back pain in the adolescent: Differential diagnosis. *Am. J. Sports Med.* 7:362.

CHAPTER 11 Hip Injuries

Akermark, C. and C. Johansson. 1992. Tenotomy of the adductor longus tendon in the treatment of chronic groin pain in athletes. *Am. J. Sports Med.* 20: 640-643.

American College of Rheumatology Subcommittee on Osteoarthritis Guidelines. 2000. Recommendations for the medical management of osteoarthritis of the hip and knee. *Arthritis Rheum.* 43(9): 1905-1915.

Anderson K., S.M. Strickland, and R. Warren. 2001. Hip and groin injuries in athletes. *Am. J. Sports Med.* 29:521-533.

Braddom, R.L. 2000. *Physical medicine and rehabilitation* (2nd ed.). Philadelphia: Saunders.

Cook, J.L. 2003. Rehabilitation of lower limb tendinopathies. *Clin. Sports Med.* 22(4):777-789.

Czerny, C., J. Kramer, A. Neuhold, M. Urban, C. Tschauner, S. Hofmann. 2001. Magnetic resonance imaging and magnetic resonance arthrography of the acetabular labrum: Comparison with surgical findings. *Roto Fortschr Geb Rontgenstr Neuen Bildgeb Verfahr* 173:702-707.

Defrin, R. 2005. Conservative correction of leg-length discrepancies of 10mm or less for the relief of chronic low back pain. *Arch. Phys. Med. Rehabil.* 86(11):2075-2080.

DeLee, J.C. and D. Drez. 2003. *DeLee and Drez's orthopaedic sports medicine* (2nd ed.). Philadelphia: Saunders.

Frontera, W.R. 2002. *Essentials of physical medicine and rehabilitation.* Philadelphia: Hanley & Belfus.

Gorsline, R.T. and C.C. Kaeding. 2005. The use of NSAIDs and nutritional supplements in athletes with osteoarthritis: Prevalence, benefits, and consequences. *Clin. Sports Med.* 24(1):71-82.

Gupta, K.B., J. Duryea, and B.N. Weissman. 2004. Radiographic evaluation of osteoarthritis. *Radiol. Clin. North Am.* 42(1):11-41.

Holmich P., P. Uhrskou P, and L. Ulnits. 1999. Effectiveness of active physical training as treatment for long-standing adductor-related groin pain in athletes: Randomised trial. *Lancet* 353:439-443.

Kelly, B.T., R.J. Williams, and M.J. Philippon. 2003. Hip arthroscopy: Current indications, treatment options, and management issues. *Am. J. Sports Med.* 31:1020-1037.

Klingele, K.E. and P.I. Sallay. 2002. Surgical repair of complete proximal hamstring tendon rupture. *Am. J. Sports Med.* 30:742-747.

Lawrence, R.C., C.G. Helmick, F.C. Arnett, R.A. Deyo, D.T. Felson, E.H. Giannini, S.P. Heyse, R. Hirsch, M.C. Hochberg, G.G. Hunder, M.H. Liang, S.R. Pillemer, V.D. Steen, and F. Wolfe. 1998. Estimates of the prevalence of arthritis and selected musculoskeletal disorders in the United States. *Arthritis Rheum.* 41(5):778-799.

McCarthy, J.C. and B. Busconi. 1995. The role of hip arthroscopy in the diagnosis and treatment of hip disease. *Orthopedics* 18:753-756.

Melamed, H. and M.R. Hutchinson. 2002. Soft tissue problems of the hip in athletes. *Sports Med. Arthrosc. Rev.* 10:168-175.

Meyers, W.C., D.P. Foley, W.E. Garrett, J.H. Lohnes, B.R. Mandelbaum, and PAIN (Performing Athletes with Abdominal or Inguinal Neuromuscular Pain Study Group). 2000. Successful management of severe lower abdominal or inguinal pain in high performance athletes. *Am. J. Sports Med.* 28:2-8.

Morelli, V. and V. Weaver. 2005. Groin injuries and groin pain in athletes: Part 1. *Prim. Care* 32(1):163-183.

Orchard, J., J. Marsden, S. Lord, and D. Garlick. 1997. Preseason hamstring muscle weakness associated with hamstring muscle injury in Australian footballers. *Am. J. Sports Med.* 25:81-85.

Reid, D.C. 1992. Soft tissue injures of the thigh. In *Sports injury assessment and rehabilitation.* Philadelphia: Churchill Livingstone.

Scopp, J.M. and C.T. Moorman. 2001. The assessment of athletic hip injury. *Clin. Sports Med.* 20:647-659.

Topol, G.A. 2005. Efficacy of dextrose prolotherapy in elite male kicking-sport athletes with chronic groin pain. *Arch. Phys. Med. Rehabil.* 86(4):697-702.

Vingard, E, L. Alfredsson, I. Goldi, and C. Hogstedt. 1993. Sports and osteoarthritis of the hip: An epidemiological study. *Am. J. Sports Med.* 21(2):195.

CHAPTER 12 Thigh and Hamstring Injuries

Aronen, J.G. and R.D. Chronister. 1992. Quadriceps contusions: Hastening the return to play. *Physician and Sportsmed.* 20(7):130-136.

Brunet, M.E. and R.B. Hontas, 1994. The thigh. In *Orthopaedic sports medicine: Principles and practice.* Edited by J.C. DeLee and D. Drez. Philadelphia: Saunders.

Clough, T.M. 2002. Femoral neck stress fracture: The importance of clinical suspicion and early review. *Br. J. Sports Med.* 36:308-309.

Colosimo, A.J., H.M. Wyatt, K.A. Frank, and R.E. Mangine. 2005. Hamstring avulsion injuries. *Operative Techniques in Sports Med.* 13:80-88.

Crosier, J.L. 2004. Factors associated with recurrent hamstring injuries. *Sports Med.* 34(10):681-695.

Cross, T.M., N. Gibbs, M.T. Houang, and M. Cameron. 2004. Acute quadriceps muscle strains MRI features and prognosis. *Am. J. Sports Med.* 32(3):710-719.

Diaz, J.A., D.A. Fischer, A.C. Rettig, T.J. Davis, and K.D. Shelbourne. 2003. Severe quadriceps muscle contusions in athletes. *Am. J. Sports Med.* 31(2):289-293.

Drezner, J.A. 2003. Practical management: Hamstring muscle injuries. *Clin. J. Sports Med.* 13:48-52.

Fredericson, M., W. Morre, M. Guillet, and C. Beaulieu. 2005. High hamstring tendinopathy in runners. *Physician and Sportsmed.* 33(5):1-14.

Hoskins, W. and H. Pollard. 2004. The management of hamstring injury—part 1: Issues in diagnosis. *Manual Therapy*. 10:96-107.

Hoskins, W. and H. Pollard. 2005. The management of hamstring injury—part 2: Hamstring injury management—part 2: Treatment. *Manual Therapy* 10:180-190.

Konin, J.G. 2004. Functional rehabilitation for hamstring strains: Emphasizing rotation. *Athl. Therapy Today*. 34-35.

Larson, C.M., L.C. Almekinders, S.G. Karas, and W.E Garrett. 2002. Evaluating and managing muscle contusions and myositis ossificans. *Physician and Sportsmed*. 2002: 30(2):41-50.

Levine, W.N., J.A. Bergfeld, W. Tessendorf, and C.T. Moorman. 2000. Intramuscular corticosteroid injection for hamstring injuries. *Am. J. Sports Med.* 28(3):297-300.

Malliaropoulos, N., S. Papalexandris, A. Papalada, and E. Papacostas. 2004. The role of stretching in rehabilitation of hamstring injuries: 80 athletes follow-up. *Med. Sci. Sports Exerc*. 36(5):756-759.

Nicholas, S.J. and T.F. Tyler. 2002. Adductor muscle strains in sport. *Sports Med.* 32(5):339-344.

Orchard, J.W., P. Farhart, C. Leopold, and T.M. Best. 2003. Lumbar spine region pathology and hamstring and calf injuries in athletes: Is there a connection? *Br. J. Sports Med.* 38:502-504.

Petersen, J. and P. Holmich. 2005. Evidence based prevention of hamstring injuries in sport. *Br. J. Sports Med.* 39:319-323.

Provencher, M.T., A.J. Baldwin, J.D. Gorman, M.T. Gould, and A.Y. Shin. 2004. Atypical tensile-sided femoral neck stress fractures. *Am. J. Sports Med.* 32(6):1528-1534.

Salminen, S.T., H.K. Pihlajamaki, T.I. Visuri, and O.M. Bostman. 2003. Displaced fatigue fractures of the femoral shaft. *Clin. Ortho and Related Research.* 409:250-259.

Sherry, M.A. and T.M. Best. 2004. A comparison of 2 rehabilitation programs in the treatment of acute hamstring strains. *J. Ortho. Sports Phys. Therapy* 34:116-125.

Verrall, G.M., J.P. Slavotinek, and P.G. Barnes. 2005. The effect of sports specific training on reducing the incidence of hamstring injuries in professional Australian rules football players. *Br. J. Sports Med.* 39:363-368.

Wang, S.Y., L.M. Lomasney, T.C. Demos, and W.J. Hopkinson. 1999. Radiologic case study: Traumatic myositis ossificans. *Orthopedics* 22(10):991-1000.

Weistroffer, J.K., M.P. Muldoon, D.D. Duncan, E.H. Fletcher and D.E. Padgett. 2003. Femoral neck stress fractures: Outcome analysis at minimum five-year follow-up. *J. Orthopaedic Trauma* 17(5):334-337.

Wen, D.Y., T. Propeck, and A. Singh. 2003. Femoral neck stress injury with negative bone scan. *JABFP* 16(2):170-174.

CHAPTER 13 **Knee Injuries**

Callaghan, J.J., A.G. Rosenberb, H.E. Rubash, P.T. Simonian, and T.L. Wickiewicz. 2002. *The adult knee*. Philadelphia: Lippincott Williams and Wilkins.

Fulkerson, J.P. 2004. *Disorders of the patellofemoral joint*. Philadelphia: Lippincott Williams and Wilkins.

Safran, M.R., S.P. Van Camp, D.B. McKeag. 1998. *Manual of sports medicine*. Philadelphia: Lippincott Williams and Wilkins.

Thompson, J.C. 2001. *Netter's concise atlas of orthopedic anatomy*. Philadelphia: Saunders.

Yurko Griffin, L. (ed.) 2005. *Essentials of musculoskeletal care* Rosemont, IL: American Academy of Orthopedic Surgeons.

CHAPTER 14 **Lower-Leg and Ankle Injuries**

Bare, A.A. and S.L. Haddad. 2001. Tenosynovitis of the posterior tibial tendon. *Foot Ankle Clin.* 6(1): 37-66.

Bates, P. 1985. Shin splints—a literature review. *Br. J. Sports Med.* 19(3):132-137.

Bong, M.R., D.B. Polatsch, L.M. Jazrawi, and A.S. Rokito. 2005. Chronic exertional compartment syndrome: diagnosis and management. *Bull. Hosp. Jt. Dis.* 62(3-4):77-84.

Chao, W. 2004. Os trigonum. *Foot Ankle Clin.* 9(4): 787-796, vii.

Chiodo, C.P. and S.A. Herbst. 2004. Osteonecrosis of the talus. *Foot Ankle Clin.* 9(4): 745-755, vi.

Clanton T.O. and P. Paul. 2002. Syndesmosis injuries in athletes. *Foot Ankle Clin.* 7(3): 529-549.

Hamilton, W.G. 1982a. Sprained ankles in ballet dancers. *Foot Ankle* 3:99-102.

Hamilton, W.G. 1982b. Stenosing tenosynovitis of the flexor hallucis longus tendon and posterior impingement upon the os trigonum in ballet dancers. *Foot Ankle* 3:74-80.

Hamilton, W.G. 1985. Surgical anatomy of the foot and ankle. *Ciba. Clinical Symposia.* 37(3):1-32.

Hamilton, W.G. 1988. Foot and ankle injuries in dancers. *Clin Sports Med.* 7:143-173.

Hamilton, W.G., F.M. Thompson, and S.W. Snow. 1993. The Bröstrom/Gould repair for lateral ankle instability. *Foot Ankle* 14(1):1-7, 1993. (Published erratum appears in *Foot Ankle* 14(3):180.)

Hamilton, W.G., M.J. Geppert, and F.M. Thompson 1996. Pain in the posterior aspect of the ankle in dancers: Differential diagnosis and operative treatment. *J. Bone Joint Surg. Am.* 78(10):1491-1500.

Horst, F., B.J. Gilbert, and Nunley, J.A. 2004. Avascular necrosis of the talus: Current treatment options. *Foot Ankle Clin.* 9(4):757-773.

Jarvinen, T.A., P. Kannus, N. Maffulli, and K.M. Khan. 2005. Achilles tendon disorders: Etiology and epidemiology. *Foot Ankle Clin.* 10(2):255-266.

Movin T., A. Ryberg, D.J. McBride, and N. Maffulli. 2005. Acute rupture of the Achilles tendon. *Foot Ankle Clin.* 10(2):331-356.

Richie, D.H. Jr. 2001. Functional instability of the ankle and the role of neuromuscular control: a comprehensive review. *J Foot Ankle Surg.* 40(4):240-251.

Saltzman, C.L. and D.S Tearse. 1998. Achilles tendon injuries. *J. Am. Acad. Orthop. Surg.* 6(5):316-325.

Schachter, A.K., A.L. Chen, P.D. Reddy, and N.C. Tejwani. 2005. Osteochondral lesions of the talus. *J. Am. Acad. Orthop. Surg.* 13(3):152-158.

Schepsis, A.A., H. Jones, and A.L. Haas. 2002. Achilles tendon disorders in athletes. *Am. J. Sports Med.* 30(2):287-305.

Schon, L.C. 1993. Foot and ankle problems in dancers. *Md. Med. J.* 42(3):267-269.

Touliopolous S. and E.B. Hershman. 1999. Lower leg pain. Diagnosis and treatment of compartment syndromes and other pain syndromes of the leg. *Sports Med.* 27(3):193-204.

van Dijk, C.N. 2002. Management of the sprained ankle. *Br. J. Sports Med.* 36(2):83-84.

Wilder, R.P. and S. Sethi. 2004. Overuse injuries: Tendinopathies, stress fractures, compartment syndrome, and shin splints. *Clin. Sports Med.* 23(1):55-81, vi.

CHAPTER 15   **Foot and Toe Injuries**

Berkowitz, M.J. and D.H. Kim. 2005. Process and tubercle fractures of the hindfoot. *J. Am. Acad. Orthop. Surg.* 13(8):492-502.

Buchbinder, R. 2004. Clinical practice. Plantar fasciitis. *N. Engl. J. Med.* 350(21):2159-2166.

Coughlin, M.J. 2000. Common causes of pain in the forefoot in adults. *J. Bone Joint Surg. Br.* 82(6):781-790.

Coughlin, M.J. and P.S. Shurnas. 2003. Hallux rigidus: Demographics, etiology, and radiographic assessment. *Foot Ankle Int.* 24(10):731-743.

Cole, C., Seto, C., and J. Gazewood. 2005. Plantar fasciitis: Evidence-based review of diagnosis and therapy. *Am. Fam. Physician.* 72(11):2237-2242.

Coris, E.E., C.C. Kaeding, and J.V. Marymont 2003. Tarsal navicular stress injuries in athletes. *Orthopedics.* 26(7):733-737; quiz 738-789.

Fetzer, G.B. and R.W. Wright. 2006. Metatarsal shaft fractures and fractures of the proximal fifth metatarsal. *Clin. Sports Med.* 25(1):139-50, x.

Grace, D.L. 2000. Sesamoid problems. *Foot Ankle Clin.* 5(3):609-627.

Hamilton, W.G. 1985. Surgical anatomy of the foot and ankle. *Ciba. Clinical Symposia.* 37(3):1-32.

Hamilton, W.G. 1988. Foot and ankle injuries in dancers. *Clin Sports Med.* 7:143-173.

Jones, M.H. and A.S. Amendola. 2006. Navicular stress fractures. *Clin. Sports Med.* 25(1):151-158, x-xi.

Kay, D. and G.L. Bennett. 2003. Morton's neuroma. *Foot Ankle Clin.* 8(1):49-59.

Mann, R.A. and J.A. Mann. 2004. Keratotic disorders of the plantar skin. *Instr. Course Lect.* 53:287-302.

Mantas J.P. and R.T. Burks. 1994. Lisfranc injuries in the athlete. *Clin. Sports Med.* 13(4):719-730.

Mullen, J.E. and M.J. O'Malley. 2004. Sprains—residual instability of subtalar, Lisfranc joints, and turf toe. *Clin. Sports Med.* 23(1):97-121.

Nunley, J.A. 2001. Fractures of the base of the fifth metatarsal: The Jones fracture. *Orthop. Clin. North Am.* 32(1):171-180.

Pfeffer, G.B. 2001. Plantar heel pain. *Instr. Course Lect.* 50:521-531.

Rammelt, S., J. Heineck, and H. Zwipp. 2004. Metatarsal fractures. Injury. 35 Suppl.2:SB77-86.

Richardson, E.G. 1999. Hallucal sesamoid pain: Causes and surgical treatment. *J. Am. Acad. Orthop. Surg.* 7(4):270-278.

Robinson, A.H. and J.P Limbers. 2005. Modern concepts in the treatment of hallux valgus. *J. Bone Joint Surg. Br.* 87(8):1038-1045.

Ugolini, P.A. and S.M. Raikin 2004. The accessory navicular. *Foot Ankle Clin.* 9(1):165-180.

Vanore, J.V., J.C. Christensen, S.R. Kravitz, J.M. Schuberth, J.L. Thomas, L.S. Weil, H.J. Zlotoff, R.W. Mendicino, and S.D. Couture. 2003. Clinical Practice Guideline First Metatarasophalangeal Joint Disorders Panel of the American College of Foot and Ankle Surgeons. Diagnosis and treatment of first metatarsophalangeal joint disorders. Section 2: Hallux rigidus. *J. Foot Ankle Surg.* 42(3):124-136. (Erratum in *J. Foot Ankle Surg.* 42(6):394.)

Weinfeld, S.B., S.L. Haddad, and M.S. Myerson. 1997. Metatarsal stress fractures. *Clin. Sports Med.* 16(2):319-338.

Wu, K.K. 1996. Morton's interdigital neuroma: A clinical review of its etiology, treatment, and results. *J. Foot Ankle Surg.* 35(2):112-119; discussion 187-188.

CHAPTER 16 **Integrative Medicine**

Assendelft, W.J., L.M. Bouter, and G.P. Knipschild. 1996. Complications of spinal manipulation: A comprehensive review of the literature. *J. Fam. Pract.* 42:475-480.

Barnes, P., E. Powell-Griner, K. McFann, and R. Nahin. 2004. Complementary and alternative medicine use among adults: United States. *Advance Data From Vital and Health Statistics* (343):1-19.

Chantre, P., A. Cappelaere, D. Lebilan, D. Guedon, J. Vandermander, and B. Fournie. 2000. Efficacy and tolerance of *Harpagophytum procumbens* vs. diacerhein in treatment of osteoarthritis. *Phytomedicine* 7:177-184.

Cho, Z.H., T.D. Oleson, D. Alimi, and R.C. Niemtzow. 2002. Acupuncture: the search for biologic evidence with functional magnetic resonance imaging and positron emission tomography techniques. *J. Altern. Complement Med.* 8:399-401.

Coulter, I.D., E.L. Hurwitz, A.H. Adams, W. Meeker, D.T. Hansen, R. Mootz, P. Aker, B. Genovese, and P.G. Shekelle. 1996. *The appropriateness of manipulation and mobilization of the cervical spine.* Santa Monica, CA: RAND, MR-781-CCR.

Eisenberg, D.M., R.C. Kessler, C. Foster, F.E. Norlock, D.R. Calkins, and T.L. Delbanco. 1993. Unconventional medicine in the United States: Prevalence, costs and patterns of use. *NEJM* 328:246-252.

Evans, S. 2004. Performance-enhancing supplements threaten sports. www.scripps.org/News.asp?ID=5.

Fahey, T.D., and M.S. Pearl. 1998. The hormonal and perceptive effects of phosphatidylserine administration during two weeks of resistive exercise induced overtraining. *Biol. Sport* 15:135-144.

Greenfield, R. 2002. Yoga. In *Complementary and Alternative Medicine Secrets.* Philadelphia: Hanley & Belfus: 54-58.

Greenman, P. 1996. *Principles of manual medicine.* Baltimore: Williams & Wilkins.

Grimshaw, D. 2002. Osteopathic medicine. In *Complementary and alternative medicine secrets.* Edited by W. Kohatsu. Philadelphia: Hanley & Belfus.

Helms, J. 1996. *Acupuncture energetics.* Berkeley, CA: Medical Acupuncture.

Helms, J. 1998. An overview of medical acupuncture. *Altern. Ther. Health Med.* 4:35-45.

Kaptchuk, T. 2002. Acupuncture: Theory, efficacy, and practice. *Ann Intern Med* 136:374-383.

Kelly, G. and P. Bongiorno 2006. Sports nutrition. In *Textbook of natural medicine* (3rd ed.). Edited by J. Pizzorno Jr. and M. Murray. Philadelphia: Churchill Livingstone.

McPartland, J. 2004. Travell trigger points—molecular and osteopathic perspectives. *JAOA.* 104(6):244-249.

Monteleone, P., M. Maj, L. Beinat, M. Natale, and D. Kemali. 1992. Blunting by chronic phosphatidylserine administration of the stress induced activation of the hypothalamic-pituitary–adrenal axis in healthy men. *Eur. J. Clin. Pharmacol.* 42:385-388.

Mootz, R. and I. Coulter. 2002. Chiropractic. In *Complementary and alternative medicine secrets.* Edited by W. Kohatsu. Philadelphia: Hanley & Belfus.

National Center for Complementary and Alternative Medicine. 2002. *Acupuncture.* Publication No. D003.

Pomeranz, B. and G. Stux. 1989. *Scientific bases of acupuncture.* Berlin: Springer-Verlag.

Randall, C., H. Randall, F. Dobbs, C. Hutton, and H. Sanders. 2000. Randomized controlled trial of nettle sting for treatment of base-of- thumb pain. *J. R. Soc. Med.* 93:305-309.

Roy, S. and R. Irvin. 1983. *Sports medicine: Prevention, evaluation, management, and rehabilitation.* Englewood Cliffs, NJ: Prentice-Hall.

Sierpina, V. and M. Frenkel. 2005. Acupuncture: A clinical review. *Southern Med. Journal* 98(3).

Srivastava, K.C. and T. Mustafa T. 1992. Ginger (Zingiber officinale) and rheumatism and musculoskeletal disorders. *Med. Hypotheses* 39:342-348.

Srivastava, K.C. and T. Mustafa. 1989. Ginger (Zingiber officinale) and rheumatic disorders. *Med. Hypotheses* 29:25-28.

Takahashi, T., E. Yamaguchi, K. Furuya, and Y. Kawakami. 2001. *Respir. Med.* 95(2):130-135.

Vincent, C. 2001. The safety of acupuncture. *BMJ* 323:467-468.

Weil, A. 2001. On integrative medicine and the nature of reality. *Alter. Ther. Health Med.* 7(4):96-104.

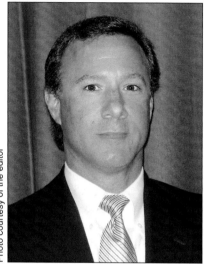

Robert S. Gotlin, DO, is the director of orthopaedic and sports rehabilitation in the department of orthopaedic surgery and the coordinator of the musculoskeletal and sports rehabilitation fellowship training program at Beth Israel Medical Center. He is also an assistant professor of physical medicine and rehabilitation at the Albert Einstein College of Medicine of Yeshiva University.

Gotlin hosts the "Dr. Rob Says . . . Sports Health and Fitness Show," which airs every Saturday from 7 to 8 a.m. on 1050 ESPN Radio. He has been a guest host for television's "ABC Now, Healthy Living," a daily television program that features breaking medical news and practical health advice. As a consultant, he has served on the medical team with Dr. W. Norman Scott, team physician for the New York Knicks (NBA basketball) and New York Liberty (WNBA basketball), and as physiatric consultant to Dr. Michael Kelly, team physician for the New Jersey Nets (NBA basketball), and to Dr. Stuart Hershon, team physician for the New York Yankees (MLB baseball). He is also a team physician for U.S. women's Rugby and the chief medical officer for the JCC Maccabi Games.

Gotlin is board certified by both the American Board of Physical Medicine and Rehabilitation and the American Osteopathic Board of Physical Medicine and Rehabilitation. He is also a past program chairman for the New York State Society of Physical Medicine and Rehabilitation. Gotlin earned his medical degree from the Southeastern University of the Health Sciences in Miami, Florida, in 1987.

ABOUT THE CONTRIBUTORS

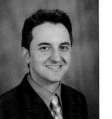

Arjang Abbasi, DO, is an attending physiatrist at Long Island Spine Specialists, PC, in Commack, New York. He specializes in nonoperative care for neck and back disorders as well as interventional pain management. He completed his specialty training at UMDNJ/Kessler Institute in New Jersey and is fellowship trained in interventional spine and sports rehabilitation. He has completed extensive research in the fields of spine, sports, and electrodiagnostic medicine. Dr. Abbasi is a certified diplomat of the American Board of Physical Medicine and Rehabilitation. He has authored numerous publications and presented at local and national conferences.

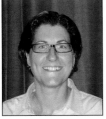

Lisa M. Bartoli, DO, MS, is the team doctor for the U.S. women's rugby team and the New York rugby team. In addition to her medical degree, Dr. Bartoli has fellowship training in interventional spine care and sports medicine. Her practice includes medical acupuncture, osteopathic manual therapy, and musculoskeletal medicine with a special focus on rehabilitation of women's sports injuries. She is board certified in physical medicine and rehabilitation and is clinical adjunct professor at the New York College of Osteopathic Medicine. Dr. Bartoli lectures extensively on musculoskeletal medicine and sports medicine and on her approach as a team physician.

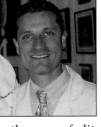

Andrew Brief, MD, is a surgeon at North Jersey Orthopaedic Specialists, PA, in Englewood and Teaneck. During his surgical internship and orthopaedic residency at the NYU Hospital for Joint Diseases in New York, Dr. Brief worked at Shea Stadium in the care and management of injuries to both spectators and professional athletes. While fulfilling an additional year of orthopaedic fellowship training in foot and ankle reconstruction at the Hospital for Special Surgery in New York, Dr. Brief was involved in the care of elite athletes as well as professional ballet dancers with the New York City Ballet and the American Ballet Theatre.

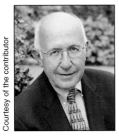

Daniel A. Brzusek, DO, is the medial director of Northwest Rehabilitation Associates Inc., located in Bellevue, Washington. He is board certified in physical medicine and rehabilitation and an active member of the American College of Sports Medicine and the American Association of Electrodiagnostic Medicine. Dr. Brzusek has lectured throughout the world and has served on several committees both nationally and internationally. He is a clinical assistant professor of rehabilitation medicine at the University of Washington. Dr. Brzusek graduated from the Philadelphia College of Osteopathic Medicine and received his specialty training at the University of Washington Medical School.

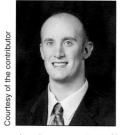

Evan Chait, PT, is founder and president of Elite Athletic Performance Institute (EAPI), a cutting-edge corrective exercise and performance conditioning center, and founder of Kinetic Physical Therapy, an integrated approach to rehabilitation, which combines physical therapy, chiropractic, massage therapy, kinesiology, and integrated manual therapy. Chait studied from the best in his field, including Dr. Michael Leahy, the founder of Active Release Techniques, and Gary Gray, the father of functional biomechanics. An internationally renowned physical therapist, Chait has lectured on and taught his unique blend of manual therapy techniques and sport conditioning concepts to coaches and teams all over the world. He has been featured in ESPN magazine and on ESPN radio and has worked with more than 50 NBA players, including as a rehabilitation and performance consultant to the New York Knicks and New Jersey Nets.

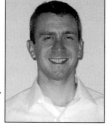

Grant Cooper, MD, is currently a fellow in sports, spine, and musculoskeletal rehabilitation at Beth Israel Medical Center in New York City. The author of numerous articles on a range of musculoskeletal pathologies, he has received national and international recognition for his research. Dr. Cooper is also the author and editor of several scientific medical texts. In 2008, his latest work, The Arthritis Book (DiaMed) is scheduled to be released. He is also the co-chief editor of the book series Musculoskeletal Medicine (Humana Press) and the scientific journal Current Reviews in Musculoskeletal Medicine (Springer, scheduled to be released in summer 2008).

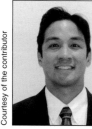

Edmund S. Evangelista, MS, is board certified in physical medicine and rehabilitation and in pain medicine. He is in private practice at Community Orthopedic Medical Group in Mission Viejo, California, where he specializes in nonoperative spine care and sports medicine. Dr. Evangelista also serves as team physician for Tesoro High School in Mission Viejo and is the medical advisor and a volunteer ski instructor for Disabled Sports USA-Orange County Chapter. Dr. Evangelista received a BS from Boston College in 1992 and an MD from Tufts University School of Medicine in 1996. He completed residency training in physical medicine and rehabilitation at UC Irvine Medical Center in 2000.

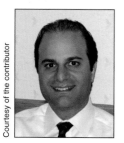

Ferdinand J. Formoso, DO, is currently an attending physician in private practice at the Florida Spine, Sports and Pain Center in Jacksonville, Florida. He completed fellowship training in interventional spine and pain medicine at Temple University/Mid-Atlantic Spine in Delaware. He completed residency training at Temple University in physical medicine and rehabilitation. Dr. Formoso graduated from the New York College of Osteopathic Medicine, where he also completed an undergraduate fellowship with the department of anatomy.

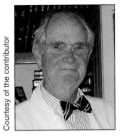

Courtesy of the contributor

William G. Hamilton, MD, is a clinical professor of Orthopedic Surgery at Columbia University College of Physicians and Surgeons. He is a senior attending orthopedic surgeon at St. Luke's Roosevelt Hospital (NY), an associate attending surgeon at the Hospital for Special Surgery (NY), and an attending orthopedic surgeon at The Keller Army Hospital, West Point (NY). Dr. Hamilton has served as president of The American Orthopedic Foot & Ankle Society and The New York Medical & Surgical Society. He is the orthopedic consultant to the New York City Ballet (1972-2007), the American Ballet Theatre (1980-2007) and a part-time foot and ankle consultant to the New York Knicks basketball team, and the NY Yankees baseball team.

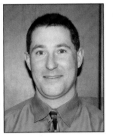

Courtesy of the contributor

Todd D. Hirsch, MS, ATC, is a certified athletic trainer at Governor Livingston High School in Berkeley Heights, New Jersey. He received a BSE in sport science and athletic training from the University of Kansas (1997) and an MS in exercise science from the University of Massachusetts (1999). Todd is the president of the New York State Athletic Trainers' Association (2006-08) and was awarded the New York State Athletic Trainers' Association Joseph Abraham Award (2005) and the Eastern Athletic Trainers' Association Micro Bio-Medics/Henry Schein Award (2006).

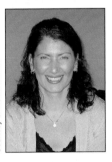

Courtesy of the contributor

Yvonne Johnson, PT, is the director of physical therapy at the Continuum Center for Health and Healing at Beth Israel Medical Center. She has been practicing since 1992 and has extensive expertise in musculoskeletal assessment and treatment and routinely treats both amateur and professional athletes. She has developed therapeutic paradigms for the treatment of several complex sport-related injuries and has been the physical therapist for the New York Knicks, the New York Liberty, and the U.S. national women's rugby team.

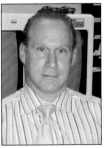

Courtesy of the contributor

Stuart Kahn, MD, is the director of the Spine Institute Pain Rehabilitation at Beth Israel Medical Center. He is a pain management specialist who diagnoses and treats painful conditions of the spine not requiring surgery. Through a multimodality approach, Dr. Kahn assists acute and chronic pain patients with pain management. He joined Beth Israel in 1992 as the physician in charge of the inpatient rehabilitation unit before moving on to lead ambulatory departments in physical medicine and rehabilitation. After becoming a pain management specialist, Dr. Kahn was named director of spine pain and rehabilitation at the Spine Institute in 1999. Dr. Kahn is a board-certified physician in physical medicine and rehabilitation with a subspecialty in pain management.

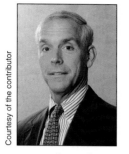

Michael Kelly, MD, is a director of Insall Scott Kelly Institute, a full-service orthopaedic center in New York City. His specialty is all aspects of knee surgery. He is also chairman of the department of orthopaedic surgery at Hackensack University Medical Center in New Jersey. Kelly has lectured worldwide on topics related to sports medicine and knee reconstruction and is active in clinical research on knee disorders. The author of numerous professional articles on many aspects of knee surgery, he also coedited the textbook *Surgery of the Knee, Second Edition.* Kelly is a member of many professional organizations, including the American Orthopaedic Society of Sports Medicine and the American Orthopaedic Association. He is currently president of the prestigious American Knee Society.

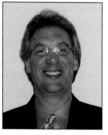

Joshua S. Krassen, DO, is a physiatrist (physical medicine and rehabilitation) at Valley Sports & Arthritis Surgeons in Allentown and Bethlehem, Pennsylvania, where he provides care for non-operative and postoperative musculoskeletal and spine injuries. Krassen is board certified by the Academy of Physical Medicine and Rehabilitation and American Osteopathic Congress of Rehabilitation Medicine. He is also a board-certified subspecialist in spinal cord injury medicine.

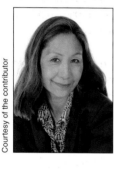

Roberta Lee, MD, is medical director of the Center for Health and Healing, director of continuing medical education, and codirector of the fellowship in integrative medicine at Beth Israel's Continuum Center for Health and Healing (CCHH). She is a board-certified internist and is the codirector of the Healer's Art Course, an elective in self-care taught at Albert Einstein College of Medicine. Dr. Lee is a contributing editor to the journal *Explore: The Journal of Science and Healing,* on the advisory board of the American Botanical Council, and a coauthor of the recently released text *Integrative Medicine: Principles for Practice.*

Ian B. Maitin, MD, MBA, is the chair of the department of physical medicine and rehabilitation at Temple University School of Medicine and Temple Hospital. After graduating Phi Beta Kappa in biochemistry from Rutgers University and earning an MD from Jefferson Medical College, Maitin completed a residency in physical medicine and rehabilitation at the Robert Wood Johnson Rehabilitation Institute at the University of Medicine and Dentistry of New Jersey. In 1993 he joined the Temple University faculty and in 2002 received an MBA in health care management from Temple's Fox School of Business.

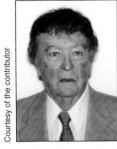

Frank McCue III, MD, held the Alfred R. Shands, Jr., Professorship of Orthopaedics and Rehabilitation and directed the orthopaedic department's Divisions of Sports Medicine and Hand Surgery at the University of Virginia's Health Sciences Center until his retirement in 2003. Dr. McCue is a founding member of the American Orthopaedic Society for Sports Medicine and a fellow of the American Society for Surgery of the Hand, American College of Surgeons, American Academy of Orthopaedic Surgery, and the American Orthopaedic Association. Dr. McCue is the first recipient of the Frank C. McCue III, MD, Sports Medicine Award given annually by the Virginia High School Coaches Association, a merit award from the American Society for Sports Medicine.

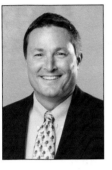

Gregory A. Rowdon, MD, is the head team physician at Purdue University. He attended medical school at the University of Kansas and completed residency training in internal medicine at Indiana University Medical School and then a sports medicine fellowship also at IU. Rowdon was in private practice at Methodist Sports Medicine Center in Indianapolis for 11 years and director of the Primary Care Sports Medicine Fellowship at IU. He has served on the Sports Medicine Advisory Committee for the National Federation of High Schools, the Sports Medicine Board Certification Examination Committee, and the Indiana State Medical Society Sports Medicine Commission.

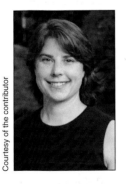

Susan Foreman Saliba, PhD, is a senior associate athletic trainer and a clinical instructor at the University of Virginia in Charlottesville, where she has taught therapeutic modalities for over 12 years. A certified athletic trainer and licensed physical therapist, Dr. Saliba also taught therapeutic modalities at James Madison University in Harrisonburg, Virginia. She is chairperson of the National Athletic Trainers' Association Clinical Education Committee and a member of its Education Executive Committee. She earned a master's degree in athletic training and a PhD in sports medicine from the University of Virginia.

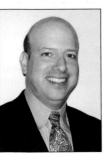

Andrew L. Sherman, MD, MS, is the associate professor of clinical rehabilitation medicine and vice chairman of the department of rehabilitation medicine at the University of Miami Miller School of Medicine in Florida. He received a BS from Cornell University (1989) and an MD from SUNY Buffalo Medical School (1993). Dr. Sherman completed his residency in physical medicine and rehabilitation (physiatry) from the University of Washington at Seattle in 1997 and a sports and spine medicine fellowship at Beth Israel Hospital in New York in 1998. He has more than nine years of experience in treating sports and spine injuries.

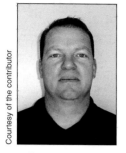

Hank Sherman, MD, is a staff physician at Habif Health & Wellness Center, the Student Health Services at Washington University in St. Louis, Missouri. After completing his family practice residency, Dr. Sherman was in private family practice for four years. He then trained in primary care sports medicine. He has been a high school team physician and assisted in the care of multiple college and professional teams, including Purdue University, Indiana State University, Butler University, the University of Indianapolis, and the Indianapolis Colts. Dr. Sherman is board certified in family medicine and has certification of added qualifications in sports medicine.

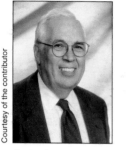

Paul Steingard, DO, is widely recognized as a pioneer in the field of sports medicine. He was the original team physician for the Phoenix Suns and served in that capacity for 23 years. He continues to serve as team physician emeritus. Dr. Steingard has also served as team physician for Grand Canyon University, Phoenix Community College, and numerous high schools in the Phoenix area. He was the team physician for Kenya in the 1984 Olympic Games. Dr. Steingard is vice president of the Grand Canyon State Games and a member of the Fiesta Bowl Committee. He is the founder and leader of the group TOPS (Team of Physicians for Students), a group that is dedicated to identifying high school athletes prone to sudden death syndrome.

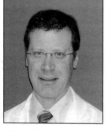

Michael M. Weinik, DO, is associate chairman of the department of physical medicine and rehabilitation at Temple University Hospital, where he is also the director of musculoskeletal and sports rehabilitation. Dr. Weinik is also an associate professor in physical medicine and rehabilitation at Temple University School of Medicine. He has served as a team physician for the Philadelphia Flyers (NHL), Philadelphia Eagles (NFL), Philadelphia Phantoms (AHL), Philadelphia KIxxs (NISL), and the U.S. rowing team. Dr. Weinik has also been an event physician for the Women's World Cup soccer and a ring physician for boxing with the Pennsylvania State Athletic Commission.

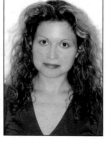

Elise Weiss, MD, specializes in musculoskeletal medicine, sports medicine, and electrodiagnostics. She currently is in private practice in New York City. Dr. Weiss is particularly interested in the role of nutrition and exercise in maintaining and enhancing health. She has coauthored numerous publications on sports injury, nutrition, athletic training, arthritis, and the use of Botox in the treatment of migraines, neuropathic pain, and spasticity. Dr. Weiss received a BS with honors from Cornell University and returned to New York City to attend medical school at Columbia University's College of Physicians and Surgeons.